Update on Management of Pain

Guest Editor

KAROL A. MATHEWS, DVM, DVSc

VETERINARY CLINICS OF NORTH AMERICA: SMALL ANIMAL PRACTICE

www.vetsmall.theclinics.com

November 2008 • Volume 38 • Number 6

SAUNDERS an imprint of ELSEVIER, Inc.

W.B. SAUNDERS COMPANY
A Division of Elsevier Inc.

1600 John F. Kennedy Blvd. • Suite 1800 • Philadelphia, PA 19103-2899

http://www.vetsmall.theclinics.com

VETERINARY CLINICS OF NORTH AMERICA: Volume 38, Number 6
SMALL ANIMAL PRACTICE
November 2008 ISSN 0195-5616, ISBN-13: 978-1-4160-6375-9, ISBN-10: 1-4160-6375-7

Editor: John Vassallo; j.vassallo@elsevier.com

Veterinary Clinics of North America: Small Animal Practice (ISSN 0195-5616) is published bimonthly (For Post Office use only: volume 38 issue 6 of 6) by Elsevier Inc., 360 Park Avenue South, New York, NY 10010-1710. Months of issue are January, March, May, July, September, and November. Business and Editorial Offices: 1600 John F. Kennedy Blvd., Suite 1800, Philadelphia, PA 19103-2899. Customer Service Office: 11830 Westline Industrial Drive, St. Louis, MO 63146. Periodicals postage paid at New York, NY and additional mailing offices. Subscription prices are $229.00 per year (domestic individuals), $366.00 per year (domestic institutions), $114.00 per year (domestic students/residents), $303.00 per year (Canadian individuals), $450.00 per year (Canadian institutions), $336.00 per year (international individuals), $450.00 per year (international institutions), and $165.00 per year (international and Canadian students/residents). To receive student/resident rate, orders must be accompanied by name of affiliated institution, date of term, and the *signature* of program/residency coordinator on institution letterhead. Orders will be billed at individual rate until proof of status is received. Foreign air speed delivery is included in all *Clinics* subscription prices. All prices are subject to change without notice. **POSTMASTER:** Send address changes to *Veterinary Clinics of North America: Small Animal Practice*, Elsevier Periodicals Customer Service, 11830 Westline Industrial Drive, St. Louis, MO 63146. Customer Service (orders, claims, online, change of address): Elsevier Periodicals Customer Service, 11830 Westline Industrial Drive, St. Louis, MO 63146. Tel: 1-800-654-2452 (U.S. and Canada). Fax: 314-523-5170. E-mail: journalscustomerservice-usa@elsevier.com (for print support); journalsonlinesupport-usa@elsevier.com (for online support).

Reprints. For copies of 100 or more of articles in this publication, please contact the Commercial Reprints Department, Elsevier Inc., 360 Park Avenue South, New York, NY 10010-1710. Tel.: 212-633-3812; Fax: 212-462-1935; E-mail: reprints@elsevier.com.

Veterinary Clinics of North America: Small Animal Practice is also published in Japanese by Inter Zoo Publishing Co., Ltd., Aoyama Crystal-Bldg 5F, 3-5-12 Kitaaoyama, Minato-ku, Tokyo 107-0061, Japan.

Veterinary Clinics of North America: Small Animal Practice is covered in *Current Contents/Agriculture, Biology and Environmental Sciences, Science Citation Index, ASCA, MEDLINE/PubMed (Index Medicus), Excerpta Medica, and BIOSIS.*

Printed in the United States of America.

Contributors

GUEST EDITOR

KAROL A. MATHEWS, DVM, DVSc
Diplomate, American College of Veterinary Emergency and Critical Care; Professor and Service Chief, Emergency and Critical Care Medicine, Department of Clinical Studies, Ontario Veterinary College, University of Guelph, Guelph, Ontario, Canada

AUTHORS

STEVEN C. BUDSBERG, DVM, MS
Diplomate, American College of Veterinary Surgeons; Professor of Small Animal Surgery, and Director of Clinical Research, Department of Small Animal Medicine and Surgery, College of Veterinary Medicine, University of Georgia, Athens, Georgia

CATHERINE M. CREIGHTON, DVM
Department of Companion Animals, Atlantic Veterinary College, University of Prince Edward Island, Charlottetown, Prince Edward Island, Canada

DORIS H. DYSON, DVM, DVSc
Diplomate, American College of Veterinary Anesthesiologists; Associate Professor of Anesthesia, Department of Clinical Studies, Ontario Veterinary College, University of Guelph, Guelph, Ontario, Canada

JAMES S. GAYNOR, DVM, MS
Diplomate, American College of Veterinary Anesthesiologists; Diplomate, American Academy of Pain Management; Medical Director, Peak Performance Veterinary Group, Colorado Springs, Colorado

BERNIE HANSEN, DVM, MS
Diplomate, American College of Veterinary Emergency and Critical Care; Diplomate, American College of Veterinary Internal Medicine; Associate Professor, Department of Clinical Sciences, North Carolina State University, College of Veterinary Medicine, Raleigh, North Carolina

SPENCER A. JOHNSTON, VMD
Diplomate, American College of Veterinary Surgeons; Edward H. Gunst Professor of Small Animal Surgery, Department of Small Animal Medicine and Surgery, College of Veterinary Medicine, University of Georgia, Athens, Georgia

LEIGH A. LAMONT, DVM, MS
Diplomate, American College of Veterinary Anesthesiologists; Assistant Professor of Anesthesiology, Department of Companion Animals, Atlantic Veterinary College, University of Prince Edward Island, Charlottetown, Prince Edward Island, Canada

KIP A. LEMKE, DVM, MS
Diplomate, American College of Veterinary Anesthesiologists; Professor of Anesthesiology, Department of Companion Animals, Atlantic Veterinary College, University of Prince Edward Island, Charlottetown, Prince Edward Island, Canada

KAROL A. MATHEWS, DVM, DVSc
Diplomate, American College of Veterinary Emergency and Critical Care; Professor and Service Chief, Emergency and Critical Care Medicine, Department of Clinical Studies, Ontario Veterinary College, University of Guelph, Guelph, Ontario, Canada

RONALD M. McLAUGHLIN, DVM, DVSc
Diplomate, American College of Veterinary Surgeons; Professor and Head, Department of Clinical Sciences, Mississippi State University, College of Veterinary Medicine, Mississippi State, Mississippi

MARK G. PAPICH, DVM, MS
Diplomate, American College of Veterinary Clinical Pharmacology; Professor of Clinical Pharmacology, Department of Molecular Biomedical Sciences, North Carolina State University College of Veterinary Medicine, Raleigh, North Carolina

SHEILAH A. ROBERTSON, BVMS, PhD, MRCVS
Diplomate, American College of Veterinary Anesthesiologists; Diplomate, European College of Veterinary Anesthesia and Analgesia; Professor, Department of Large Animal Clinical Sciences, College of Veterinary Medicine, University of Florida, Gainesville, Florida

NANCY SHAFFRAN, CVT, VTS(ECC)
Senior Nursing Specialist, Veterinary Specialty Team, Pfizer Animal Health, Erwinna, Pennsylvania

ALEXANDER VALVERDE, DVM, DVSc
Diplomate, American College of Veterinary Anesthesiologists; Associate Professor, Section of Anesthesiology, Department of Clinical Studies, Ontario Veterinary College, University of Guelph, Guelph, Ontario, Canada

Contents

Preface **xi**

Karol A. Mathews

Multimodal Pain Management in Veterinary Medicine: The Physiologic Basis of Pharmacologic Therapies **1173**

Leigh A. Lamont

Multimodal analgesia refers to the practice of combining multiple analgesic drug classes or techniques to target different points along the pain pathway in an effort to improve analgesia. This strategy requires an understanding of pain physiology and pathophysiology so pharmacologic interventions can be tailored to meet the needs of the patient. This article reviews the physiologic basis of pain as it relates to analgesic treatments and also introduces new developments in molecular biology that may guide analgesic drug development in the future.

Adjunctive Analgesic Therapy in Veterinary Medicine **1187**

Leigh A. Lamont

Adjunctive analgesic therapies are interventions for pain that involve agents or techniques other than the traditional analgesics (opioids, nonsteroidal anti-inflammatory drugs, and local anesthetics). Adjunctive therapies may be pharmacologic or nonpharmacologic in nature. The focus of this article is on pharmacologic interventions with potential utility as adjunctive analgesics in veterinary medicine. Pharmacology of selected agents, including medetomidine, ketamine, amantadine, gabapentin, systemic lidocaine, and pamidronate, is discussed in addition to evidence for their safety and efficacy and guidelines for their use in veterinary patients.

Epidural Analgesia and Anesthesia in Dogs and Cats **1205**

Alexander Valverde

Current knowledge of drugs administered epidurally has allowed an effective way of providing analgesia for a wide variety of conditions in veterinary patients. Proper selection of drugs and dosages can result in analgesia of specific segments of the spinal cord with minimal side effects. Epidural anesthesia is an alternative to general anesthesia with inhalation anesthetics, although the combination of both techniques is more common and allows for reduced doses of drugs used with each technique. Epidural anesthesia and intravenous anesthetics can also be used without inhalation anesthetics in surgical procedures caudal to the diaphragm.

Paravertebral Blockade of the Brachial Plexus in Dogs **1231**

Kip A. Lemke and Catherine M. Creighton

Local anesthetic techniques have the unique ability to block peripheral nociceptive input associated with surgical trauma and inflammation and to prevent sensitization of central nociceptive pathways and the development of pathologic pain. Complete neural blockade of the canine brachial plexus is difficult to achieve using the traditional axillary technique. This article describes paravertebral blockade of the brachial plexus in dogs and a new modified paravertebral technique. Both techniques are relatively easy to perform and produce complete blockade of the forelimb, including the shoulder. A review of relevant clinical anatomy and guidelines for using electrical nerve locators are also included.

An Update on Nonsteroidal Anti-Inflammatory Drugs (NSAIDs) in Small Animals **1243**

Mark G. Papich

There are several choices of nonsteroidal anti-inflammatory drugs (NSAIDs) for treating dogs that have osteoarthritis. However, fewer drugs are available for cats. Like people, there may be greater differences among individuals in their response than there are differences among the drugs. In past practice, veterinarians often selected aspirin or phenylbutazone as an initial drug, and then progressed to off-label human drugs or other agents as an alternative. Now we have the advantage of several approved NSAIDs for which there are excellent published studies and US Food and Drug Administration or foreign approval to guide clinical use and safe dosages.

Managing Pain in Feline Patients **1267**

Sheilah A. Robertson

This article reviews the current knowledge of pain assessment in cats and the most effective methods for its alleviation. Excellent acute pain management is achievable in cats by using opioids, nonsteroidal anti-inflammatory drugs (NSAIDs), α_2-agonists, and local anesthetics. A multimodal approach using agents that work at different places in the pain pathway is encouraged because this can have added benefits. Management of chronic pain in cats can be challenging, but there is now an approved NSAID for long-term use. As we gain experience with less traditional analgesics, such as gabapentin, and critically evaluate complimentary therapies, our ability to provide comfort to this population of cats should improve.

Pain Management for the Pregnant, Lactating, and Neonatal to Pediatric Cat and Dog **1291**

Karol A. Mathews

Little information on the approach to analgesia in pregnant, nursing, or extremely young animals is available in the veterinary literature. Various analgesics and analgesic modalities are discussed, with emphasis placed on preference and caution for each group. Management of pain is extremely important in all animals but especially in the extremely young, in which a permanent hyperalgesic response to pain may exist with inadequate therapy. Inappropriate analgesic selection in pregnant and nursing mothers may result in congenital abnormalities of the fetus or neonate.

Inadequate analgesia in nursing mothers may cause aggressive behavior toward the young. Review of the human and veterinary literature on the various analgesics available for use in this group of patients is discussed.

Perioperative Pain Management in Veterinary Patients **1309**

Doris H. Dyson

Pain exists; however, we can prevent it, and we can treat it. The fallacy that pain is protective and must be allowed to avoid risk for damage after surgery needs to be eradicated. Preoperative and postoperative analgesia is directed at aching pain, whereas sharp pain associated with inappropriate movements persists. Analgesia provides much more benefit than concern. This article provides suggestions for development of an analgesic plan from the point of admission to discharge. These guidelines can then be adjusted according to the patient's needs and responses.

Analgesia and Chemical Restraint for the Emergent Veterinary Patient **1329**

Doris H. Dyson

Frequently, analgesics are withheld in the emergent patient based on common misconceptions. Concerns expressed are that analgesics "mask" physiologic indicators of patient deterioration or that potential toxicity and adverse reactions associated with drug administration outweigh the benefits gained. Appropriate selection of drugs and doses as described in this article allow the veterinarian to achieve analgesia, in addition to sedation or restraint when needed, without unwarranted fears. Guidelines are provided for typical situations encountered in trauma patients to provide a safe starting point for providing analgesia. Caution required in these cases is also discussed, with emphasis on individualization of the approach to analgesia and chemical restraint.

Analgesia for the Critically Ill Dog or Cat: An Update **1353**

Bernie Hansen

Acute pain reliably accompanies severe illness and injury, and when sufficiently severe, it can complicate the recovery of critically ill patients. Because acute pain is closely tied to the neurologic process of nociception, pharmacologic therapy is often essential and effective. This update focuses on two methods of treatment of acute pain—local anesthetic infusion and continuous intravenous infusion of multimodal agents—that can be layered on top of standard care with other drugs.

Neuropathic Pain in Dogs and Cats: If Only They Could Tell Us If They Hurt **1365**

Karol A. Mathews

Neuropathic pain is difficult to diagnose in veterinary patients because they are unable to verbalize their pain. By assuming that neuropathic pain may exist based on the history of events that each patient has experienced, a focused client history and neurologic examination may identify a lesion resulting in persistent or spontaneous pain. Once neuropathic pain is diagnosed, a trial analgesic or acupuncture session(s) should be prescribed with instructions for owners to observe behavior. Dosing of the analgesic can be titrated to the patient's needs while avoiding adverse effects. When a particular analgesic may be ineffectual, an alternate class should be tried. As research into the neurobiologic mechanisms of neuropathic pain continues, specific therapies for its management should eventually appear in the human clinical setting and subsequently be investigated for veterinary clinical use.

Pain Management: The Veterinary Technician's Perspective **1415**

Nancy Shaffran

In veterinary medicine, technicians provide primary nursing care and function as patient advocates. In this role, veterinary technicians have great influence over animal pain management. This article focuses on assessing patients for comfort, providing appropriate nonpharmacologic and pharmacologic therapy, and general concepts of providing optimal analgesia. The communication necessary for successful implementation of pain management strategies is discussed in detail.

Control of Cancer Pain in Veterinary Patients **1429**

James S. Gaynor

Control of cancer pain is within the capabilities of most veterinarians and is achievable in most animal patients that have cancer with techniques that are currently available. Great satisfaction can be derived from not only treating the pet's cancer but its pain. Incorporating pain management into oncology practice is good for the well-being of the pet, the owner, the staff, the veterinarians, and the practice.

Nonsurgical Management of Osteoarthritis in Dogs **1449**

Spencer A. Johnston, Ronald M. McLaughlin, and Steven C. Budsberg

Osteoarthritis (OA), although superficially considered to be deterioration of the joint associated with pain and dysfunction, is actually quite a complex condition. When considering treatment of OA, a multitude of biochemical, physical, and pathologic alterations must be recognized. This article presents a review of the published material regarding various nonsurgical treatments for OA. When there are no data regarding a specific treatment or when a statement is the opinion of the authors, such a deficiency is identified.

Index **1471**

FORTHCOMING ISSUES

January 2009

Changing Paradigms in Diagnosis and Treatment of Urolithiasis

Carl A. Osborne, DVM, PhD
and Jody P. Lulich, DVM, PhD
Guest Editors

March 2009

Veterinary Public Health

Rosalie Trevejo, DVM, MPVM, PhD
Guest Editor

May 2009

Hepatology

P. Jane Armstrong, DVM, PhD
and Jan Rothuizen, DVM, PhD,
Guest Editors

RECENT ISSUES

September 2008

Practical Applications and New Perspectives in Veterinary Behavior

Gary M. Landsberg, DVM
and Debra F. Horwitz, DVM,
Guest Editors

July 2008

Emerging and Reemerging Viruses of Dogs and Cats

Sanjay Kapil, DVM, MS, PhD
and Catherine G. Lamm, DVM
Guest Editors

May 2008

Advances in Fluid, Electrolyte, and Acid-Base Disorders

Helio Autran de Morais, DVM, PhD
and Stephen P. DiBartola, DVM
Guest Editors

RELATED INTEREST

Veterinary Clinics of North America: Exotic Animal Practice May 2007 (Vol. 10, No. 2)
Emergency and Critical Care
Marla Lichtenberger, DVM, Dipl. ACVECC, *Guest Editor*

Preface

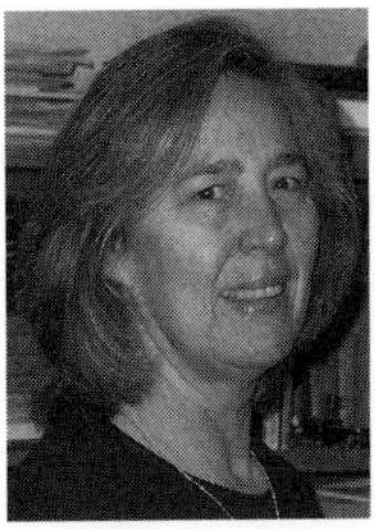

Karol A. Mathews, DVM, DVSc
Guest Editor

> *We must all die. But that I can save him from days of torture, that is what I feel is my great and ever new privilege. Pain is a more terrible lord of mankind than even death itself.*
>
> *Albert Schweitzer, 1931*

This update on the management of pain is designed to build on the information presented in the July 2000 issue of this series. I thank the authors for sharing their experience, scientific contributions, and expertise with us, and for devoting an extensive amount of time in preparing their articles. We are extremely fortunate that these extremely busy and well-sought experts of pain management have contributed to this very practical, yet educational issue. Combined, the current issue and the July 2000 issue on pain management provide a comprehensive library of managing all causes of pain in cats and dogs.

Dr. Lamont's article, "Multimodal Pain Management in Veterinary Medicine: The Physiologic Basis of Pharmacologic Therapies," introduces the various pharmaceutical agents available to manage pain at different sites in the nervous system and sets the stage for managing pain of any origin. Her following article on adjuvant analgesics and their mechanism of action presents the "not so commonly used" analgesics that complement the "more commonly used" agents to ensure optimal analgesia in all patients. Dr. Valverde, who I have the pleasure of working with on a daily basis, gives a detailed report on the technique of and the pharmaceutical agents used in epidural anesthesia/analgesia, a method that is essential for managing moderate to severe pain in many situations. To add to the many local blockade techniques presented in the July 2000 issue titled "Management of Pain," Drs. Lemke and Creighton contribute details on performing the brachial plexus blockade for procedures of the forelimbs.

Dr. Papich, a world-renowned expert in clinical pharmacology, keeps us all well-informed on the latest information through reviews and scientific studies on nonsteroidal anti-inflammatory analgesics, a class of analgesics used extensively in veterinary medicine. Dr. Robertson has dedicated much of her time to the management of pain in cats. She realized that many veterinarians experience apprehension when administering analgesics in this species, and she is determined to prove the safety and efficacy

Vet Clin Small Anim 38 (2008) xi–xiii
doi:10.1016/j.cvsm.2008.09.003

of various analgesics when used appropriately in cats through scientific study. We are very fortunate to have Dr. Robertson contribute her article titled "Managing Pain in Feline Patients." Dr. Dyson, a long-time colleague and friend, is a very knowledgeable yet practical anesthetist who has a strong interest in pain management for compromised and healthy patients. Her articles titled "Perioperative Pain Management in Veterinary Patients" and "Analgesia and Chemical Restraint for the Emergent Veterinary Patient" are detailed and applicable for any situation. Dr. Hansen, who is dedicated to managing pain of all causes in critically ill patients, provides a detailed application of continuous local anesthetic infiltration of wounds and a practical delivery of several other analgesics.

To raise awareness of the needs for pain management in pregnant and lactating cats and dogs and their offspring, and patients who may experience neuropathic pain, I have added two articles providing various aspects of clinical presentation, diagnosis, and management. To complete the sections on acute management of pain, Dr. Shaffran has provided us with information on the important role of the technician and nursing staff in caring for our patients. To complete the issue, the final two articles, again written by experts in their field, cover the ongoing chronic care management of animals experiencing pain caused by cancer (Dr. Gaynor) and osteoarthritis (Drs. Johnston, McLaughlin, and Budsberg).

We have learned that nociception activates various pathways to the cortex where pain is perceived. However, along the way, the sensory process delivers signals to various areas in the brain, which activates the adrenergic and endocrine systems, which in turn, have a significant impact on disruption of homeostasis and energy consumption. In addition, limbic structures are activated, resulting in the affective dimension of pain—the associated emotions that are different from the "pain experience."[1] Together, this "stress" on the individual results in a great expenditure of biological resources and associated homeostatic dysfunction. When the biological cost of stress is sufficient to divert biological resources away from functions that are critical to the animal's well-being, stress then becomes "distress." During distress, the stress-induced changes in biological function are sufficient to place the animal in an immunocompromised state and make it vulnerable to secondary infection, reduced wound healing, and potential multiple organ dysfunction. The animal will remain "distressed" until the stressors (pain, uncomfortable environment, excessive noise, inappropriate handling, and lack of good nursing care and nourishment) are eliminated, and the biological resources expended during the stress response are replenished sufficiently to the pre-stressed condition.[2] I hope the contents of this issue will provide the practitioner with the tools to eliminate the stress and distress associated with the emotional and actual experience associated with pain.

I thank John Vassallo for his patience and expertise and the editorial staff of Elsevier for their assistance in the preparation of the articles.

Karol A. Mathews, DVM, DVSc
Emergency and Critical Care Medicine
Department of Clinical Studies
Ontario Veterinary College
University of Guelph
Guelph, Ontario N1G 2W1, Canada

E-mail address:
kmathews@uoguelph.ca

REFERENCES

1. Chapman RC. Limbic process and the affective dimension of pain. In: Carli G, Zimmerman M, editors. Progress in brain research. Vol 10. Elsevier Science B.V.; 1996. p. 63–81.
2. Moberg GP. When does stress become distress? Lab Animal 1999;28(4):22–6.

Multimodal Pain Management in Veterinary Medicine: The Physiologic Basis of Pharmacologic Therapies

Leigh A. Lamont, DVM, MS

KEYWORDS

- Multimodal analgesia • Nociception • Pain

Multimodal analgesia refers to the practice of combining multiple analgesic drug classes or techniques to target different points along the pain pathway. This approach has become widely accepted in veterinary medicine for two reasons. First, it takes advantage of additive or synergistic analgesic effects that optimize analgesia and improve patient comfort. Second, lower doses of individual analgesic agents are typically required, which reduces the potential for development of undesirable side effects associated with treatment.

Although this strategy seems simple on the surface, effective multimodal pain management plans go beyond the philosophy that more drugs equal better analgesia. A rational multimodal approach to treating pain must be based on an understanding of physiology and pathophysiology. With this foundation, pharmacologic interventions can be tailored to meet the needs of the patient. This article reviews the physiologic basis of pain as it relates to analgesic treatments (**Box 1**) and also introduces new developments in molecular biology that may guide analgesic drug development in the future (**Box 2**).

DEFINITIONS

Pain: a sensory event involving the peripheral and central nervous systems in addition to an unpleasant experience arising from, and reciprocally affecting, processes of higher consciousness

Department of Companion Animals, Atlantic Veterinary College, University of Prince Edward Island, 550 University Avenue, Charlottetown, Prince Edward Island, Canada C1A 4P3
E-mail address: llamont@upei.ca

Vet Clin Small Anim 38 (2008) 1173–1186
doi:10.1016/j.cvsm.2008.06.005 vetsmall.theclinics.com

Box 1
Analgesic drugs and their targets along the nociceptive pathway

Drugs acting at peripheral nociceptors

- Capsaicin
- Local anesthetics

Drugs acting at primary afferent fibers

- Local anesthetics
- α_2-Agonists

Drugs acting at the dorsal horn

- Opioids
- Nonsteroidal anti-inflammatory drugs (NSAIDs)
- α_2-Agonists
- Local anesthetics

Drugs acting at thalamocortical structures

- Opioids
- α_2-Agonists

Drugs acting at descending antinociceptive pathways

- Opioids
- α_2-Agonists

Drugs minimizing development of or showing efficacy during peripheral sensitization

- NSAIDs
- Opioids

Drugs minimizing development of or showing efficacy during central sensitization

- Ketamine
- Amantadine
- Gabapentin
- Cyclooxygenase (COX)-2–specific NSAIDs

Analgesia: the absence of pain sensation

Nociception: the physiologic component of pain processing involving the transduction, transmission, and modulation of signals generated by stimulation of peripheral nociceptors

Noxious: a stimulus that damages or threatens to damage tissue; it may be mechanical, chemical, or thermal

Allodynia: pain that is produced by a stimulus that does not normally provoke pain (ie, by a nonnoxious stimulus)

Hyperalgesia: increased pain response to a noxious stimulus at the site of injury (primary) or in surrounding undamaged tissue (secondary)

Box 2
Potential targets for development of novel analgesic drugs

Drugs acting at peripheral nociceptors

- Transient receptor potential (TRP) V1 antagonists
- TRPV1 desensitizers

Drugs acting at primary afferent fibers

- $Na_v1.8$ antagonists
- Downregulation of $Na_v1.8$ activity by gene therapy

Drugs minimizing development of peripheral sensitization

- Peripheral-acting opioids
- Bradykinin or protein kinase C (PKC) antagonists
- Nerve growth factor (NGF)–capturing drugs
- TrkA antagonists

Drugs minimizing development of central sensitization

- Specific *N*-methyl-D-aspartate (NMDA) antagonists
- Glial antagonists or immunomodulators
- Cytokine or chemokine antagonists

NOCICEPTION

There is a tendency when discussing the physiology of pain to paint a simple stimulus-response picture similar to that of the other somatosensations, such as touch or pressure. Although there are certainly fundamental similarities between the pathways that produce pain and those that lead to other types of sensations, the perception of pain in human beings or domestic animals is much more complex than the sum of these nociceptive processes alone. This complexity is exemplified in the chronic and neuropathic pain syndromes that continue to challenge our current understanding of pain, requiring new theories to explain these phenomena better. One such theory, proposed by Melzack,[1,2] states that the multidimensional experience we call pain is produced by characteristic neurosignature patterns of nerve impulses generated by a widely distributed neural network in the brain that he calls the "body-self neuromatrix." These neurosignature patterns may be triggered by sensory inputs but, notably, may also be generated independently of them. By recognizing that injury and pain may not always have a simple one-to-one relation, this theory provides a template to explore factors that determine or modulate the body-self neuromatrix, including genetic influences, the stress system, and cognitive brain functions, in addition to traditional sensory inputs.

Thus, although it is understood that a discussion of nociceptive pathways and acute pain is inherently limited in its ability to explain the complexities of the pain experience, a basic understanding of these pathways remains a prerequisite for designing effective clinical pain management strategies. With this in mind, the following sections outline these pathways, beginning in the periphery.

Peripheral Nociceptors

In cutaneous tissues, muscle, and visceral tissues, transduction of high-threshold (ie, noxious) stimuli into electrical impulses occurs at specialized free nerve endings of certain primary afferent fibers known as nociceptors.[3,4] Most nociceptors are nonselective ion channels that are gated not by voltage but by temperature, chemical ligands, or mechanical shearing forces.[5] Once they are activated, the channels open and Na^+ and Ca^{2+} ions flow into the nociceptor peripheral terminal, producing an inward current that depolarizes the membrane.[6] The presence, specificity, and threshold of these nociceptor transducers constitute the first and most important filter in nociceptive processing and define the different classes of primary afferent fibers.[4] Most fibers are considered polymodal, responding to multiple types of noxious stimuli, whereas some are unimodal and respond to only one form of stimulus. There has been considerable progress in the past decade in identifying the molecular structure and function of various nociceptor ion channels.

Of all of these "transducers," the TRP ion channels have emerged as the major family involved in generating thermally and chemically evoked pain.[7–9] All TRP receptors are considered to be primarily thermoreceptors, but they may also respond to mechanical and chemical activators. Within the TRP family are several subfamilies, including TRPV, TRPM, and TRPA. In the TRPV subfamily, the most important member is TRPVI (also known as the vanilloid receptor-1).[10] It is located on C and Aδ fibers, responds to noxious heat (>42°C), and is also capsaicin-sensitive.[3,6,7] Another type, TRPV2, is capsaicin-insensitive and has a higher thermal threshold (approximately 52°C). Two additional TRPV members, TRPV3 and TRPV4, respond to lower thermal ranges and other chemical mediators.[7] The TRPM and TRPA subfamilies have receptors that respond to cold, with TRPM8 responding at <28 °C and TRPA1 responding at <18 °C.[11,12]

Another potentially important transducer is TREK-1, a member of the 2P-domain K^+ channel family.[4,9] The TREK-1 receptor is located on C and Aδ fibers and responds to mechanical and thermal stimuli. Interestingly, TREK-1 receptors seem to be extensively colocalized with TRPV1 receptors in dorsal root ganglia neurons.[13] In addition, other transducer channels, such as the acid-sensing ion channels (ASICs), have been identified on nociceptive (Aδ) and nonnociceptive (Aβ fibers) and are involved in transducing mechanical and chemical stimuli.[9]

Analgesic Drugs Acting at Nociceptors

At present, there are few pharmacologic interventions that specifically target the process of transduction in the nonsensitized nociceptor. One exception is capsaicin, an algogenic substance found in hot peppers. As mentioned previously, capsaicin binds to TRPV1 receptors and activates them, which initiates a pain response. Prolonged application of a topical preparation of capsaicin, however, has been shown to desensitize TRPV1 and, ultimately, to produce analgesia. TRPV1 desensitization seems to depend on calcium and may be mediated by calmodulin.[14] There are commercial preparations of topical capsaicin available that have been used to treat human patients who have postherpetic neuralgia and other types of neuropathic pain. Resiniferatoxin is a capsaicin analogue, and one recent veterinary study has demonstrated that intrathecal administration of resiniferatoxin produced clinically significant analgesic effects in dogs with spontaneously occurring bone cancer.[15]

On the horizon for the future, the pharmaceutical industry is currently pursuing development of specific TRPV1 antagonists for potential use as clinical analgesics. Other groups are looking at development of new synthetic capsaicin-like drugs to induce TRPV1 desensitization and produce analgesia.

Primary Afferent Fibers

As discussed previously, the transduction of noxious stimuli is manifested by influx of Na^+ and K^+ ions into the peripheral terminal of the nociceptor, which initiates depolarization. If the depolarizing current is of sufficient magnitude, voltage-gated Na^+ channels are activated, further depolarizing the membrane and causing a burst of action potentials.[5] These action potentials are conducted from the periphery to the central nervous system along the axons of primary afferent nociceptive fibers. There are several isoforms of Na^+ channels that have been recognized for their specific role in nociception, including the nociceptor-specific $Na_v1.7$, $Na_v1.8$, and $Na_v1.9$ channels.[3,16] Under normal conditions, most of these channels are of the tetrodotoxin (TTX)-sensitive type; however, neural insult, inflammation, and exposure to algogenic substances cause increased expression of a TTX-resistant (TTX-R) isoform, which may subserve lowered threshold Na^+ conductance.[17]

It is now well recognized that multiple small-fiber afferents can transmit nociceptive impulses, based on their expression of transductive receptors and TTX-R type Na^+ channels. Aδ and C fibers are still regarded as the principal nociceptive primary afferents, however, and their differential activity is responsible for the unique sensory qualities of fast and slow pain.

Type I and type II Aδ fibers range in size from 1 to 5 μm in diameter, are myelinated, and conduct impulses rapidly at a rate of 5 to 30 m/sec. The conduction rate is correlated to the initial sensation of pain, often referred to as "first pain," which is sharp, localized, and transient. These afferents have small receptive fields and specific high-threshold ion channels that are activated by noxious thermal or mechanical input.[3]

C-fibers constitute most cutaneous nociceptive innervation. They are small, ranging in size from 0.25 to 1.5 μm in diameter, are unmyelinated with conduction velocities of only 0.5 to 2 m/sec, and have larger receptive fields compared with Aδ fibers.[3] These characteristics contribute to "second pain," which is the poorly localized, burning, gnawing sensation that persists after termination of the noxious stimulus. C fibers are polymodal and may be activated by thermal, mechanical, or chemical stimuli. In addition to their cutaneous locations, C fibers are also found extensively throughout muscle and viscera.

Analgesic Drugs Acting at Primary Afferent Fibers

The local anesthetics, such as lidocaine and bupivacaine, are classic Na^+ channel blockers and are considered to be primary analgesic agents. Their principal effect in the nociceptive pathway is to inhibit nerve impulse conduction along Aδ and C fibers, thereby blocking the transmission of nociceptive signals to the central nervous system. Physicians and veterinarians exploit this class of drugs extensively by using them in local and regional nerve block techniques to prevent and actively manage pain. Techniques like peripheral nerve blocks and epidural anesthesia are extremely effective components of a multimodal pain management plan, and the reader is referred elsewhere in this issue for a detailed discussion of their use.

Another class of drugs, the α_2-agonists, may also possess some ability to inhibit nerve impulse conduction when applied perineurally and may potentiate the intensity and duration of blockade when coadministered with a local anesthetic.[18]

Despite the clinical utility of the currently available Na^+ channel blockers, such as lidocaine, to inhibit nociceptive transmission, these drugs are all nonselective, and thus have relatively narrow therapeutic indices. Because of the restricted expression patterns of voltage-gated Na^+ channels associated with nociceptive primary afferents, notably $Na_v1.8$, this channel has become a target for future drug development.[5,16] Isoform-specific channel antagonists or gene therapy approaches targeted at downregulating these specific isoforms could, in theory, block only fibers transmitting pain input while leaving those transmitting innocuous sensations and motor and autonomic outputs intact.

Dorsal Horn Neurons and Ascending Spinal Tracts

The dorsal horn represents the first relay point for somatic sensory information, including nociceptive input, en route to the brain. Aδ and C fibers enter the spinal cord by way of the dorsal roots of spinal nerves and synapse in specific laminae (layers) of the dorsal horn. Aδ fibers terminate in laminae I, II, and IIa, whereas C fibers terminate in laminae II, IIa, and V.[3] Primary afferents may synapse with local interneurons (which may be excitatory or inhibitory), with propriospinal neurons, or with projection neurons that extend beyond the spinal cord to transmit nociceptive input to supraspinal structures. The primary synaptic transmitter present in all types of primary afferents is glutamate. Most transmission between primary afferents and dorsal horn neurons occurs through postsynaptically located ionotropic α-amino-3-hydroxyl-5-methyl-4-isoxazole propionic acid (AMPA) receptors with a small NMDA component.[19] In addition to neurotransmitters, there is a long and growing list of other substances that can also modulate synaptic transmission in the dorsal horn.

There are two major types of nociceptive projection neurons located in the dorsal horn, wide dynamic range (WDR) and nociceptive-specific (NS) neurons. Most of these neurons extend axons contralaterally to form the spinothalamic tract (STT). WDR neurons predominate in lamina V and receive innocuous input from low-threshold Aα and Aβ fibers in addition to nociceptive input from Aδ and C fibers.[20] WDR neurons respond in a graded manner over large receptive fields and often receive convergent deep and visceral input. NS neurons are concentrated in lamina I and respond to input from Aδ and C fibers only. They have smaller receptive fields compared with WDR neurons and function in stimulus localization and discrimination.

WDR and NS neurons project to the reticular formation and thalamus of the brain stem by way of multiple parallel pathways called tracts, including the STT, the spinocervicothalamic tract (SCT), the spinoreticular tract (SRT), the spinomesencephalic tract (SMT), and the postsynaptic dorsal column pathway.[21] Although there is considerable species variation in the relative importance of these tracts with regard to nociception, the STT and SCT seem to be most important in domestic species, with the SCT being of particular note in carnivores.[22] In human beings, the sensory discriminative aspects of pain seem to be mediated by projections to the lateral thalamocortical system, whereas the motivational and affective aspects seem to be mediated by projections to the medial thalamocortical system.[23]

Analgesic Drugs Acting at the Dorsal Horn

In the nonsensitized nervous system, the principal analgesic drugs that act in the dorsal horn are the opioids, the α_2-agonists, and the NSAIDs. The opioids and the α_2-agonists are used extensively in veterinary medicine to manage pain, and opioids, in particular, remain among the most effective analgesics currently available. Dense populations of opioid receptors exist in the dorsal horn, and activation of these receptors may have pre- and postsynaptic effects. At the presynaptic level, decreased Ca^{2+} influx reduces the release of excitatory transmitter substances, such as substance P, from primary afferents, which inhibits nociceptive transmission.[20] Postsynaptically, enhanced K^+ efflux causes hyperpolarization of projection neurons, which also inhibits ascending nociceptive pathways. Because α_2-adrenoceptors belong to the same superfamily as do opioid receptors, the α_2-agonists have a similar mechanism of analgesic action within the dorsal horn.

The NSAIDs are also widely used in veterinary medicine to manage various types of pain. Although their peripheral antiprostaglandin effects make them obvious choices for minimizing development of peripheral sensitization of nociceptors, they also inhibit cyclooxygenase (COX) within the spinal cord dorsal horn, and thus are also considered to have central-acting analgesic effects.

Although there are numerous other drugs that may have an impact on dorsal horn modulation of nociceptive input, the role of most of these agents is to suppress or inhibit the development of central sensitization rather than to induce analgesia in the nonsensitized state. As such, these agents are discussed in a later section.

Thalamocortical System

As mentioned previously, the sensory discriminative aspects of pain are produced in the lateral thalamocortical system, which consists of relay nuclei in the lateral thalamus and the primary and secondary somatosensory cortices. The motivational and affective aspects of the pain experience arise in the medial thalamocortical system, which includes relay nuclei in the medial thalamus that send projections to limbic structures, such as the anterior cingulate gyrus and prefrontal cortex, but that also includes spinal projections to the hypothalamus and amygdala.

Analgesic Drugs Acting at Thalamocortical Structures

Drugs like opioids and α_2-agonists also have analgesic effects that are mediated at the supraspinal level through their effects on descending inhibitory nociceptive pathways. In addition, the sedative effects induced by these drugs, although not producing analgesia, may act to modify certain aspects of pain perception.

Other drug classes, such as benzodiazepines, phenothiazines, and general anesthetics, have no primary analgesic activity. They are able to decrease or, in the case of general anesthetics, completely obliterate the perception of pain, however, by altering the state of consciousness. Despite the fact that an individual may be totally unaware of pain while under the influence of such drugs, nociceptive processing continues virtually unabated during this time. Consequently, it is universally recognized that patients undergoing painful procedures while under general anesthesia require a multimodal approach to pain management involving analgesic therapy before, during, and after the procedure is completed.

Descending Antinociceptive Pathways

In addition to the ascending nociceptive pathways outlined previously, it is equally important to recognize that there are powerful descending pathways that are able to modulate the pain response, upregulating it or downregulating it. This system has four different tiers: (1) the dorsal horn, (2) the periaqueductal gray matter (PAG) of the midbrain, (3) the rostroventral medulla (RVM) and pons of the brain stem, and (4) thalamocortical structures.[3,24,25] Of these, the PAG and the RVM are generally viewed as the core of this important system.

Within the RVM, there are unique populations of cells referred to as "on" and "off" cells.[26] Predictably, off cells hyperpolarize in response to STT activation and reduce the transmission of nociceptive volleys in the brain stem.[3] Conversely, on cells are excited by nociceptive input from the STT and engage parabrachial, hypothalamic, cingulate, insular, and septohippocampal pathways subserving arousal and aversive reactions to pain.[27] These cells, it now seems, are critical in producing hyperalgesia after peripheral tissue injury by maintaining central sensitization.

At the level of the midbrain, the PAG has long been recognized as a key structure in the endogenous analgesia system. Afferent input from the STT, efferent projections from the cingulate gyrus, and nuclei of the limbic forebrain and hypothalamus all activate endorphin-, enkephalin- and nociception-containing neurons of the PAG.[27] Projections extending from the PAG to the brain stem are inhibitory and excitatory. Opioids from the PAG act postsynaptically to suppress GABAergic interneurons in the brain stem, thereby disinhibiting tonic and burst activity of descending serotonergic and adrenergic bulbospinal pathways.[3]

Analgesic Drugs Acting at Descending Antinociceptive Pathways

Obviously, the opioids are the class of drugs that play the most significant and best known role in descending nociceptive modulatory pathways through their actions at multiple levels, including the PAG and the dorsal horn. Despite the potential for adverse side effects associated with their administration, physicians and veterinarians continue to use exogenous opioids extensively because they remain among the most powerful and efficacious analgesics available.

Although the analgesic effects of the α_2-agonists have traditionally been attributed to their effects at the level of the spinal cord, analgesia may also be mediated at the supraspinal level through descending antinociceptive pathways. The α_2-agonists bind receptors in a group of catecholaminergic nuclei in the pons known as the locus ceruleus (LC), which receives noradrenergic efferents from the PAG and also extends noradrenergic axons to the spinal cord. Activation in the LC seems to contribute indirectly to analgesia at the level of the dorsal horn through these descending projections.[28,29]

NERVOUS SYSTEM SENSITIZATION

In the clinical setting, physicians and veterinarians are often called on to manage pain associated with substantial tissue injury. If a noxious stimulus is sufficiently intense to produce such injury, prolonged poststimulus sensory disturbances may be observed, including continued pain, increased sensitivity to noxious stimuli (hyperalgesia), and pain after innocuous stimuli (allodynia). These clinical findings are a result of changes in nervous system processing occurring peripherally and centrally.

Peripheral Sensitization

Injury to tissues causes inflammation that results in profound changes to the chemical environment of nociceptor peripheral terminals. Damaged cells release their intracellular contents, such as ATP and K^+ ions; local pH decreases; and cytokines, chemokines, and growth factors are produced by inflammatory cells that are recruited to the site of damage.[30] Many of these chemicals act on G-protein–coupled receptors or tyrosine kinase (TrK) receptors expressed on nociceptor terminals. Intracellular signaling pathways are then activated, which, by means of phosphorylating receptors and ion channels within the terminal, actually modify nociceptor threshold and kinetics.[5]

Inflammatory mediators may be broadly classified into two categories: direct or indirect acting. Of the direct-acting mediators, some are considered nociceptor activators because they directly stimulate the nociceptor, whereas others are nociceptor sensitizers because they sensitize the terminal, making it hyperresponsive to subsequent inputs.[5] A discussion of all the relevant inflammatory mediators that play a part in peripheral sensitization is beyond the scope of this article; thus, instead, a few selected mediators are presented.

Prostaglandins are considered the prototypic nociceptor sensitizers. Prostaglandin E_2 (PGE_2), for example, can cause changes in TRPV1 by means of activation of cyclic adenosine monophosphate (cAMP)–dependent protein kinase A (PKA) and Ca^{2+}-dependent protein kinase C (PKC), resulting in phosphorylation of TRPV1 and radically lowering its thermal threshold (from approximately 42°C to 35°C).[5,31]

Bradykinin is an example of a direct-acting mediator capable of nociceptor activation and sensitization. Like PGE_2, the TRPV1 receptor seems to be responsible for most bradykinin-induced nociceptive activity.[32] Bradykinin seems to work through multiple signaling pathways to reduce TRPV1 thermal thresholds, including phospholipase C (PLC), PKC, phospholipase A (PLA), and, downstream of this, lipoxygenase (LOX).[33] In addition to its ability to reduce TRPV1 thermal thresholds dramatically, bradykinin can also activate TRPA1 in a PLC-dependent manner to enhance noxious cold sensitivity.[11]

A relatively new discovery is the importance of neurotrophic factors as key players in the process of peripheral sensitization. Traditionally, the role of neurotrophic factors, such as NGF, was thought to be regulation of neuronal survival in the developing nervous system. As its contribution to the pain response continues to be unraveled, however, it seems that NGF may soon be recognized primarily for its role as a pain mediator.

NGF is the founding member of the neurotrophin family of proteins, which includes brain-derived neurotrophic factor (BDNF), neurotropin 3 (NT-3), and neurotropin 4 (NT-4).[34] The receptor tyrosine kinase known as TrkA and the receptor p75 NTR bind NGF.[35,36] Evidence indicates that TrkA receptors are mandatory for the nociceptive actions of NGF but that p75 NTR may also play a role.[37]

Induction of expression of NGF is an early event in injured and inflamed tissues, and elevated levels are sustained throughout chronic inflammation. Increased levels of NGF may contribute to peripheral sensitization directly or indirectly. First, NGF can sensitize TRPV1 channels directly through PKC signaling. Second, retrograde NGF signaling from nociceptor peripheral terminals triggers altered gene expression in the cell bodies to produce substance P, the $Na_v1.8$ channel, the ASIC3 channel, the TRPV1 channel, and BDNF. These proteins further sensitize the primary afferents and contribute to the phenomenon of primary hyperalgesia.[35,36] Finally, NGF released under conditions of tissue injury and inflammation can also sensitize nociceptors indirectly by activating mast cells.[38]

Analgesic Drugs that Inhibit Peripheral Sensitization

The NSAIDs, through their antiprostaglandin effects, are the classic group of drugs with efficacy at inhibiting peripheral sensitization. NSAIDs are widely used in veterinary medicine for the management of acute perioperative pain and various types of chronic pain. Because they focus on COX pathways only, numerous other sensitizers, such as bradykinin and NGF, are still able to alter nociceptor function significantly during tissue injury and inflammation. Thus, the currently available NSAIDs always have a ceiling effect that limits their analgesic potential.

Opioids have traditionally been considered the prototype class of centrally acting analgesics, although evidence has emerged over the past decade suggesting that these drugs have peripheral effects as well. Opioid receptors of all three major types have been identified on the processes of sensory neurons, and they respond to peripherally applied opioids and locally released endogenous opioid peptides when upregulated during inflammation.[39,40] Currently available opioid analgesics bind central and peripheral opioid receptors nonselectively; however, there is the theoretic potential to develop selective ligands for peripheral opioid receptors, which would offer the possibility of analgesia without centrally mediated adverse side effects.

Other future drug discovery approaches to inhibit peripheral sensitization include the following: (1) drugs that reduce bradykinin production, (2) drugs that block binding of bradykinin or one or more of its signaling pathways (eg, PKC), (3) NGF-capturing drugs that could effectively remove free NGF, (4) drugs that prevent NGF binding to TrkA, and (5) drugs that inhibit TrkA signaling.[32,34]

Central Sensitization

In the same way that the peripheral terminal of the nociceptor can become sensitized, dorsal horn nociceptive neurons can also exhibit increased excitability. Initially, central sensitization is considered to depend on activity; that is, it is triggered by nociceptor input into the spinal cord.[5] Later, it is sustained beyond the initiating stimulus by transcriptional changes in the molecular machinery of the cell and is referred to as transcription dependent.[41] Within seconds of major nociceptive inputs, dorsal horn neurons begin to exhibit hyperresponsiveness and the ensuing clinical manifestations become evident. Exaggerated pain responses are noted within the injured area (called primary hyperalgesia) and also well outside the site of injury (called secondary hyperalgesia). As well, low-threshold Aβ fibers that, under normal circumstances, do not respond to noxious inputs are recruited and contribute to the pain response. This means that normally innocuous stimuli, such as a light touch to the skin, now elicit pain (called tactile allodynia).

In general, many of the alterations underlying central sensitization are similar to those that produce peripheral sensitization. Mechanistically, numerous intracellular signaling pathways are activated in the dorsal horn by the neurotransmitter glutamate in addition to other neuromodulators, including substance P and BDNF. Increased synaptic efficacy seems to result from two primary mechanisms: (1) alterations in ion channel or receptor activity arising from posttranslational processing and (2) mobilization of receptors to neuronal membranes. One key receptor involved in these changes is the glutamate-activated NMDA receptor. Phosphorylation of this receptor stimulates its mobilization from intracellular stores to the synaptic membrane and increases its responsiveness to glutamate by removal of the voltage-dependent Mg^{2+} ion block, thereby favoring the open-state configuration.[5]

Recent investigations into the basis of central sensitization have revealed the central neuroimmune response as a driving force, with particular relevance in chronic pain states after peripheral nerve injury.[42] Traditionally, nonneuronal glial cells were thought to function mainly as "housekeepers," whose role was to provide support and nutrition to neurons while acting as passive bystanders of neuronal transmission. Within the past decade, considerable evidence has accrued to support the notion that glial cells are in fact key players in the creation and maintenance of pathologic pain states.[43] Glial cell activation occurs secondary to nerve trauma or inflammation, which results in the production of numerous proinflammatory mediators.[43,44] Important proinflammatory cytokines include interleukin (IL)-1β, tumor necrosis factor-α (TNFα), and IL-6.[44] Chemokines (ie, chemoattractant cytokines), such as macrophage inflammatory protein-2 and monocyte chemoattractant protein-1, recruit macrophages and neutrophils from the circulation into nerves.[43] Together, these neuroexcitatory substances released after glial cell activation can create and maintain the state of augmented pain facilitation known as central sensitization.

Furthermore, these immune cells also seem to compromise opioid efficacy for management of clinical pain.[45,46] It is now clear that glial cells regulate morphine analgesia, tolerance, and dependence and withdrawal.[47] Although it is also clear that such effects are not limited to morphine, it is as yet unknown how pervasive this glial regulation may turn out to be.

Analgesic Drugs that Inhibit Central Sensitization

Because of the importance of the NMDA receptor in central sensitization, inhibition of this receptor is a rational analgesic strategy. Ketamine has NMDA antagonistic properties and is a drug well known to veterinary medicine, wherein it has been used traditionally as a short-acting anesthetic. Ketamine has been shown to reduce the early phase of central sensitization and the resultant hypersensitivity to pain.[48,49] Unfortunately, because of the widespread distribution of the NMDA receptor throughout the brain, psychomimetic side effects may accompany ketamine's analgesic effects, which limits its clinical utility. Amantadine is another drug with anti-NMDA effects that has been shown to produce analgesia. Because amantadine's predominant inhibitory mechanism is stabilization of NMDA channels in the closed state[50] rather than blockade of current flow through open channels like ketamine, amantadine seems to have a more favorable clinical safety profile. Development of new anti-NMDA drugs that are able to block central sensitization without other central nervous system side effects is being actively pursued at this time.

The anticonvulsant gabapentin is another drug used increasingly by veterinarians as an adjunctive and occasionally primary analgesic agent. Evidence suggests that this drug works by binding to the α_2-δ_1 subunit of presynaptic voltage-gated calcium channels that are upregulated during central sensitization.[51] The intensity of the analgesic effect achieved with gabapentin seems to be proportional to the magnitude of sensitization within the dorsal horn.[52,53]

The NSAIDs, as discussed previously, have effects at numerous locations along nociceptive pathways, peripherally and centrally. COX-2 begins to be expressed by neurons in many areas of the central nervous system several hours after localized peripheral tissue injury.[54] The resultant COX-2–mediated increase in PGE_2 production contributes to a late-onset, prolonged, and diffuse phase of central sensitization.[54] Thus, COX-2–specific NSAIDs are likely to continue to be important components of multimodal pain management strategies because of their ability to dampen central sensitization.

The new appreciation of the importance of immune glial cells in the pain response is currently driving the search for antiglial drugs, or drugs with anticytokine or antichemokine effects, as novel analgesic agents. Such agents have significant potential to reduce opioid tolerance and improve analgesic efficacy in chronic neuropathic pain states.

NEW DIRECTIONS IN UNDERSTANDING THE BIOCHEMICAL BASIS OF PAIN

A group of investigators has recently proposed an interesting theory that the origin of all pain is inflammation and the inflammatory response.[55] Furthermore, they suggest that pain syndromes should be reclassified and treated based on their inflammatory profiles. Specifically, they recommend following four general principles for the treatment of all types of pain: (1) determination of the inflammatory profile of the pain syndrome, (2) inhibition or suppression of production of the appropriate inflammatory mediators, (3) inhibition or suppression of neuronal afferent and efferent (motor) transmission, and (4) modulation of neuronal transmission.[55,56] This theory is appealing in that it supports development of rational multimodal analgesic strategies tailored to the individual patient rather than empiric trial-and-error approaches. Whether this theory proves to be true or not, a transition to mechanism-specific pharmacologic management of pain seems to be the way of the future.

REFERENCES

1. Melzack R. From the gate to the neuromatrix. Pain 1999;(Suppl 6):S121–6.
2. Melzack R. Evolution of the neuromatrix theory of pain. The Prithvi Raj Lecture. Presented at the Third World Congress of the World Institute of Pain. Barcelona, 2004. Pain Pract 2005;5:85–94.
3. Giordano J. The neurobiology of nociceptive and anti-nociceptive systems. Pain Physician 2005;8:277–90.
4. Woolf CJ, Ma Q. Nociceptors—noxious stimulus detectors. Neuron 2007;55: 353–64.
5. Woolf CJ, American College of Physicians, American Physiological Society. Pain: moving from symptom control toward mechanism-specific pharmacologic management. Ann Intern Med 2004;140:441–51.
6. Caterina MJ, Rosen TA, Tominaga M, et al. A capsaicin-receptor homologue with a high threshold for noxious heat. Nature 1999;398:436–41.
7. Wang H, Woolf CJ. Pain TRPs. Neuron 2005;46:9–12.
8. Levine JD, Alessandri-Haber N. TRP channels: targets for the relief of pain. Biochim Biophys Acta 2007;1772:989–1003.
9. Xie W. Ion channels in pain transmission. Int Anesthesiol Clin 2007;45:107–20.
10. Greffrath W. The capsaicin receptor. "TRPing" transduction for painful stimuli. Schmerz 2006;20:219–25.
11. Bandell M, Story GM, Hwang SW, et al. Noxious cold ion channel TRPA1 is activated by pungent compounds and bradykinin. Neuron 2004;41:849–57.
12. Peterlin Z, Chesler A, Firestein S. A painful TRP can be a bonding experience. Neuron 2007;53:635–8.
13. Alloui A, Zimmermann K, Mamet J, et al. TREK-1, a K+ channel involved in polymodal pain perception. EMBO J 2006;25:2368–76.
14. Lambers TT, Weidema AF, Nilius B, et al. Regulation of the mouse epithelial Ca2(+) channel TRPV6 by the Ca(2+)-sensor calmodulin. J Biol Chem 2004; 279:28855–61.
15. Brown DC, Iadarola MJ, Perkowski SZ, et al. Physiologic and antinociceptive effects of intrathecal resiniferatoxin in a canine bone cancer model. Anesthesiology 2005;103:1052–9.
16. Cummins TR, Sheets PL, Waxman SG. The roles of sodium channels in nociception: implications for mechanisms of pain. Pain 2007;131:243–57.
17. Amaya F, Decosterd I, Samad TA, et al. Diversity of expression of the sensory neuron-specific TTX-resistant voltage-gated sodium ion channels SNS and SNS2. Mol Cell Neurosci 2000;15:331–42.
18. Eisenach JC, De Kock M, Klimscha W. Alpha(2)-adrenergic agonists for regional anesthesia. A clinical review of clonidine (1984–1995). Anesthesiology 1996;85: 655–74.
19. Doubell TP, Mannion RJ, Woolf CJ. The dorsal horn: state dependent sensory processing, plasticity and the generation of pain. In: Wall PD, Melzack R, editors. The textbook of pain. 4th edition. Edinburgh (UK): Churchill Livingstone; 1999. p. 165–78.
20. Inturrisi CE. Clinical pharmacology of opioids for pain. Clin J Pain 2002;18:S3–13.
21. Willis WD Jr. The somatosensory system, with emphasis on structures important for pain. Brain Res Rev 2007;55:297–313.
22. Kajander KC, Giesler GJ Jr. Responses of neurons in the lateral cervical nucleus of the cat to noxious cutaneous stimulation. J Neurophysiol 1987;57:1686–704.

23. Youell PD, Wise RG, Bentley DE, et al. Lateralisation of nociceptive processing in the human brain: a functional magnetic resonance imaging study. Neuroimage 2004;23:1068–77.
24. Tracey I, Mantyh PW. The cerebral signature for pain perception and its modulation. Neuron 2007;55:377–91.
25. Yoshimura M, Furue H. Mechanisms for the anti-nociceptive actions of the descending noradrenergic and serotonergic systems in the spinal cord. J Pharmacol Sci 2006;101:107–17.
26. Mason P. Ventromedial medulla: pain modulation and beyond. J Comp Neurol 2005;493:2–8.
27. Fields HL, Basbaum AI. Central nervous system mechanisms of pain modulation. In: Wall PD, Melzack R, editors. Textbook of pain. 4th edition. Edinburgh (UK): Churchill Livingstone; 1999. p. 309–30.
28. Budai D, Harasawa I, Fields HL. Midbrain periaqueductal gray (PAG) inhibits nociceptive inputs to sacral dorsal horn nociceptive neurons through alpha2-adrenergic receptors. J Neurophysiol 1998;80:2244–54.
29. Guo TZ, Jiang JY, Buttermann AE, et al. Dexmedetomidine injection into the locus ceruleus produces antinociception. Anesthesiology 1996;84:873–81.
30. Levine JD, Reichling DB. Peripheral mechanisms of inflammatory pain. In: Wall PD, Melzack R, editors. Textbook of pain. 4th edition. Edinburgh (UK): Churchill Livingstone; 1999. p. 59–84.
31. Velazquez KT, Mohammad H, Sweitzer SM. Protein kinase C in pain: involvement of multiple isoforms. Pharmacol Res 2007;55:578–89.
32. Wang H, Ehnert C, Brenner GJ, et al. Bradykinin and peripheral sensitization. Biol Chem 2006;387:11–4.
33. Ferreira J, da Silva GL, Calixto JB. Contribution of vanilloid receptors to the overt nociception induced by B2 kinin receptor activation in mice. Br J Pharmacol 2004;141:787–94.
34. Hefti FF, Rosenthal A, Walicke PA, et al. Novel class of pain drugs based on antagonism of NGF. Trends Pharmacol Sci 2006;27:85–91.
35. Huang EJ, Reichardt LF. Trk receptors: roles in neuronal signal transduction. Annu Rev Biochem 2003;72:609–42.
36. Nicol GD, Vasko MR. Unraveling the story of NGF-mediated sensitization of nociceptive sensory neurons: ON or OFF the Trks? Mol Interv 2007;7:26–41.
37. Fang X, Djouhri L, McMullan S, et al. TrkA is expressed in nociceptive neurons and influences electrophysiological properties via Nav1.8 expression in rapidly conducting nociceptors. J Neurosci 2005;25:4868–78.
38. Kawamoto K, Aoki J, Tanaka A, et al. Nerve growth factor activates mast cells through the collaborative interaction with lysophosphatidylserine expressed on the membrane surface of activated platelets. J Immunol 2002;168:6412–9.
39. Fields HL, Emson PC, Leigh BK, et al. Multiple opiate receptor sites on primary afferent fibres. Nature 1980;284:351–3.
40. Stein C, Schafer M, Machelska H. Attacking pain at its source: new perspectives on opioids. Nat Med 2003;9:1003–8.
41. Woolf CJ, Salter MW. Neuronal plasticity: increasing the gain in pain. Science 2000;288:1765–9.
42. DeLeo JA. Basic science of pain. J Bone Joint Surg Am. 2006;88(Suppl 2):58–62.
43. Watkins LR, Hutchinson MR, Milligan ED, et al. "Listening" and "talking" to neurons: implications of immune activation for pain control and increasing the efficacy of opioids. Brain Res Rev 2007;56(1):148–59.

44. Verri WA Jr, Cunha TM, Parada CA, et al. Hypernociceptive role of cytokines and chemokines: targets for analgesic drug development? Pharmacol Ther 2006;112: 116–38.
45. Watkins LR, Hutchinson MR, Johnston IN, et al. Glia: novel counter-regulators of opioid analgesia. Trends Neurosci 2005;28:661–9.
46. Hansson E. Could chronic pain and spread of pain sensation be induced and maintained by glial activation? Acta Physiol (Oxf) 2006;187:321–7.
47. Hutchinson MR, Bland ST, Johnson KW, et al. Opioid-induced glial activation: mechanisms of activation and implications for opioid analgesia, dependence, and reward. ScientificWorldJournal 2007;7:98–111.
48. South SM, Kohno T, Kaspar BK, et al. A conditional deletion of the NR1 subunit of the NMDA receptor in adult spinal cord dorsal horn reduces NMDA currents and injury-induced pain. J Neurosci 2003;23:5031–40.
49. Stubhaug A, Breivik H, Eide PK, et al. Mapping of punctuate hyperalgesia around a surgical incision demonstrates that ketamine is a powerful suppressor of central sensitization to pain following surgery. Acta Anaesthesiol Scand 1997;41: 1124–32.
50. Blanpied TA, Clarke RJ, Johnson JW. Amantadine inhibits NMDA receptors by accelerating channel closure during channel block. J Neurosci 2005;25:3312–22.
51. Field MJ, Cox PJ, Stott E, et al. Identification of the alpha2-delta-1 subunit of voltage-dependent calcium channels as a molecular target for pain mediating the analgesic actions of pregabalin. Proc Natl Acad Sci U S A 2006;103:17537–42.
52. Gottrup H, Juhl G, Kristensen AD, et al. Chronic oral gabapentin reduces elements of central sensitization in human experimental hyperalgesia. Anesthesiology 2004;101:1400–8.
53. Curros-Criado MM, Herrero JF. The antinociceptive effect of systemic gabapentin is related to the type of sensitization-induced hyperalgesia. J Neuroinflammation 2007;4:15.
54. Samad TA, Moore KA, Sapirstein A, et al. Interleukin-1beta-mediated induction of COX-2 in the CNS contributes to inflammatory pain hypersensitivity. Nature 2001; 410:471–5.
55. Omoigui S. The biochemical origin of pain—proposing a new law of pain: the origin of all pain is inflammation and the inflammatory response. Part 1 of 3—a unifying law of pain. Med Hypotheses 2007;69:70–82.
56. Omoigui S. The biochemical origin of pain: the origin of all pain is inflammation and the inflammatory response. Part 2 of 3—inflammatory profile of pain syndromes. Med Hypotheses 2007;69:1169–78.

Adjunctive Analgesic Therapy in Veterinary Medicine

Leigh A. Lamont, DVM, MS

KEYWORDS

• Adjunctive • Analgesic • Pain

Until fairly recently, most standard pain management protocols used in veterinary medicine have been based on administration of pharmacologic agents known as "traditional analgesics." All traditional analgesics share one thing in common: their primary indication is for the management of pain. Historically, the traditional analgesics have included three distinct classes of drugs: opioids, nonsteroidal anti-inflammatory drugs (NSAIDs), and local anesthetics. Although these agents continue to figure prominently in most pain management protocols, ongoing research in pain pathophysiology and clinical experience involving human and veterinary patients has demonstrated that there are numerous other therapeutic options beyond the traditional analgesics. These other treatment options are broadly referred to as "adjunctive analgesic therapies."

TYPES OF ADJUNCTIVE ANALGESIC THERAPIES

Adjunctive analgesic therapies may be separated into two categories: pharmacologic and nonpharmacologic. Within the pharmacologic category, therapies most often involve drugs that have primary indications other than pain but that seem to contribute to analgesia in certain painful conditions. Alternatively, pharmacologic therapy may also involve a traditional analgesic agent that is administered by way of a novel route.

PHARMACOLOGIC ADJUNCTIVE ANALGESIC THERAPY

As the name implies, adjunctive analgesic agents are often, but not exclusively, coadministered with traditional analgesics. They have been used most often in the management of chronic pain states; however, their use in acute pain settings is increasing, and certain adjunctive agents have become common analgesic supplements during the perioperative period. In the chronic pain setting, adjunctive analgesics may be administered to (1) manage pain that is refractory to the traditional analgesics, (2) allow

Department of Companion Animals, Atlantic Veterinary College, University of Prince Edward Island, 550 University Avenue, Charlottetown, Prince Edward Island, Canada C1A 4P3
E-mail address: llamont@upei.ca

Vet Clin Small Anim 38 (2008) 1187–1203
doi:10.1016/j.cvsm.2008.06.002 vetsmall.theclinics.com
0195-5616/08/$ – see front matter

a reduction in the dose of traditional analgesics to lessen side effects, and (3) concurrently treat a symptom other than pain. In some clinical settings, such as chronic neuropathic pain syndromes, adjunctive analgesics have become so well accepted that they are administered as the first-line therapy in human patients.

There is a long and diverse list of adjunctive analgesic drugs that may have utility in veterinary medicine (**Table 1**). Some of these, such as ketamine and the α_2-agonists, are familiar to practitioners, whereas others have not been historically used in veterinary medicine. Although their use is rapidly increasing, controlled clinical trials evaluating most of these agents in dogs and cats are currently lacking. At this time, most treatment recommendations have been extrapolated from human medicine or are based on anecdotal reports in small numbers of veterinary patients. The following section briefly reviews the current state of knowledge regarding selected adjunctive analgesics in veterinary medicine.

Table 1
Selected adjunctive analgesic agents

Class of Drug and Representative Agents	Multipurpose	Neuropathic Pain	Musculoskeletal Pain	Malignant Bone Pain
α_2-Agonists Medetomidine Dexmedetomidine	X	X	—	—
Atypical opioids Tramadol	X	—	—	—
NMDA antagonists Ketamine Amantadine	X	X	—	—
Anticonvulsants Gabapentin	X	X	—	—
Systemic local anesthetics Lidocaine (intravenous) Mexiletine (oral)	X	X	—	—
Bisphosphonates Pamidronate Zoledronate	—	—	—	X
Topical local anesthetics Lidocaine Lidocaine or prilocaine	X	X	—	—
Antidepressants Amitriptyline	X	X	—	—
Corticosteroids Prednisone Dexamethasone	X	—	—	—
Capsaicin	X	X	—	—
Radiopharmaceuticals Strontium-89 Samarium-153	—	—	—	X
Calcitonin	X	X	—	X

Abbreviation: NMDA, *N*-methyl-D-aspartate.

α_2-Agonists: Medetomidine and Dexmedetomidine

This group of sedative-analgesic drugs is well known to most veterinarians and includes medetomidine, detomidine, romifidine, and dexmedetomidine. They exert their clinical effects by interacting with α_2-adrenergic receptors in the central nervous system, specifically the dorsal horn of the spinal cord and the locus ceruleus in the brain stem.[1,2] Although not considered first-line analgesics like opioids or NSAIDs, α_2-agonists are commonly used as adjunctive analgesics. Because their mechanism of action is similar to that of opioids, coadministration of these two classes of drugs is thought to produce synergistic analgesic effects. The major factor that limits their use in pain management protocols is their significant cardiovascular side effects, which have been reviewed in detail elsewhere.[3,4]

Of the available α_2-agonists, medetomidine is currently the most commonly used α_2-agonist for adjunctive analgesia in veterinary medicine. In North America, it is labeled as a sedative-analgesic agent for use in dogs only, whereas it is also approved for use in cats in other parts of the world. Dexmedetomidine is the pharmacologically active enantiomer found in the racemic preparation of medetomidine. It is approved for use in human beings, in whom it is being used increasingly as an adjunctive analgesic; more recently, it has also begun to appear in the veterinary literature.[4,5] Whether it offers any benefits in veterinary patients compared with medetomidine remains unclear at this time. The other α_2-agonists currently available to veterinarians, romifidine and detomidine, are not commonly used as analgesics in small animal patients.

Medetomidine and dexmedetomidine may be used as adjunctive analgesics in a variety of clinical settings. Perhaps most commonly, medetomidine is used in relatively low doses in combination with an opioid before inducing general anesthesia in dogs and cats. The perceived value of this well-accepted clinical practice is twofold: to capitalize on the significant anesthetic-sparing effects of medetomidine and to induce analgesia superior to that obtained with an opioid alone. From an analgesic standpoint, there is emerging evidence to support this practice in human patients, in whom studies have shown that perioperative dexmedetomidine administration decreases postoperative analgesic requirements.[6–8] In veterinary patients, similar studies documenting decreased postoperative opioid requirements in animals receiving α_2-agonists have not been performed to date. In a canine study using a tail clamp as a noxious stimulus, however, Grimm and colleagues[9] demonstrated that the combination of medetomidine and butorphanol produced longer and more consistent analgesia than either drug alone.

Recent attention in veterinary medicine has focused on administration of continuous rate infusions (CRIs) of α_2-agonists during the intraoperative and postoperative periods to supplement anesthesia and analgesia. This interest stems largely from experience in human patients, in whom dexmedetomidine infusions are used to provide sedation, supplement analgesia, and reduce the stress response. There is little evidence evaluating medetomidine or dexmedetomidine infusions in veterinary patients, despite their growing use in clinical practice.

In one study by Pascoe and colleagues,[10] dexmedetomidine was infused intravenously in isoflurane-anesthetized dogs at 0.1, 0.5, and 3 μg/kg/h. This would be equivalent to administering medetomidine at dosages of 0.2, 1, and 6 μg/kg/h. Reductions in isoflurane minimum alveolar concentration (MAC) of 18% and 59% were noted with the 0.5 and 3 μg/kg/h infusion rates, and hemodynamic effects at the 0.5 μg/kg/h infusion rate were considered minimal. It is difficult to translate the MAC reduction effect documented in this experimental study to improved analgesia after surgery in clinical patients, so although α_2-agonist infusions may prove to be useful in providing balanced anesthesia, their contribution to clinically relevant analgesia requires further clarification.

Another study by Grimm and colleagues[11] evaluated the cardiopulmonary effects of medetomidine in combination with fentanyl as a continuous infusion without the influence of concurrent inhalant anesthesia. A dose of 1.5 μg/kg/h administered intravenously was infused with 15 μg/kg boluses of fentanyl. The investigators documented significant adverse hemodynamic effects, including reductions in heart rate and cardiac index and increases in pulmonary arterial pressure. Although sedative and analgesic effects were not evaluated, these results caution the use of extended-duration medetomidine CRIs in conscious dogs until more data are available.

In addition to systemic administration, α_2-agonists may be administered by novel routes. In particular, the spinal site of action seems to be important in mediating α_2-agonist–induced analgesia.[12–15] Although intrathecal administration is not routinely used in veterinary medicine, epidural administration is common. It has been demonstrated that incorporation of a low dose of medetomidine into an epidural protocol in dogs produces additive or synergistic analgesic effects when combined with opioids or local anesthetics.[16] Medetomidine has typically been combined with standard epidural doses of morphine, hydromorphone, buprenorphine, fentanyl, lidocaine, or bupivacaine and injected into the epidural space at the lumbosacral junction. Medetomidine's lipophilicity means that it is rapidly cleared from cerebrospinal fluid in the vicinity of the spinal injection site, which anatomically restricts the drug's action and results in significant systemic absorption. Consequently, when the total dose administered approaches that which would otherwise be given systemically, the specificity of the regional analgesic effect may be lost. The regional spinal analgesic effects of medetomidine can be optimized by administering a CRI through an indwelling epidural catheter using microdoses delivered directly to the desired segment of spinal cord while minimizing medetomidine plasma levels. Unfortunately, clinical use of epidural medetomidine by means of CRI in veterinary patients remains anecdotal at this time.

In addition to the epidural route, α_2-agonists may be administered by means of other peripheral routes to supplement analgesia, such as intra-articularly or perineurally. α_2-Adrenoceptors have been identified in the peripheral nervous system on terminals of primary afferent nociceptive fibers, and they seem to contribute to analgesia by inhibition of norepinephrine release.[12] Several studies in human beings have demonstrated a peripheral analgesic effect after intra-articular administration of α_2-agonists to patients undergoing arthroscopic knee surgery that is unrelated to vascular uptake of the drug and redistribution to central sites.[17] Furthermore, additive and synergistic analgesic effects have also been documented for intra-articular combinations of α_2-agonists with local anesthetics and opioids.[18] Although there are currently no veterinary studies evaluating medetomidine administered by means of this route, extrapolation from human patients suggests that animals undergoing routine arthrotomy may benefit from low doses of medetomidine combined with morphine, bupivacaine, or both injected into the joint at the end of surgery.

In human patients, there is also clinical evidence to suggest that α_2-agonists enhance peripheral nerve block intensity and duration when added to local anesthetics administered perineurally. Enhanced perineural blockade with α_2-agonists may be a result of hyperpolarization of C fibers through blockade of a specific type of potassium channel or local vasoconstriction, which decreases vascular removal of local anesthetic surrounding neural structures and prolongs the duration of action.[12] A recent study has demonstrated that the addition of medetomidine, systemically or perineurally, to radial nerve blockade with mepivacaine in dogs significantly prolonged sensory and motor blockade compared with mepivacaine alone. Although there was a trend toward prolonged sensory blockade with the perineural medetomidine group relative to the systemic medetomidine group, the difference was not significant.[19] These results suggest that medetomidine may be a useful adjunct to peripheral nerve blockade with a local anesthetic, but further work is needed to determine if the perineural route of administration offers any specific advantages over systemic administration.

Tramadol

Tramadol is a synthetic codeine analogue that is a weak μ-receptor agonist.[20] Because it is not classified as a controlled substance, it is often referred to as an "atypical opioid." In addition to its μ-agonist activity, tramadol inhibits neuronal reuptake of norepinephrine and 5-hydroxytryptamine (serotonin) and may facilitate 5-hydroxytryptamine release.[21,22] It is thought that these effects on central catecholaminergic pathways contribute significantly to the drug's analgesic efficacy.[22] Tramadol is recommended for the management of acute and chronic pain of moderate intensity associated with a variety of conditions, including osteoarthritis, fibromyalgia, diabetic neuropathy, neuropathic pain, and even perioperative pain in human patients.[23–28] It is considered a step 2 analgesic under the World Health Organization's guidelines for the treatment of cancer pain.

Tramadol use in veterinary clinical practice has increased significantly in the past several years as veterinarians seek new and better pain management alternatives for their patients. There is considerable interest in using tramadol to manage acute perioperative pain and chronic pain in dogs and cats. Although animal models were used extensively during the preclinical phase of drug approval for the human market, there is little published in the veterinary literature addressing tramadol efficacy or safety in clinical situations. One recent study has compared the effects of intravenous tramadol and morphine administered before ovariohysterectomy in dogs.[29] The investigators concluded that tramadol was comparable to morphine in its analgesic efficacy for this type of surgical pain. In North America, only oral formulations of tramadol are commercially available at this time. In the United States, tramadol is available in various tablet strengths in addition to an extended-release version and in combination with acetaminophen. In Canada, only the extended-release preparation and the combination with acetaminophen are currently available. Many veterinarians have elected to have tramadol prepared for them by a local compounding pharmacy in an attempt to access more convenient forms of dosing.

Dosing guidelines at this time are based on extrapolation from human beings and clinical experience with animal patients. One study by KuKanich and Papich[30] investigated the pharmacokinetics of tramadol in dogs. These investigators reported that a simulated oral dosing regimen of 5 mg/kg administered every 6 hours resulted in plasma concentrations of tramadol and its principle metabolite that were consistent with levels associated with analgesia in human beings. At this time, the safety and efficacy of this dosing schedule have not been evaluated in clinical trials. Based on anecdotal experience, however, a dose range of 3 to 10 mg/kg administered orally every 8 to 12 hours for the immediate-release tablets is recommended for dogs. Because dysphoria has been a common side effect in cats, dose recommendations for this species are more conservative (3–5 mg/kg administered orally every 12 hours). Titration of the dose is often necessary to minimize sedation or dysphoria in both species. Dosing guidelines for the extended-release formulations are more difficult to estimate; at this time, there are no published pharmacokinetic data in dogs or cats to guide recommendations for this formulation. When using the tramadol-acetaminophen combination product in dogs, it is recommended to dose the patient based on the acetaminophen (ie, approximately 10–15 mg/kg administered every 8–12 hours), which tends to underdose the tramadol. Higher doses are not recommended because they increase the risk for adverse side effects related to acetaminophen. It is crucial to remember that acetaminophen is toxic to cats; thus, this combination product should never be used in this species at any dose.

Common side effects associated with tramadol administration include sedation and dysphoria, especially in cats. It is also been reported to decrease the seizure threshold in certain human patients.[31] Because of its inhibitory effect on 5-hydroxytryptamine uptake, tramadol should not be used in patients that may have received monoaminoxidase inhibitors, such as selegiline (Anipryl).

N-Methyl-D-Aspartate Receptor Antagonists: Ketamine and Amantadine

The contribution of the *N*-methyl-D-aspartate (NMDA) glutamate receptor to central nervous system sensitization and hyperalgesia in pain syndromes was recognized more than 20 years ago.[32,33] Since that time, the search for pharmacologic NMDA antagonists has been ongoing as investigators have sought to identify therapies to minimize "windup" of dorsal horn neurons and improve pain management in the clinical setting. At the moment, there are two agents with significant NMDA antagonist activity that have relevance in veterinary medicine: ketamine and amantadine.

Ketamine is a drug that has been used by veterinarians in clinical practice for more than 30 years. Traditionally, it has been referred to as a dissociative anesthetic and used in relatively high doses, in combination with other agents, to produce effects ranging from chemical restraint to general anesthesia. In the early 1980s, ketamine's antagonistic effects at spinal cord NMDA receptors were established.[34,35] Since that time, ketamine use as an adjunctive analgesic in human beings and, to a lesser extent, animals has increased dramatically.

In people, there seems to be good data to support the use of low-dose ketamine as an analgesic supplement in many clinical situations, including: acute postoperative pain,[36,37] acute posttraumatic pain,[38] and neuropathic pain.[39,40] Several studies also present evidence to suggest a preemptive analgesic effect of ketamine administration in human surgical patients.[41,42]

In veterinary medicine, use of low-dose ketamine infusions for adjunctive analgesia has become a common practice in the perioperative setting. There are two studies evaluating the effects in ketamine infusions during surgery on the MAC of isoflurane in dogs, and both documented significant dose-dependent MAC-sparing effects.[43,44] In the study by Muir and colleagues,[43] an infusion rate of ketamine alone of 0.6 mg/kg/h resulted in a MAC reduction of 25%, whereas the combination of ketamine, morphine, and lidocaine resulted in a MAC reduction of 45%. In a feline study by Pascoe and colleagues,[45] higher infusion rates of ketamine were used (ranging from approximately 1.4–6.9 mg/kg/h administered intravenously by CRI), which decreased the isoflurane MAC by 45% to 75%, respectively. These rates also resulted in increases in heart rate and arterial blood pressure, however, and significantly prolonged recoveries. Clearly, the canine MAC reduction studies suggest that ketamine CRIs may contribute to balanced anesthesia protocols in this species (and perhaps lower infusion rates may prove to be useful in cats), but they do not address the question of postoperative analgesia per se.

At present, there are limited studies in the veterinary literature that evaluate the analgesic effects of ketamine in the perioperative period in dogs. The first of these reports is a study by Slingsby and Waterman-Pearson[46] that involved administration of a single dose of ketamine (2.5 mg/kg administered intramuscularly) before anesthetic induction or after extubation in dogs undergoing routine ovariohysterectomy.

Results demonstrated that ketamine administration decreased pain scores, rescue analgesic requirements, and postoperative wound hyperalgesia compared with control dogs. In a study by Wagner and colleagues,[47] dogs undergoing forelimb amputation received saline or a 0.5 mg/kg intravenous bolus before surgery, a 0.6 mg/kg/h intravenous CRI during surgery, and a 0.12 mg/kg/h intravenous CRI for 18 hours after surgery. Dogs that received ketamine infusions had significantly lower pain scores 12 and 18 hours after surgery, and were significantly more active on postoperative day 3 than dogs that received saline infusions, although opioid requirements were not significantly different between the groups. In a recent study by Sarrau and colleagues,[48] female dogs undergoing mastectomy received saline or one of two infusion rates of ketamine (0.15 mg/kg intravenous bolus with a 0.12 mg/kg/h intravenous CRI or 0.7 mg/kg intravenous bolus followed by a 0.6 mg/kg/h intravenous CRI). These investigators found that although the dogs receiving ketamine showed improved postoperative feeding behavior, a difference in opioid requirements could not be documented. Although the evidence remains limited at this time, these studies suggest that low doses of ketamine, especially administered by means of CRI throughout the perioperative period, may effectively augment analgesia in dogs. Although further work is necessary to clarify the role of ketamine in the perioperative period better, it seems that infusion rates of between 0.1 and 0.6 mg/kg/h administered by means of intravenous CRI may be useful adjunctive analgesics in dogs.

In addition to systemic administration, ketamine may be administered by means of several other novel routes to supplement analgesia. In human beings, the epidural,[49] intra-articular,[50] topical,[51] and even infiltrative[52] routes have been used. There are a limited number of veterinary studies that have evaluated the analgesic effects of epidural ketamine in dogs,[53–55] and the results suggest a potential, although probably limited, role for ketamine in select epidural protocols. Other novel routes of administration for ketamine, including the intra-articular route, have not been reported in dogs or cats at this time.

Amantadine is an antiviral drug that was originally approved to treat influenza A in people. It is also used clinically to reduce symptoms of Parkinson's disease and other drug-induced extrapyramidal syndromes. Its ability to block NMDA receptors came to light in the 1990s,[56,57] and its potential as an analgesic agent was recognized. More recently, specific details regarding precisely how amantadine inhibits NMDA responses have been discovered that distinguish this drug from other organic NMDA antagonists, like ketamine. It has been shown that amantadine's predominant inhibitory mechanism is not blockade of current flow through open channels but stabilization of channels in the closed state.[58] This key difference in NMDA channel-blocking properties is thought to contribute to its clinical safety profile.

Although there are numerous laboratory animal studies suggesting that amantadine's NMDA antagonist activities may make it a useful adjunctive analgesic agent, there are a limited number of controlled trials documenting its safety and efficacy. In one human study, perioperative amantadine administration in patients undergoing radical prostatectomy resulted in significantly decreased opioid consumption, but there was evidence to suggest this may have been related to pharmacokinetic mechanisms.[59]

In the field of chronic pain management, amantadine seems to hold more promise. In a study by Kleinbohl and colleagues,[60] amantadine reduced experimental sensitization and clinical pain perception in human patients who had chronic back pain. In the veterinary world, a recent abstract by Lascelles and colleagues[61] presented data evaluating amantadine as part of a multimodal analgesic regimen for the alleviation of refractory canine osteoarthritis pain. In this randomized, blind, placebo-controlled study, dogs receiving amantadine (3–5 mg/kg administered orally every 24 hours) in addition to meloxicam (0.1 mg/kg administered orally every 24 hours after a 0.2 mg/kg oral loading dose) had better activity scores (as assessed by the owner) and better lameness scores (as assessed by a veterinarian). These investigators concluded that in dogs with osteoarthritis that continue to have mobility impairment despite NSAID therapy, the ability to perform everyday activities is improved by the addition of amantadine. This study suggests that amantadine may come to play a key role in managing chronic pain in dogs in the future.

In the United States and Canada, amantadine is available commercially as 100 mg capsules and as 10 mg/mL oral syrup. A 100 mg tablet formulation is also available in the United States.

Anticonvulsants: Gabapentin

Gabapentin is a human anticonvulsant drug that has been approved by the United States Food and Drug Administration since 1993. Several years later, reports of its antihyperalgesic effects in rodent experimental pain models in addition to case reports and uncontrolled clinical trials involving human patients who had neuropathic pain began to appear in the literature. Recent studies have shown that the analgesic mechanism of action of gabapentin and pregabalin (its successor) seems to be mediated by binding to the α_2-δ_1 subunit of presynaptic voltage-gated calcium channels, which are upregulated in the dorsal root ganglia and spinal cord after a noxious insult.[62] It is speculated that gabapentin contributes to antinociception by inhibiting calcium influx by way of these channels and subsequently inhibiting release of excitatory neurotransmitters (eg, substance P and calcitonin gene-related peptide) from primary afferent nerves fibers.[63]

In human beings, gabapentin has emerged as an established first-line treatment for chronic neuropathic pain during the past decade. More recent interest has focused on expanding its use for other types of pain, notably perioperative pain. There are numerous clinical trials documenting its efficacy for a wide range of surgical-related pain in human beings.[63–71] One study has even documented its ability to decrease postoperative nausea and vomiting in a subset of patients undergoing laparoscopic cholecystectomy.[72] Gabapentin-related side effects occur in approximately 25% of patients and are usually mild and self-limiting. They include drowsiness, fatigue, and weight gain, especially with chronic administration.

Gabapentin use, like some of the other adjunctive analgesic agents, has increased significantly in veterinary medicine over the past several years. It has anecdotally been used to treat chronic cancer pain, chronic osteoarthritis pain, chronic neuropathic pain, and, increasingly, perioperative pain in dogs and cats. At this time, there are no clinical trials evaluating its safety and efficacy as an analgesic agent in dogs and cats. There is, however, one recent study that has evaluated the effects of another α_2-δ ligand chemically related to gabapentin in dogs with experimentally induced osteoarthritis, and it was found that this compound was able to slow the progression of cartilage structural changes.[73] Whether or not these findings can be extrapolated to gabapentin in clinical canine patients that have osteoarthritis remains to be seen. Veterinary dosing guidelines for gabapentin have been largely based on human recommendations despite some key species differences in pharmacokinetics. In the mouse, rat, monkey, and human being, gabapentin is essentially excreted unchanged into the urine.[74,75] In contrast, in the dog, the drug undergoes significant hepatic metabolism to *N*-methyl-gabapentin before renal elimination.[74,75] Gabapentin disposition in the cat has not been studied to date. Based on collective clinical experience, doses in the range of 3 to 10 mg/kg administered orally every 8 to 12 hours are recommended to start, and most regimens typically require adjustments to achieve the desired analgesic effect without significant sedation. In the United States, gabapentin is available commercially as capsules and tablets in 100 mg, 300 mg, 400 mg, 600 mg, and 800 mg sizes. It is also supplied as a 250 mg/5-mL oral solution. In Canada, the same capsule sizes are available; however, only large-dose tablet formulations (600 mg and 800 mg) are available, and there is currently no oral solution.

Systemic Local Anesthetics: Intravenous Lidocaine

Lidocaine, like other sodium channel–blocking drugs classified as local anesthetics, is considered to be a traditional analgesic when administered perineurally to produce nerve conduction blockade. Local anesthetics may also be administered systemically (orally or intravenously) to supplement analgesia, however. Because this approach is considered a novel route of administration for this class of drugs, it is discussed here as an adjunctive analgesic technique. Although there are other options for systemic local anesthetic therapy, such as oral mexiletine, the only one with relevance to veterinary medicine currently is intravenous lidocaine.

Although lidocaine's mechanism of nerve conduction blockade has been thoroughly elucidated, its analgesic mechanism of action when administered intravenously is not known. At the moment, there is evidence to support peripheral[76] and central[77] sites of action. Despite this lack of understanding, clinical evidence supporting the use of intravenous lidocaine infusions to manage perioperative pain in human patients is mounting. Several studies have shown that lidocaine infusions are associated with improved bowel function, decreased postoperative pain and reduced opioid consumption, shortened hospital stays, and earlier rehabilitation in patients undergoing major abdominal surgery.[78–80]

In veterinary medicine, one study has documented the safety of lidocaine infusion rates in isoflurane-anesthetized dogs at intravenously administered doses up to 0.12 mg/kg/min.[81] Other studies have reported isoflurane MAC reductions associated with intravenously administered 0.05 mg/kg/min lidocaine infusions ranging from approximately 19% to 29%.[43,82] Although these studies suggest that lidocaine infusions seem to be safe in isoflurane-anesthetized dogs and that they may be valuable anesthetic adjuncts, they do not address the issue of analgesia directly. In another recent canine study, investigators explored a totally noninvasive method of delivery to achieve systemic lidocaine concentrations. They applied 5% lidocaine transdermal patches to the dogs' ventral midlines and demonstrated detectable drug levels by 12 hours after application and steady-state levels between 24 and 48 hours after application.[83] Once again, the analgesic potential of this technique is unclear at this time.

Only one study has investigated the analgesic effects of systemic lidocaine infusions in dogs in a clinical setting. The study, by Smith and colleagues,[84] demonstrated that intra- and postoperative lidocaine (1.0 mg/kg intravenously administered bolus followed by 0.025 mg/kg/min intravenously administered CRI) produced comparable postoperative analgesia to morphine (0.15 mg/kg intravenously administered bolus followed by 0.1 mg/kg/h intravenously administered CRI). Although the number of dogs in this study was small, this pilot study encourages further investigation of this technique. In cats, the effects of lidocaine in isoflurane-anesthetized patients have been reported. Pypendop and Ikliw[85] used a target-directed plasma concentration model and documented significant dose-dependent isoflurane MAC reductions with intravenous lidocaine infusions; however, these MAC reductions were associated with a greater degree of cardiovascular depression than the equipotent dose of isoflurane alone.[86] Another study describing the pharmacokinetics of lidocaine and its active metabolite demonstrated significant differences in kinetic variables in conscious versus isoflurane-anesthetized cats.[87] There is one study performed in conscious cats that has evaluated the effects of lidocaine infusions on a model of thermal antinociception, and it failed to illustrate any beneficial effects despite documenting moderate plasma lidocaine levels.[88] Taken together, these studies caution against the use of intravenous lidocaine infusions in feline patients until more data are available.

Bisphosphonates: Pamidronate and Zoledronate

Bisphosphonates are a family of drugs characterized by their ability to inhibit bone resorption. They are classified according to their chemical structure as nonaminobisphosphonates or aminobisphosphonates. The aminobisphosphonates, such as pamidronate and zoledronate, represent a newer generation of drugs and are characterized by greater antiresorptive capabilities. The primary mechanism of action of bisphosphonates is inhibition of osteoclast activity. For the aminobisphosphonates, this inhibition occurs by means of inhibition of the mevalonate pathways, resulting in disruption of intracellular signaling and induction of apoptosis.[89] The net result of this includes inhibition of cancer cell proliferation, induced apoptosis in in vitro cultures, inhibition of angiogenesis, inhibition of matrix metalloproteinase, effects on cytokine and growth factors, and immunomodulation.[89] Although they have been used extensively to manage nonneoplastic bone disorders, such as osteoporosis, in human beings for many years, interest in oncologic applications has increased dramatically in the past decade. Clinical applications for the bisphosphonates in oncology are broad and include therapy for hypercalcemia of malignancy, inhibition of bone metastasis, and therapy for bone pain. For a subset of veterinary patients that have cancer, these drugs may have significant potential as adjunctive analgesics.

There are numerous studies evaluating the effects of the oral bisphosphonate alendronate on bone in vitro and in vivo, but there is little evidence evaluating its analgesic efficacy in clinical patients. One case report describes the apparently successful use of alendronate for palliation in two dogs with osteosarcoma.[90] More recently, oncologists in human and veterinary medicine have moved to the intravenous aminobisphosphonates, such as pamidronate or zoledronate, which hold more promise as adjunctive analgesics. There are several studies that have recently been published addressing the safety and efficacy of pamidronate in dogs. Intravenous pamidronate was evaluated by Fan and colleagues[91] in 33 tumor-bearing dogs and demonstrated what these investigators classified as a modest ability to reduce homeostatic and pathologic osteoclastic activity while observing that this reduction seemed to correlate with bone pain relief in dogs showing subjective clinical improvement. In another study that focused on the potential analgesic effects of the drug, single-agent pamidronate administered intravenously with NSAID therapy was shown to relieve pain and diminish pathologic bone turnover associated with appendicular osteosarcoma in a subset of dogs.[92] Currently, the recommended pamidronate protocol for dogs is 1 to 2 mg/kg administered intravenously over 2 hours in 250 mL of 0.9% sodium chloride (NaCl) administered every 21 to 28 days. There are also two studies evaluating zoledronate, although they involve healthy dogs only. Both studies demonstrated significant inhibition of homeostatic osteolytic activity associated with single-dose intravenous administration (0.25 mg/kg).[93,94] Although zoledronate may possess similar bone pain–relieving properties as pamidronate, its use in veterinary oncology is limited because of the substantial cost associated with the drug. Based on these initial studies, it seems that further investigation into the efficacy of intravenous aminobisphosphonates in canine patients that have cancer is clearly warranted.

Table 2
Dosage ranges for selected adjunctive analgesic agents

Analgesic Adjuvant	Dogs	Cats
Medetomidine	0.002–0.015 IV, IM	0.005–0.02 IV, IM
Tramadol (immediate-release)	3–10 PO q 8–12 hours	3–5 PO q 12 hours
Ketamine	0.5 IV loading dose0.1–0.6/h IV CRI	0.5 IV loading dose0.1–0.6/h IV CRI
Amantadine	3–5 PO q 24 hours	3–5 PO q 24 hours
Gabapentin	3–10 PO q 8–12 hours	3–10 PO q 8–12 hours
Lidocaine	1.0 IV loading dose1.5/h IV CRI	?

All doses are presented in mg/kg.
Abbreviations: IM, intramuscular; IV, intravenous; PO, orally; q, every.

NONPHARMACOLOGIC ADJUNCTIVE ANALGESIC THERAPIES

In addition to drug interventions, there are numerous and diverse nonpharmacologic methods that may be used to supplement analgesia. Many of these physical methods have been used anecdotally in veterinary patients, although little has been published regarding their analgesic efficacy in dogs and cats. Although a comprehensive discussion of these techniques is well beyond the scope of this article, **Table 2** contains a list of the more common techniques and a brief definition of each. The reader is referred to other articles in this issues in which selected techniques are presented in the context of specific pain syndromes.

GUIDELINES FOR PRESCRIBING ADJUNCTIVE ANALGESIC THERAPIES TO VETERINARY PATIENTS

Although pharmacologic and nonpharmacologic adjunctive analgesic therapies have the potential to relieve pain and greatly improve patient comfort in veterinary patients, all the therapies discussed in this article are not approved specifically for this purpose in dogs and cats. In most cases, large-scale clinical trials have not been conducted; thus, it becomes the veterinarian's sole responsibility to become educated and carefully weigh the advantages and disadvantages of a particular therapy for a particular patient. In the case of a pharmacologic agent, the veterinarian must have a basic understanding of the drug's clinical pharmacology, including: (1) approved indications, (2) unapproved indications (eg, for analgesia) that are widely accepted in veterinary medical practice, (3) common side effects and uncommon but potentially severe adverse effects, (4) important pharmacokinetic features, and (5) specific dosing guidelines for pain. With this information, the veterinarian can communicate potential risks to pet owners and make rationale therapeutic decisions for patients.

REFERENCES

1. Buerkle H, Yaksh TL. Pharmacological evidence for different alpha 2-adrenergic receptor sites mediating analgesia and sedation in the rat. Br J Anaesth 1998;81: 208–15.
2. Guo TZ, Jiang JY, Buttermann AE, et al. Dexmedetomidine injection into the locus ceruleus produces antinociception. Anesthesiology 1996;84:873–81.
3. Sinclair MD. A review of the physiological effects of alpha2-agonists related to the clinical use of medetomidine in small animal practice. Can Vet J 2003;44:885–97.

4. Murrell JC, Hellebrekers LJ. Medetomidine and dexmedetomidine: a review of cardiovascular effects and antinociceptive properties in the dog. Vet Anaesth Analg 2005;32:117–27.
5. Granholm M, McKusick BC, Westerholm FC, et al. Evaluation of the clinical efficacy and safety of intramuscular and intravenous doses of dexmedetomidine and medetomidine in dogs and their reversal with atipamezole. Vet Rec 2007; 160:891–7.
6. Del Angel Garcia R, Castellanos Olivares A, Munguia Miranda C. Dexmedetomidine as preventive postoperative analgesia in inguinal hernioplasty. Gac Med Mex 2006;142:9–12.
7. Gurbet A, Basagan-Mogol E, Turker G, et al. Intraoperative infusion of dexmedetomidine reduces perioperative analgesic requirements. Can J Anaesth 2006;53: 646–52.
8. Unlugenc H, Gunduz M, Guler T, et al. The effect of pre-anaesthetic administration of intravenous dexmedetomidine on postoperative pain in patients receiving patient-controlled morphine. Eur J Anaesthesiol 2005;22:386–91.
9. Grimm KA, Tranquilli WJ, Thurmon JC, et al. Duration of nonresponse to noxious stimulation after intramuscular administration of butorphanol, medetomidine, or a butorphanol-medetomidine combination during isoflurane administration in dogs. Am J Vet Res 2000;61:42–7.
10. Pascoe PJ, Raekallio M, Kuusela E, et al. Changes in the minimum alveolar concentration of isoflurane and some cardiopulmonary measurements during three continuous infusion rates of dexmedetomidine in dogs. Vet Anaesth Analg 2006;33:97–103.
11. Grimm KA, Tranquilli WJ, Gross DR, et al. Cardiopulmonary effects of fentanyl in conscious dogs and dogs sedated with a continuous rate infusion of medetomidine. Am J Vet Res 2005;66:1222–6.
12. Eisenach JC, De Kock M, Klimscha W. Alpha(2)-adrenergic agonists for regional anesthesia. A clinical review of clonidine (1984–1995). Anesthesiology 1996;85: 655–74.
13. Eisenach JC, Hood DD, Curry R. Intrathecal, but not intravenous, clonidine reduces experimental thermal or capsaicin-induced pain and hyperalgesia in normal volunteers. Anesth Analg 1998;87:591–6.
14. De Kock M, Eisenach J, Tong C, et al. Analgesic doses of intrathecal but not intravenous clonidine increase acetylcholine in cerebrospinal fluid in humans. Anesth Analg 1997;84:800–3.
15. Sabbe MB, Penning JP, Ozaki GT, et al. Spinal and systemic action of the alpha 2 receptor agonist dexmedetomidine in dogs. Antinociception and carbon dioxide response. Anesthesiology 1994;80:1057–72.
16. Branson KR, Ko JC, Tranquilli WJ, et al. Duration of analgesia induced by epidurally administered morphine and medetomidine in dogs. J Vet Pharmacol Ther 1993;16:369–72.
17. Gentili M, Juhel A, Bonnet F. Peripheral analgesic effect of intra-articular clonidine. Pain 1996;64:593–6.
18. Joshi W, Reuben SS, Kilaru PR, et al. Postoperative analgesia for outpatient arthroscopic knee surgery with intraarticular clonidine and/or morphine. Anesth Analg 2000;90:1102–6.
19. Lamont LA, Lemke KA. The effects of medetomidine on radial nerve blockade with mepivacaine in dogs. Vet Anaesth Analg 2008;35(1):62–8.

20. Gutstein HB, Akil H. Opioid analgesics. In: Harman JG, Limbird LE, Goodman Gilman A, editors. Goodman and Gilman's: the pharmacological basis of therapeutics. 10th edition. New York: McGraw-Hill; 2001. p. 569.
21. Dayer P, Desmeules J, Collart L. Pharmacology of tramadol. Drugs 1997; 53(Suppl 2):18–24.
22. Desmeules JA, Piguet V, Collart L, et al. Contribution of monoaminergic modulation to the analgesic effect of tramadol. Br J Clin Pharmacol 1996;41:7–12.
23. Arbaiza D, Vidal O. Tramadol in the treatment of neuropathic cancer pain: a double-blind, placebo-controlled study. Clin Drug Investig 2007;27:75–83.
24. But AK, Erdil F, Yucel A, et al. The effects of single-dose tramadol on postoperative pain and morphine requirements after coronary artery bypass surgery. Acta Anaesthesiol Scand 2007;51:601–6.
25. Buvanendran A, Kroin JS. Useful adjuvants for postoperative pain management. Best Pract Res Clin Anaesthesiol 2007;21:31–49.
26. Cepeda MS, Camargo F, Zea C, et al. Tramadol for osteoarthritis: a systematic review and metaanalysis. J Rheumatol 2007;34:543–55.
27. Prommer EE. Tramadol: does it have a role in cancer pain management? J Opioid Manag 2005;1:131–8.
28. Pyati S, Gan TJ. Perioperative pain management. CNS Drugs 2007;21:185–211.
29. Mastrocinque S, Fantoni DT. A comparison of preoperative tramadol and morphine for the control of early postoperative pain in canine ovariohysterectomy. Vet Anaesth Analg 2003;30:220–8.
30. KuKanich B, Papich MG. Pharmacokinetics of tramadol and the metabolite O-desmethyltramadol in dogs. J Vet Pharmacol Ther 2004;27:239–46.
31. Gardner JS, Blough D, Drinkard CR, et al. Tramadol and seizures: a surveillance study in a managed care population. Pharmacotherapy 2000;20:1423–31.
32. Davies SN, Lodge D. Evidence for involvement of N-methylaspartate receptors in 'wind-up' of class 2 neurones in the dorsal horn of the rat. Brain Res 1987;424: 402–6.
33. Dickenson AH, Sullivan AF. Evidence for a role of the NMDA receptor in the frequency dependent potentiation of deep rat dorsal horn nociceptive neurones following C fibre stimulation. Neuropharmacology 1987;26:1235–8.
34. Lodge D, Anis NA, Burton NR. Effects of optical isomers of ketamine on excitation of cat and rat spinal neurones by amino acids and acetylcholine. Neurosci Lett 1982;29:281–6.
35. Zukin SR, Fitz-Syage ML, Nichtenhauser R, et al. Specific binding of [3H]phencyclidine in rat central nervous tissue: further characterization and technical considerations. Brain Res 1983;258:277–84.
36. Bell RF, Dahl JB, Moore RA, et al. Perioperative ketamine for acute postoperative pain. Cochrane Database Syst Rev 2006;(1):CD004603.
37. Michelet P, Guervilly C, Helaine A, et al. Adding ketamine to morphine for patient-controlled analgesia after thoracic surgery: influence on morphine consumption, respiratory function, and nocturnal desaturation. Br J Anaesth 2007; 99:396–403.
38. Galinski M, Dolveck F, Combes X, et al. Management of severe acute pain in emergency settings: ketamine reduces morphine consumption. Am J Emerg Med 2007;25:385–90.
39. Chizh BA, Headley PM. NMDA antagonists and neuropathic pain—multiple drug targets and multiple uses. Curr Pharm Des 2005;11:2977–94.

40. Correll GE, Maleki J, Gracely EJ, et al. Subanesthetic ketamine infusion therapy: a retrospective analysis of a novel therapeutic approach to complex regional pain syndrome. Pain Med 2004;5:263–75.
41. Aida S, Yamakura T, Baba H, et al. Preemptive analgesia by intravenous low-dose ketamine and epidural morphine in gastrectomy: a randomized double-blind study. Anesthesiology 2000;92:1624–30.
42. Fu ES, Miguel R, Scharf JE. Preemptive ketamine decreases postoperative narcotic requirements in patients undergoing abdominal surgery. Anesth Analg 1997;84:1086–90.
43. Muir WW 3rd, Wiese AJ, March PA. Effects of morphine, lidocaine, ketamine, and morphine-lidocaine-ketamine drug combination on minimum alveolar concentration in dogs anesthetized with isoflurane. Am J Vet Res 2003;64:1155–60.
44. Solano AM, Pypendop BH, Boscan PL, et al. Effect of intravenous administration of ketamine on the minimum alveolar concentration of isoflurane in anesthetized dogs. Am J Vet Res 2006;67:21–5.
45. Pascoe PJ, Ilkiw JE, Craig C, et al. The effects of ketamine on the minimum alveolar concentration of isoflurane in cats. Vet Anaesth Analg 2007;34:31–9.
46. Slingsby LS, Waterman-Pearson AE. The post-operative analgesic effects of ketamine after canine ovariohysterectomy—a comparison between pre- or post-operative administration. Res Vet Sci 2000;69:147–52.
47. Wagner AE, Walton JA, Hellyer PW, et al. Use of low doses of ketamine administered by constant rate infusion as an adjunct for postoperative analgesia in dogs. J Am Vet Med Assoc 2002;221:72–5.
48. Sarrau S, Jourdan J, Dupuis-Soyris F, et al. Effects of postoperative ketamine infusion on pain control and feeding behaviour in bitches undergoing mastectomy. J Small Anim Pract 2007;48(12):670–6.
49. Wang X, Xie H, Wang G. Improved postoperative analgesia with coadministration of preoperative epidural ketamine and midazolam. J Clin Anesth 2006;18:563–9.
50. Borner M, Burkle H, Trojan S, et al. Intra-articular ketamine after arthroscopic knee surgery: optimisation of postoperative analgesia. Anaesthesist 2006;18(8):563–9.
51. Lynch ME, Clark AJ, Sawynok J, et al. Topical amitriptyline and ketamine in neuropathic pain syndromes: an open-label study. J Pain 2005;6:644–9.
52. Tan PH, Cheng JT, Kuo CH, et al. Preincisional subcutaneous infiltration of ketamine suppresses postoperative pain after circumcision surgery. Clin J Pain 2007;23:214–8.
53. Acosta AD, Gomar C, Correa-Natalini C, et al. Analgesic effects of epidurally administered levogyral ketamine alone or in combination with morphine on intraoperative and postoperative pain in dogs undergoing ovariohysterectomy. Am J Vet Res 2005;66:54–61.
54. Duque JC, Valadao CA, Farias A, et al. Pre-emptive epidural ketamine or S(+)-ketamine in post-incisional pain in dogs: a comparative study. Vet Surg 2004;33:361–7.
55. Hamilton SM, Johnston SA, Broadstone RV. Evaluation of analgesia provided by the administration of epidural ketamine in dogs with a chemically induced synovitis. Vet Anaesth Analg 2005;32:30–9.
56. Lupp A, Lucking CH, Koch R, et al. Inhibitory effects of the antiparkinsonian drugs memantine and amantadine on N-methyl-D-aspartate-evoked acetylcholine release in the rabbit caudate nucleus in vitro. J Pharmacol Exp Ther 1992;263:717–24.

57. Blanpied TA, Boeckman FA, Aizenman E, et al. Trapping channel block of NMDA-activated responses by amantadine and memantine. J Neurophysiol 1997;77:309–23.
58. Blanpied TA, Clarke RJ, Johnson JW. Amantadine inhibits NMDA receptors by accelerating channel closure during channel block. J Neurosci 2005;25:3312–22.
59. Snijdelaar DG, Koren G, Katz J. Effects of perioperative oral amantadine on postoperative pain and morphine consumption in patients after radical prostatectomy: results of a preliminary study. Anesthesiology 2004;100:134–41.
60. Kleinbohl D, Gortelmeyer R, Bender HJ, et al. Amantadine sulfate reduces experimental sensitization and pain in chronic back pain patients. Anesth Analg 2006;102:840–7.
61. Lascelles BD, Gaynor J, Smith ES, et al. Evaluation of amantadine as part of a multimodal analgesic regimen for the alleviation of refractory canine osteoarthritis pain. J Vet Intern Med 2008;22(1):53–9.
62. Field MJ, Cox PJ, Stott E, et al. Identification of the alpha2-delta-1 subunit of voltage-dependent calcium channels as a molecular target for pain mediating the analgesic actions of pregabalin. Proc Natl Acad Sci U S A 2006;103:17537–42.
63. Tiippana EM, Hamunen K, Kontinen VK, et al. Do surgical patients benefit from perioperative gabapentin/pregabalin? A systematic review of efficacy and safety. Anesth Analg 2007;104:1545–56 [table of contents].
64. Mathiesen O, Moiniche S, Dahl JB. Gabapentin and postoperative pain; a qualitative and quantitative systematic review, with focus on procedure. BMC Anesthesiol 2007;7:6.
65. Peng PW, Wijeysundera DN, Li CC. Use of gabapentin for perioperative pain control—a meta-analysis. Pain Res Manag 2007;12:85–92.
66. Ho KY, Gan TJ, Habib AS. Gabapentin and postoperative pain—a systematic review of randomized controlled trials. Pain 2006;126:91–101.
67. Hurley RW, Cohen SP, Williams KA, et al. The analgesic effects of perioperative gabapentin on postoperative pain: a meta-analysis. Reg Anesth Pain Med 2006;31:237–47.
68. Seib RK, Paul JE. Preoperative gabapentin for postoperative analgesia: a meta-analysis. Can J Anaesth 2006;53:461–9.
69. Sihoe AD, Lee TW, Wan IY, et al. The use of gabapentin for post-operative and post-traumatic pain in thoracic surgery patients. Eur J Cardiothorac Surg 2006;29:795–9.
70. Turan A, Kaya G, Karamanlioglu B, et al. Effect of oral gabapentin on postoperative epidural analgesia. Br J Anaesth 2006;96:242–6.
71. Turan A, White PF, Karamanlioglu B, et al. Gabapentin: an alternative to the cyclooxygenase-2 inhibitors for perioperative pain management. Anesth Analg 2006;102:175–81.
72. Pandey CK, Priye S, Ambesh SP, et al. Prophylactic gabapentin for prevention of postoperative nausea and vomiting in patients undergoing laparoscopic cholecystectomy: a randomized, double-blind, placebo-controlled study. J Postgrad Med 2006;52:97–100.
73. Boileau C, Martel-Pelletier J, Brunet J, et al. Oral treatment with PD-0200347, an alpha2delta ligand, reduces the development of experimental osteoarthritis by inhibiting metalloproteinases and inducible nitric oxide synthase gene expression and synthesis in cartilage chondrocytes. Arthritis Rheum 2005;52:488–500.

74. Radulovic LL, Turck D, von Hodenberg A, et al. Disposition of gabapentin (Neurontin) in mice, rats, dogs, and monkeys. Drug Metab Dispos 1995;23: 441–8.
75. Vollmer KO, von Hodenberg A, Kolle EU. Pharmacokinetics and metabolism of gabapentin in rat, dog and man. Arzneimittelforschung 1986;36:830–9.
76. Devor M, Wall PD, Catalan N. Systemic lidocaine silences ectopic neuroma and DRG discharge without blocking nerve conduction. Pain 1992;48:261–8.
77. Jaffe RA, Rowe MA. Subanesthetic concentrations of lidocaine selectively inhibit a nociceptive response in the isolated rat spinal cord. Pain 1995;60:167–74.
78. Kaba A, Laurent SR, Detroz BJ, et al. Intravenous lidocaine infusion facilitates acute rehabilitation after laparoscopic colectomy. Anesthesiology 2007;106: 11–8 [discussion: 5–6].
79. Koppert W, Weigand M, Neumann F, et al. Perioperative intravenous lidocaine has preventive effects on postoperative pain and morphine consumption after major abdominal surgery. Anesth Analg 2004;98:1050–5 [table of contents].
80. Groudine SB, Fisher HA, Kaufman RP Jr, et al. Intravenous lidocaine speeds the return of bowel function, decreases postoperative pain, and shortens hospital stay in patients undergoing radical retropubic prostatectomy. Anesth Analg 1998;86:235–9.
81. Nunes de Moraes A, Dyson DH, O'Grady MR, et al. Plasma concentrations and cardiovascular influence of lidocaine infusions during isoflurane anesthesia in healthy dogs and dogs with subaortic stenosis. Vet Surg 1998;27:486–97.
82. Valverde A, Doherty TJ, Hernandez J, et al. Effect of lidocaine on the minimum alveolar concentration of isoflurane in dogs. Vet Anaesth Analg 2004;31:264–71.
83. Ko J, Weil A, Maxwell L, et al. Plasma concentrations of lidocaine in dogs following lidocaine patch application. J Am Anim Hosp Assoc 2007;43:280–3.
84. Smith LJ, Bentley E, Shih A, et al. Systemic lidocaine infusion as an analgesic for intraocular surgery in dogs: a pilot study. Vet Anaesth Analg 2004;31:53–63.
85. Pypendop BH, Ilkiw JE. The effects of intravenous lidocaine administration on the minimum alveolar concentration of isoflurane in cats. Anesth Analg 2005;100: 97–101.
86. Pypendop BH, Ilkiw JE. Assessment of the hemodynamic effects of lidocaine administered IV in isoflurane-anesthetized cats. Am J Vet Res 2005;66:661–8.
87. Thomasy SM, Pypendop BH, Ilkiw JE, et al. Pharmacokinetics of lidocaine and its active metabolite, monoethylglycinexylidide, after intravenous administration of lidocaine to awake and isoflurane-anesthetized cats. Am J Vet Res 2005;66: 1162–6.
88. Pypendop BH, Ilkiw JE, Robertson SA. Effects of intravenous administration of lidocaine on the thermal threshold in cats. Am J Vet Res 2006;67:16–20.
89. Milner RJ, Farese J, Henry CJ, et al. Bisphosphonates and cancer. J Vet Intern Med 2004;18:597–604.
90. Tomlin JL, Sturgeon C, Pead MJ, et al. Use of the bisphosphonate drug alendronate for palliative management of osteosarcoma in two dogs. Vet Rec 2000;147: 129–32.
91. Fan TM, de Lorimier LP, Charney SC, et al. Evaluation of intravenous pamidronate administration in 33 cancer-bearing dogs with primary or secondary bone involvement. J Vet Intern Med 2005;19:74–80.
92. Fan TM, de Lorimier LP, O'Dell-Anderson K, et al. Single-agent pamidronate for palliative therapy of canine appendicular osteosarcoma bone pain. J Vet Intern Med 2007;21:431–9.

93. de Lorimier LP, Fan TM. Bone metabolic effects of single-dose zoledronate in healthy dogs. J Vet Intern Med 2005;19:924–7.
94. Martin-Jimenez T, de Lorimier LP, Fan TM, et al. Pharmacokinetics and pharmacodynamics of a single dose of zoledronate in healthy dogs. J Vet Pharmacol Ther 2007;30:492–5.

Epidural Analgesia and Anesthesia in Dogs and Cats

Alexander Valverde, DVM, DVSc

KEYWORDS

- Epidural • Intrathecal • Opioids • Local anesthetics
- Alpha-2 agonists • Spinal cord

Epidural anesthesia using local anesthetic drugs has been a common technique used in veterinary medicine to perform surgical procedures since the 1950s in North America and Europe. With the advent of safer injectable and inhalational anesthetic drugs and accessibility to anesthetic equipment, the use of epidural anesthesia became less frequent in the following years. In the late 1980s, however, with the recognition of opioids' analgesic actions on the spinal cord, the use of epidural analgesia became an important tool that has re-emerged in intra- and postoperative epidural techniques to provide analgesia and anesthesia in veterinary medicine.

The ideal drug(s) for epidural use should cause analgesia or anesthesia, minimal motor blockade, and minimal systemic effects. Epidural analgesia is now most frequently provided with the combination of a local anesthetic and an opioid using a spinal needle or an epidural catheter, although depending on the dermatome to be blocked, these drugs can also be administered alone to achieve the desired analgesic or anesthetic effect without unwarranted complications. Other drugs, such as α_2-agonists, have also been used alone or combined with local anesthetics or opioids, but practitioners should expect that systemic absorption of α_2-agonists from the epidural space might result in some of their undesirable effects. Ketamine, nonsteroidal anti-inflammatory drugs (NSAIDs), and many other drugs have also been used epidurally with less success, and their effects are also summarized.

This review presents relevant information in regard to anatomy and pharmacologic behavior of drugs administered in the epidural space to provide the necessary knowledge for correct application of epidural techniques used in pain management.

ANATOMIC CONSIDERATIONS

Epidural injections are commonly performed at the lumbosacral (L7–sacrum [L-S]) intervertebral space in small animals. Other intervertebral spaces can potentially be

Section of Anesthesiology, Department of Clinical Studies, Ontario Veterinary College, University of Guelph, Guelph, Ontario, Canada N1G 2W1
E-mail address: valverde@uoguelph.ca

Vet Clin Small Anim 38 (2008) 1205–1230
doi:10.1016/j.cvsm.2008.06.004 **vetsmall.theclinics.com**

used; however, the L-S intervertebral space provides the largest access to the epidural space and in close proximity to the spinal cord in the aforementioned species.

Access to the L-S intervertebral space involves insertion of a needle through skin, subcutaneous fascia, and ligaments. In human beings, there are three ligaments: the supraspinous, interspinous, and flavum (intervertebral) ligaments. In dogs and cats, there is no supraspinous ligament at the level of the lumbar spine and the counterpart for the human collagenous interspinous ligament (ventral, middle, and dorsal parts) is rudimentary and poorly developed except dorsally. The ventral and middle parts are thin and consist of collagenous fascia arranged obliquely in a dorsocranial fashion from the cranial border of one spinous process to the lumbodorsal fascia or erector spinae tendons, whereas the dorsal part consists of (1) a thin band of elastic fibers that run longitudinally between the spinous processes and (2) oblique bands of collagen in the dog and elastic fibers in the cat that run lateral and cranially.[1] The flavum ligament consists of connective tissue that seals the L-S intervertebral space and forms the roof or dorsal wall of the epidural space; its rigid consistency is what results in the "pop" noticed as the needle pierces it during insertion. The L-S intervertebral space is only 2 to 4 mm in diameter in medium-sized dogs and less than 3 mm in cats in cadaver specimens examined by the author. This is in contrast to a larger L3-to-L4 space of 10.7 mm and 11.6 mm reported in pregnant and nonpregnant women, respectively.[2]

Within the vertebral canal, the spinal cord is surrounded by three specialized membranes: the meninges, including the dura; arachnoid; and pia mater. The dura mater consists of two laminae that are well defined in human infants; however, in adults, the external lamina cannot be identified as a separate layer and is represented by the periosteum of the vertebral canal.[3] The dura closely adheres to the skull as a fused double layer but is separated in the vertebral column, and only the internal lamina, made of fibrous tissue, surrounds the spinal cord and provides rigidity to help support the blood vessels that supply the spinal cord. The epidural space is the space between the dura mater and the vertebral column, but it actually represents an intradural space because it is located between the two dural laminae.[3] The process of injecting any substance into this space is referred as an epidural injection.

The arachnoid mater is in close contact with the inner portion of the dura mater and encloses the subarachnoid space filled with cerebrospinal fluid (CSF). The terms *subarachnoid*, *spinal*, and *intrathecal* injections are all synonyms that refer to injection of a substance into the subarachnoid space. The arachnoid mater is a membrane with tight intercellular junctions and a spider-web appearance composed also of fibrous tissue and trabeculae that extend from the arachnoid to the pia mater to secure the cord in the CSF. This membrane is the barrier that determines the passage of drugs into the CSF depending on their lipophilicity.[4] A third potential space is the subdural space between the dura and arachnoid membrane, but it is less likely to fill with blood than the cranium, as may occur in cases of head trauma and subdural hemorrhage. The pia mater is the innermost layer that surrounds the brain and spinal cord and through which blood vessels supply nutrients and oxygen.

At birth, the spinal cord extends through the vertebral canal as far caudal as the sacrum. During growth, the spinal cord shrinks into the growing vertebral column and terminates at the caudal lumbar or cranial sacral level, depending on the species. In large-breed dogs, the spinal cord terminates as the filum terminale, approximately 1 cm caudal to the fifth lumbar vertebra, whereas in smaller breeds, the filum terminale is located at the lumbosacral vertebral junction (**Fig. 1**). The dural sac and subarachnoid space extend approximately 2 cm beyond the end of the spinal cord, and the cauda equina, formed by sacral and caudal spinal roots, lies caudal to the dural sac.[5]

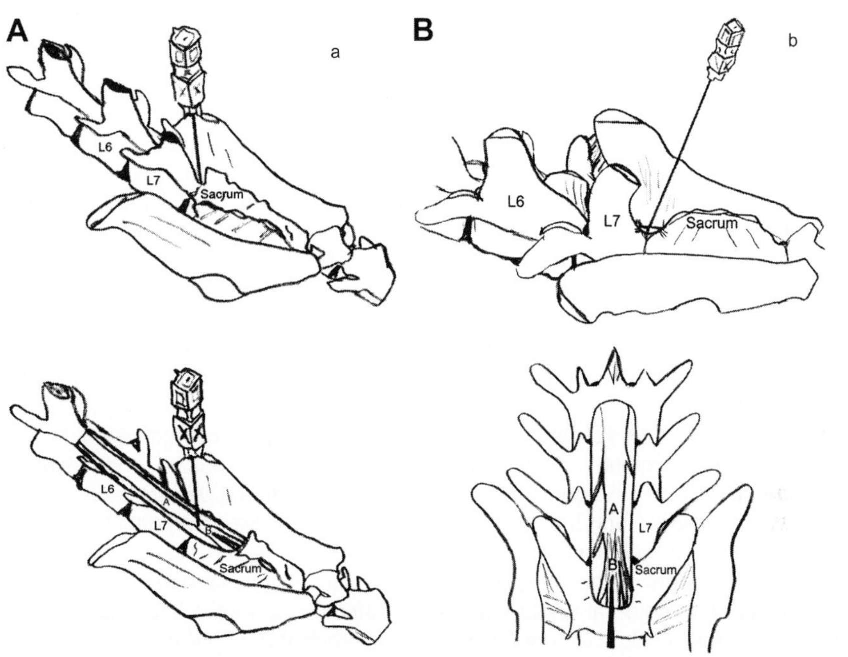

Fig. 1. Anatomic views of the lumbosacral space in the cat (*A*) and dog (*B*). L6, sixth lumbar vertebrae; L7, seventh lumbar vertebrae; a, spinal cord; b, cauda equina.

In cats, like dogs, the spinal cord is shorter than the vertebral column, and the spinal cord ends at approximately the level of the L7 vertebra in cats; however, the spinal dura mater extends further caudally and may give an initial false impression of a longer spinal cord (see **Fig. 1**).[6] Because of the spinal cord's more caudal location in small-breed dogs and in cats, the piercing of meninges and leakage of CSF during epidural attempts is likely. Because epidural drug doses are much higher than for intrathecal use, injection of an epidural dose if CSF is obtained should be avoided unless the needle is repositioned in the epidural space or the epidural dose is adjusted for intrathecal requirements.

Meningovertebral ligaments, which are present as early as the fetal stages and remain throughout adulthood, are described in the human literature at the lumbar region.[7] Although not described in animals, it is likely that they are also present. They are loose ligaments consisting of fibroelastic fibers surrounded by fat lobules that anchor the outer surface of the dura mater from the anterior (ventral for small animals), posterior (dorsal), and lateral epidural spaces to the osteofibrous walls of the lumbar canal in an irregular and discontinuous arrangement, and they are not present for every vertebra, causing partial partitioning of the epidural space as a result of the growth of the vertebral canal and their progressive stretching out along axial spinal blood vessels.[7] It has been suggested that this compartmentalization contributes to failure of epidural injections through inhomogeneous spread of the injected anesthetic drugs and may also interfere with catheter introduction, leading to lateral positioning of the catheter and an incomplete block. Trauma of the meningovertebral ligaments during needle or catheter insertion can also result in injury of the epidural vessels present in close anatomic relation to these ligaments.[7]

Epidural fat is also an important component of the epidural space. Fat fills in all irregularities of the canal walls and provides a smooth sheath for the dural surface to move within. It also provides insulation to the spinal cord against shock and mechanical injury from surrounding bony parts.[8] In cats and dogs, it has been shown that most of the fat is scanty in the cervical region and more abundant in more caudal portions of the vertebral column.[8,9] The greater part of the epidural fat is located lateral and dorsal to the spinal cord, unattached to the vertebral wall or the dura and enclosed by a delicate smooth capsule of varying thickness, whereas ventral fat can be bound to surrounding structures in the immediate vicinity of lumbar and sacral spinal nerves and large blood vessels from the epidural space.[8,9] Lipophilic drugs injected into the epidural space readily bind to fat, and actions on the spinal cord are limited because of entrapment and absorption from the well-vascularized fat and epidural vessels. Conversely, supraspinal (systemic) effects are common after epidural injection of lipophilic drugs. For hydrophilic drugs, less binding to fat provides a higher concentration gradient that enhances absorption into the CSF despite their low affinity for traversing the meninges.

The epidural venous vessels consist of valveless plexuses, located within the vertebral canal, that communicate with vessels from the bones (basivertebral veins) and from the spinal cord. Epidural veins drain into intervertebral veins that accompany the spinal nerves through the intervertebral foramina before communicating with the azygos and hemiazygos veins and the vena cava.[3]

This vascular network has the potential of transmitting intra-abdominal and intrathoracic pressure to epidural vessels and could affect drug absorption or spread within the epidural space. Studies in women have shown that during pregnancy, increased maternal blood volume and aortocaval compression cause epidural blood vessels to become engorged; in addition, the density of the vascular network within the epidural space is increased, reducing the relative volume (size) of the epidural space.[10] Although the spread of epidural anesthesia has not always been shown to be different between pregnant and nonpregnant women,[11] the potential for rostral spread and absorption of injected drugs increases the risk for overdose and toxicity; therefore, lower epidural volumes of local anesthetics have been recommended in pregnant animals.

The arterial supply to the meninges in the epidural space originates from branches of thyrocervical, subclavian, intercostal, lumbar, and sacral arteries that enter the space through the intervertebral foramina.[3]

Position and Volume

The effects of different volumes injected into the epidural space and positioning have been investigated in dogs and cats using dye techniques.[12,13] Using dog cadavers, methylene blue at a dose of 0.1 mL/kg was injected in the L-S intervertebral space with the cadavers positioned in sternal recumbency before placing them in three positions: right lateral, left lateral and rotated to right lateral 10 minutes later, and dorsal and rotated to right lateral 10 minutes later. The vertebral canal was then examined 40 minutes later for rostral spread of the dye and staining of the dura mater in all quadrants (dorsal, both lateral quadrants, and ventral). Specimens that remained in the same position (right lateral) showed the greatest migration for that same quadrant; however, there were no significant differences within groups for the staining of all quadrants,[12] although the degree of staining was not graded in this study. The rostral spread varied between 10.4 and 20.3 cm from the L-S intervertebral space for specimens weighing between 14.1 and 27.1 kg, but no indication of vertebrae level that corresponded to that distance was mentioned.[12]

Findings from that study seem to indicate that position is important for the rostral spread of the injectate and that rotation of the animal, as often happens during surgical preparation of the patient in the clinical setting, limits but does not prevent the drug from contacting the target tissue. The use of cadavers does not allow studying the effects of a dynamic circulatory system in facilitating systemic vascular absorption by epidural vessels and the effects of CSF motion, however. Cardiac function is responsible for movement of CSF in the spinal canal. During systole, anterior and caudal spinal cord movement and expansion is followed by caudal CSF flow, and during diastole, the CSF flows cranially,[14] all of which may facilitate or interfere with epidural drug spread and absorption into the CSF.

A similar study in anesthetized cats evaluated volumes of methylene blue at 0.1 to 0.4 mL/kg injected at the L-S intervertebral space while the cat was positioned in sternal recumbency and kept in this position for 20 minutes before being euthanized.[13] A linear relation between volume and vertebrae stained was established, wherein 0.1 mL/kg stained up to the L3 to L4 vertebrae, 0.2 mL/kg up stained up to the L1 to L2 vertebrae, 0.3 mL/kg stained up to the T7 to T11 vertebrae, and 0.4 mL/kg stained up to the T6 to T10 vertebrae. There was also a tendency for the dye to migrate more rostrally in the ventral quadrant because the cats were kept in a sternal position.[13]

There is controversy among veterinary anesthesiologists on whether the patient needs to be rotated to allow enough contact of the injectate with the target tissue (eg, nerve roots) for drugs that exert their actions by contact (ie, local anesthetics). Part of the controversy is related to the smaller injected volumes used in small animals. In human beings, small volumes (5–10 mL) spread under the influence of gravity to the dependent side,[15] and as the volume increases (up to 25 mL), it overcomes the effects of gravity and spreads uniformly.[16,17] Conversely, a body inclination of 15° (Trendelenburg position) and injection of lidocaine at a dose of 20 mL in women resulted in faster onset and rostral spread than for the supine position.[18] The disadvantage of larger volumes of local anesthetic to overcome the effects of gravity include blockade of numerous sympathetic fibers along the sympathetic trunk that may induce hypotension and interference with motor fibers that may affect diaphragm contractions and respiratory function. Other possible complications include discomfort from transient compression of the spinal cord.

In small animals, a total epidural volume of injectate that approximates 0.2 mL/kg but does not exceed 6 mL for animals weighing more than 30 kg has been recommended.[19] Total epidural injected volumes of different drugs that amount to 0.13 to 0.36 mL/kg have been used without adverse effects related to volume, however.[20–26] Based on the study by Lee and colleagues,[13] it seems appropriate that volumes of 0.2 mL/kg of local anesthetic be used to avoid rostral spread beyond the thoracolumbar area in cats. In dogs, volumes of methylene blue at a dose of 0.26 mL/kg spread to the T11-to-T13 vertebrae (author's unpublished data). For drugs that do not cause sympathetic or motor blockade, such as the opioids, however, it may not be necessary to adhere to this rule. In addition, the limit of 6 mL of total volume for larger animals is based on the assumption that the vertebral canal is not proportionally larger than for smaller animals; however, this has not been confirmed scientifically.

Body positioning also affects the CSF pressure in the cranium and spinal space, and therefore may facilitate or interfere with the spread of drugs injected into the epidural space and interfere with techniques used to verify proper positioning of the needle in the epidural space. Studies in cats have demonstrated that CSF pressures in the cranium and spinal space are similar (approximately 12 cm H_2O) when the cat is in the horizontal position with head and spine at the same height, whereas elevating the head to 5 or 10 cm higher than the spine linearly decreases the CSF pressure in the cranium (to 7.7 and 4.7 cm H_2O, respectively) and increases it in the spinal space (to 13.8 and 18.5 cm H_2O, respectively).[27] These changes are not related to displacement of blood or CSF from the cranium to the lower part of the body but are the result of the biophysical characteristics of the CSF system.[27]

TECHNIQUE

Proper selection of the patient is important before attempting an epidural injection to avoid complications. Patients not suitable for this technique include those with coagulation disorders and infection in area of the L-S intervertebral space. Other conditions, such as deformity of the anatomy of the area of the L-S intervertebral space from traumatic injury and obesity, can make the technique difficult, whereas cardiovascular status can be negatively affected by some drugs, such as local anesthetics, more than others because of their hypotensive actions.

Epidural injections can be performed in awake, sedated, and anesthetized animals. The choice depends on familiarity with the procedure and convenience for the clinician and patient. A recent study estimated failure of the epidural technique, as evidenced by inability to decrease the requirements for inhalant anesthesia, at 7% in dogs and 9% in cats.[28] There are multiple factors that can affect the success of this technique, which are not restricted only to lack of expertise but to anatomic and pharmacologic considerations reviewed in this article. Factors that affect epidural rostral spread are as follows:

- Lipophilic drugs have less spread.
- Hydrophilic drugs have more spread.
- Meningovertebral ligaments cause compartmentalization.
- Increased epidural space pressures prevent spread.
- Injected volume facilitates spread.
- Gravity favors spread to dependent body areas.
- Epidural fat prevents spread of lipophilic drugs.
- Leakage through intervertebral foramina.

At the author's hospital, the preemptive approach to pain management in surgical patients results in epidural injections performed after induction to general anesthesia before the start of surgery. Epidural injections and catheter placement are also performed on sedated patients in the intensive care unit (ICU), where superficial infiltration of local anesthesia to facilitate the procedure is preferred. In conscious or lightly sedated individuals, it is important to avoid cold solutions (5°C) for epidural injection, because discomfort has been reported in women when compared with solutions at room temperature.[29]

With the patient positioned in lateral or sternal recumbency, the area of the L-S intervertebral space should be clipped and aseptically prepared. Considerations for volume injected and drugs used determine if positioning is important while the drug's actions take effect. The L-S intervertebral space is located by palpation of the anterior aspect of both iliac crests with the thumb and middle finger; the imaginary line between them runs over the L6-to-L7 space, which is palpated with the index finger before moving the finger caudally along the midline over the spinous process of L7 and cranial to the sacrum (see **Fig. 1**). The diameter of the L-S intervertebral space is relatively small in dogs and cats, and some investigators recommend that the hind limbs be moved forward to enhance the L-S intervertebral space.[30] In this author's experience using cadaver specimens, moving the hind limbs forward enhances palpation of the area of the L-S intervertebral space but does not increase the size of the space because of the restricted motion of the L-S vertebrae.

Spinal needles are recommended because they have a stylet. A 22-gauge 3.8-cm (1.5 inches) needle is recommended in small-breed and young dogs and cats; a 20-gauge 3.8- to 6.35-cm (1.5–2.5 inches) needle is used for larger dogs.

Under sterile conditions, the needle is introduced perpendicular to the skin while the index finger of the palpating hand remains in the L-S intervertebral space to ensure accurate positioning. This means that depending on which side of the patient the person is standing, the needle can be immediately caudal or cranial to the finger. Adjustments to the angle of insertion can be made as required to facilitate correct placement in the epidural space. As the needle advances, a "pop" can usually be felt (but not always) when it pierces the flavum ligament, and the needle is introduced further into the epidural space. This author recommends advancing the needle all the way to the floor of the epidural space in dogs and then withdrawing 1 to 2 mm; in this way, the position of the needle is ensured in the epidural space and being off midline can be ruled out. In cats, the presence of the spinal dura mater beyond L7 makes it likely that CSF is obtained if the needle is advanced to the floor; therefore, it is best avoided. Instead, flicking of the tail, movement of the hind limbs, or twitching of the skin in the area of the L-S intervertebral space is commonly observed in cats when the needle enters the epidural space and pricks the spinal cord or cauda equina, without subsequent adverse effects; however, for this reason, smaller gauge spinal needles are recommended in cats. To verify correct placement of the needle, several tests can be performed. A glass syringe, which offers minimal resistance, can be attached to the needle, and air can be injected to detect lack of resistance on injection because of the subatmospheric pressure of the epidural space. Average pressure readings in dogs of −2.72 mm Hg have been reported within 5 to 10 minutes at steady state at the L-S intervertebral space.[31] Caution should be exercised when injecting air, and only a small volume (0.25–2 mL depending on the size of the animal) should be used because it can potentially reach the heart or brain directly through absorption from the epidural vascular network. In addition, the subatmospheric pressure rapidly becomes positive after injection of fluid or air into the space,[32] which can increase resistance on injection in subsequent attempts. Subatmospheric pressure is reestablished when the injected volume is removed from the epidural space by systemic absorption and leakage through intervertebral foramina.

If CSF is obtained during epidural attempts, withdrawing the needle slowly may reposition the needle back into the epidural space. It is not recommended to inject an epidural dose intrathecally; alternatively, the epidural dose can be adjusted to an intrathecal dose if the injection is to be completed without withdrawing the needle. Preservative-free drugs must be used for intrathecal injections to avoid adverse effects associated with the preservative. The intrathecal doses for opioids have not been established in controlled studies in small animals, and despite recommendations for reducing the dose by 40% to 50%,[19] caution is advised, because the bioavailability of morphine in CSF from an epidural dose is only 2% of that for intrathecal morphine.[33] Based on this bioavailability, the concentration achieved from an intrathecal injection using 40% to 50% of the epidural dose results in a CSF concentration that is 20 to 25 times higher than necessary and increases the incidence of side effects. In fact, the intrathecal dose of morphine used in people is approximately 30 times lower than for an epidural dose.[34–36] Similarly, epidural anesthesia with local anesthetics requires approximately 10 times the dose used by the intrathecal route. Based on these data, doses should be reduced by at least 90%.

Another method to verify correct placement is to use the "hanging drop" technique by removing the stylet before the needle penetrates the flavum ligament and to place a drop of saline or local anesthetic in the hub; once in the epidural space, the fluid is aspirated into the needle shaft by the subatmospheric epidural pressure. In dogs, this technique was 88% effective in medium-sized dogs (13 kg) in sternal recumbency using a 20-gauge spinal needle, but it was ineffective in all dogs in lateral recumbency.[37] False-negative results are most commonly associated with tissue plugs that obstruct the needle during insertion; therefore, it is advised to remove the stylet only in close proximity to the flavum ligament or once it has been pierced. Other causes that should be considered include conditions that increase central venous pressure and are paralleled by epidural pressures from epidural venous distention, which raises the epidural space pressure to positive values, such as in systemic volume overload and increased abdominal pressure; volume depletion has the opposite effect and results in more negative pressures.[31] In cats, it is also common to have a false-negative result because of the smaller epidural space and the use of smaller gauge needles.

More sophisticated ways of verifying correct placement include the measurement of pressure waves from the epidural space and the use of electrical stimulation. For the epidural pressure waveform method, the epidural needle or catheter is connected to a pressure transducer, volume is injected into the space, and waveforms are observed on the monitor. The presence of the injected fluid in the epidural space undamps transmission from CSF pressures and allows arterial pulsations to be visible[32] because of the effects of cardiac function on CSF movement.[14] This technique has been successfully used in dogs in which the synchronous epidural and arterial pressure waves were observed in 15 of 18 dogs before epidural injection and in all dogs after the injection.[38] Pressures up to 20 to 30 mm Hg can be measured.

The epidural electrical stimulation method has mostly been recommended in anesthetized people to detect motor responses and to prevent needle encroachment on neural structures or the spinal cord, which are signs otherwise manifested by pain on injection in awake patients. The cathode of the nerve stimulator is connected to the metal hub of the adapter, and the anode is connected to the patient's skin. The epidural catheter is primed with 0.2 to 1 mL of saline, and the nerve stimulator is set at 1 Hz with a pulse width of 200 milliseconds and current of up to 15 mA to evaluate the motor response.[39] The use of epidural catheters reinforced with spiral stainless-steel wire or with a stainless-steel stylet has been recommended to decrease resistance and facilitate current delivery from the nerve stimulator without affecting the desired current.[40]

In dogs undergoing hind limb or perineal surgery, a 1.0-mA current at 2 Hz with a pulse width of 200 milliseconds was used to elicit motor twitches of the tail or hind limbs and confirm correct needle placement; this method was faster to perform and resulted in better success (100% versus 88%) than the standard epidural method based on lack of sympathetic responses to surgical stimulation while maintained at a light plane of anesthesia.[41] Nevertheless, studies in 20-kg pigs with delivery of a 3.6-mA current, using an 18-gauge insulated Tuohy needle inserted along different dermatomes of the vertebral column, elicited 59% false-positive motor responses when the needle was still not in the epidural space and resistance on injection was present.[42] Decreasing the current to 2.0 mA is recommended to reduce the high false-positive predictive value by preventing intraneural or intrathecal injections, and it is suggested that confirmation of the epidural space can only be guaranteed by achieving the loss of resistance on injection.[42]

Comparison of epidural pressure waveform and epidural nerve stimulation methods in people has yielded similar results: 100% positive predictive value (no false-positive values), specificity but moderate sensitivity (around 80%), and a low negative predictive value for false-negative values (around 17%) for both methods.[43] The poor negative predictive value is in contrast to the more simple techniques, such as loss of resistance on injection, which can be successful in more than 95% of cases.

Epidural catheter placement is usually accomplished by using commercial kits that include the catheter and a Tuohy needle, which has a curved bevel that facilitates direction of the threaded catheter through it into the epidural space. The author uses epidural catheters available in 19-, 20- and 24-gauge sizes that thread through a 17-, 18-, and 20-gauge 7.6- to 8.9-cm (3–3.5-inch) Tuohy needles. Threading the catheter without resistance is indicative of correct placement in the epidural space unless the intrathecal space was inadvertently penetrated, in which case, the presence of CSF should be noticed. Studies in people have demonstrated that intended catheter placement is often not achieved because of coiling of the catheter and lateral deviation.[44,45] As mentioned previously, the presence of meningovertebral ligaments is one of the causes for lateral deviation and subsequent compartmentalization and an incomplete block.[7] Therefore, radiographic verification is recommended for epidural catheters. Of note, even though the presence of an epidural catheter decreases the likelihood of failure of epidural techniques, it does not guarantee 100% success.

Epidural catheters are inserted mainly through the L-S intervertebral space, but other intervertebral spaces have also been used, including L3 to L4. The tip of the catheter can be positioned in close proximity to dermatomes associated with the painful area and allow intermittent or continuous administration of analgesic drugs. For drugs like local anesthetics, it is possible to administer them in lower amounts than if injected at the L-S intervertebral space, because the need for rostral spread is overcome when the drug is applied directly to the desired area. Some studies in dogs under research and clinical conditions have advanced catheters cranially as far as T4 and left them in place for periods between 1 and 28 days; during that time, such drugs as opioids, local anesthetics, and α_2-agonists have been administered as frequently as once daily without inducing major microscopic or macroscopic signs of inflammation, fibrous tissue formation, or infection.[46–50] A review of major complications encountered in clinical cases requiring analgesia at different dermatomes (eg, hind limb, forelimb, thorax, abdomen, perineal, cervical), reports dislodgement of the catheter (16%), inflammation (2.4%), and contamination at the catheter site (2.4%) for catheters left in place for up to 7 days.[49]

Other Techniques

Combining an epidural and intrathecal injection is a common technique performed in people to obtain the major advantages of each technique. This technique involves intrathecal blockade and epidural catheter placement during the same procedure to provide profound blockade of fast onset with use of low doses from the intrathecal injection and prolonged duration from the epidural injection.[51] To achieve these effects, an intrathecal injection with a lipophilic drug (eg, local anesthetic) and an epidural injection with a hydrophobic drug (eg, morphine) is usually recommended. This technique has also been reported in a dog requiring invasive surgery of the hind end, using an epidural catheter inserted at L5 to L6 for morphine administration and a spinal needle inserted intrathecally at L6 to L7 for bupivacaine and fentanyl administration.[52]

PHARMACOLOGIC CONSIDERATIONS

The selection of drug(s) to be administered epidurally depends on the degree and desired duration of analgesia or anesthesia and the dermatomes to be blocked.

Absorption from the Epidural Space

Drugs administered epidurally undergo uptake by three routes: systemic absorption through the epidural vascular network, sequestration by epidural fat tissue, and absorption into the CSF and spinal cord.[53]

The degree to which each of these routes affects each drug depends on the physicochemical properties of the drug. Because the mechanism of action differs among drugs commonly administered epidurally (eg, local anesthetics, opioids, α_2-agonists), the impact of these routes is more relevant for opioids, for which it has been more thoroughly investigated. The effects of these routes should always be considered for any drug, however.

In general, lipophilicity of the drug enhances systemic absorption, sequestration by fat, and free movement between the epidural and intrathecal spaces; whereas hydrophilicity has the opposite effects. Therefore, drugs administered epidurally are expected to have effects within the spinal compartment (spinal effect) and systemically (supraspinal effect). Lipophilic drugs have marked systemic effects from rapid vascular uptake that limits the amount of drug for rostral spread in the intrathecal space. For lipophilic opioids (eg, fentanyl, sufentanil), epidural doses are similar to systemic doses and the analgesic effects of these opioids are more related to supraspinal than to spinal effects and are also accompanied by sedation.[54–58] For hydrophilic opioids, such as morphine, epidural doses are a fraction of systemic doses and their effects after epidural administration are the result of interactions at the spinal cord (spinal effect).[53] There are variations to this arrangement, because drugs like hydromorphone with intermediate lipophilicity (octanol/buffer [O/B] distribution coefficient = 525) are also dosed at a fraction of the systemic dose.

There is a positive correlation between lipophilicity, mean residence time (MRT), and terminal elimination half-life in the extracellular fluid of the lumbar epidural space and in the epidural venous plasma. Morphine (O/B = 1.0) and alfentanil (O/B = 129) had shorter MRTs and terminal elimination half-lives than the more lipophilic opioids fentanyl (O/B = 955) and sufentanil (O/B = 1737). The explanation for these differences involves sequestration of lipophilic opioids by epidural fat, which allows for slow release back into the extracellular fluid of the epidural space, prolonging the MRT and elimination time.[4,57] This constant source of lipophilic opioids in the epidural space, and subsequent systemic uptake, is the reason for supraspinal effects and a slightly more prolonged analgesic effect than after systemic administration.[57,58] The degree of analgesia and plasma concentrations of fentanyl is similar between epidural and intravenous administration.[58,59] For hydrophilic opioids (eg, morphine), plasma concentrations are rapidly achieved after epidural administration,[60] and despite use of a lower dose epidurally than systemically, morphine is more effective and remains interacting longer with opioid receptors in the spinal cord, resulting in a higher degree and duration of analgesia.[57,59,61]

Spinal absorption of epidurally administered drugs is the result of movement of the drug through the meninges from the epidural space. The specific gravity of CSF in dogs ranges between 1.005 and 1.017 (median of 1.010) and between 1.005 and 1.021 (median of 1.010) in cats.[62] The specific gravity is more important for intrathecal injections than for epidural injections because it determines how the drug is distributed within the CSF. Because positioning of the spine varies during intrathecal injection (sternal versus lateral) and the anatomy of the patient influences the areas of maximal elevation of the spine, it is possible to facilitate the spread of the drug injected intrathecally by affecting the baricity of the solution. Drugs with a high specific gravity (hyperbaric) spread toward the lower areas of the spine, whereas hypobaric solutions spread against gravity to higher areas of the spine. The specific gravity of lidocaine 1% (1.005), bupivacaine 0.5% (1.003), ropivacaine 1% (1.006), morphine (1.002), and methadone (1.006) makes them hypobaric, because the values are lower than that for CSF. Lidocaine 2% (1.010) and morphine diluted with 0.9% saline (1.009) are isobaric to CSF.[62] Combining hypobaric or isobaric drugs with 5% dextrose increases their baricity. For epidural injections, only isobaric or hypobaric solutions are used.

Hydrophilic opioids have a greater bioavailability in CSF than in the epidural space.[33,57] Morphine's terminal elimination half-life from the intrathecal space is significantly longer than its epidural elimination, and the slow clearance of high morphine concentrations from the CSF is responsible for the prolonged analgesic effect by means of a spinal mechanism.[57] For lipophilic opioids, the terminal elimination half-life does not differ significantly between the epidural and intrathecal spaces and the meninges are the rate-limiting step controlling elimination.[57] In addition, the limited rostral spread of lipophilic opioids reduces the likelihood of delayed sedation and respiratory depression that has been observed for hydrophilic opioids.

For opioids injected epidurally in the lumbosacral area, the rostral spread to the thoracic area is inversely related to the molecular weight of the opioid (morphine = 285, hydromorphone = 285, butorphanol = 327, fentanyl = 336, oxymorphone = 337, methadone = 345, sufentanil = 387, alfentanil = 417, and buprenorphine = 467), and their subsequent elimination depends more on the rate at which they spread to the thoracic area than on the rate of elimination from the thoracic epidural space.[4,57]

Opioids

Opioid receptors (μ, κ, and δ) are present in the spinal cord in high concentrations in laminae I and II of the dorsal horn. Binding of these receptors inhibits the release of substance P from C nociceptive fibers and, to a lesser extent, A-δ fibers[63] and blocks the ascending transmission to higher brain centers through excitatory pathways. Because A-δ fibers are responsible for "stabbing" sensation, surgical pain is not blocked with epidural opioids and their use is for analgesia but not anesthesia. B-sympathetic and A-β fibers are not affected; therefore, vascular tone and tactile sensory modalities (touch and pressure) remain intact, whereas opioids with μ-agonism have the potential to affect motor function from hyperpolarizing motor neurons,[47] but motor weakness is rarely seen (**Table 1**).

Based on the pharmacologic considerations mentioned previously, opioids used epidurally in small animals can be divided according to their lipophilicity. Opioids with high lipophilicity include fentanyl and sufentanil; opioids with intermediate lipophilicity include butorphanol (O/B = 180), oxymorphone, hydromorphone, buprenorphine, and methadone; and opioids with low lipophilicity (hydrophilic) include morphine.

Table 1
Actions of drugs used epidurally on different fibers

	Sympathetic Blockade (B-fibers)	Motor Blockade (A-α fibers)	Sensory Blockade (A-δ and C fibers)	Tactile Sensory Blockade (A-β fibers)
Local anesthetics	+++	+++	+++	+++
Opioids	–	±	++	–
α_2-Agonists	–	+	+++	++
Ketamine	–	++	++	++

Abbreviations: –, no effect; ±, at toxic doses; +, ++, +++, minimal, moderate, and maximal effect, respectively.

Lipophilic opioids administered epidurally are expected to cause analgesia of fast onset but of only slightly longer duration than a similar systemic dose. The dose used is similar to systemic doses, and because of the rapid vascular absorption from the epidural space, systemic effects are equal, including supraspinal analgesia, as a result of the similar plasma concentrations (**Table 2**). Their rostral spread is limited because of the vascular absorption and sequestration by fat, which, in addition to the limited spinal effect, prevents them from affecting dermatomes distant to the site of injection.

Several studies have corroborated these statements. Epidural oxymorphone (0.1 mg/kg) and butorphanol (0.25 mg/kg) have been administered in dogs and achieved plasma concentrations similar to intramuscular injections.[64,65] The rostral spread of lipophilic opioids has not been demonstrated with either drug in terms of prolonged analgesia or a segmental effect that would affect cranial areas of the body less significantly than caudal areas when a noxious stimulus is applied.[64,65] In awake cats administered epidural fentanyl (4 μg/kg), however, the analgesic duration of action of fentanyl against an electrical cutaneous stimulus, although short (20 minutes), affected the hind limb but not the forelimb.[66] A likely explanation is that the concentration gradient between the epidural and intrathecal spaces induced by the injection initially facilitated higher concentrations of fentanyl reaching the spinal cord. In people, the use of constant fentanyl epidural infusions causes analgesia by supraspinal effects, and epidural boluses can, in addition, cause a spinal effect because of the higher concentration gradient.[67]

Epidural methadone (0.3 mg/kg) was superior to the same dose administered intravenously in dogs undergoing stifle surgery for cruciate repair based on lower isoflurane requirements during the most noxious stimulating phases of surgery; however, there were no significant differences in the duration of postoperative analgesia

Table 2
Doses of drugs used by the epidural route in dogs and cats

	Drug	Dose (mg/kg)	Onset (Minutes)	Duration (Hours)	Notes
Local anesthetics	Lidocaine 2%	4–5	<10	1.5	Can be combined with α_2-agonists or opioids Adding epinephrine prolongs the duration of lidocaine
	Bupivacaine 0.25%, 0.5%, 0.75%	1–1.65	<15	2–4	
	Ropivacaine 0.5%, 0.75%	1–1.65	<15	2–4	
	IQB-9302 0.25%, 0.5%, 0.75%	0.5–1.5	<10	2–4	
Opioids	Morphine	0.1	30–60	12–24	Diluted with preservative-free saline (0.2 mL) or local anesthetic
	Hydromorphone	0.02	<30	6–12	
	Methadone	0.3	<20	7	
	Buprenorphine	0.005	NA	NA	
	Butorphanol[a]	0.25	<30	2–4	
	Fentanyl[a]	0.004	<10	0.5	
α_2-Agonists	Xylazine	0.1–0.4	<15	1–3	—
	Medetomidine	0.005–0.01	<20	4–6	

[a] Predominant supraspinal effects.

between the two routes.[68] Methadone has a relatively low O/B coefficient (55), which should result in prolonged epidural analgesia.

The combined analgesic effects of epidural buprenorphine and lidocaine were assessed in dogs undergoing ovariohysterectomy under propofol intravenous infusion.[69] Systemic buprenorphine (15 μg/kg administered intramuscularly) combined with epidural analgesia that consisted of buprenorphine (5 μg/kg) and lidocaine 2% (4.4 mg/kg) resulted in a dose of propofol to maintain surgical anesthesia that was 55% lower than the dose required in dogs receiving only systemic buprenorphine and propofol administered intravenously.[69] Buprenorphine has an O/B coefficient in excess of 100 and should provide analgesia of intermediate duration.

Epidural hydromorphone, like the other intermediate lipophilic opioids, results in analgesia of faster onset and shorter duration than morphine.[70]

Hydrophilic opioids administered epidurally are expected to cause analgesia of slow onset (30–60 minutes) and prolonged duration (6–24 hours) at lower than systemic doses. Systemic absorption occurs, but the lower dose does not usually result in systemic effects. Their rostral spread is extensive because of their prolonged presence in CSF, which facilitates their actions on dermatomes distant to the site of injection.

The segmental effect from rostral spread of epidural morphine (0.1 mg/kg) was evident by producing a significant reduction in the minimum alveolar concentration (MAC) of halothane for the forelimb (35%) and an even higher reduction in the hind limb (42%) in accordance with the proximity to the L-S intervertebral space injection.[23]

In cats, epidural morphine (0.1 mg/kg diluted to saline, 0.3 mL/kg) or buprenorphine (0.0125 mg/kg diluted to saline, 0.3 mL/kg) did not change the MAC of isoflurane,[71] which is in contrast to another study, in which a 31% reduction in the MAC isoflurane was shown.[72]

The combination of epidural morphine (0.1–0.4 mg/kg) and bupivacaine (0.6–2 mg/kg) provided analgesia of longer duration than epidural morphine alone in dogs and cats undergoing surgery.[28] Analgesia for 19.6 hours was reported in clinical cases receiving epidural morphine alone or morphine and the local anesthetic bupivacaine.[28] The advantages of combining opioids and local anesthetics include a higher percentage of reduction in inhalant requirements and longer and more complete analgesia that reduces postoperative use but may also result in prolonged motor blockade associated with the use of local anesthetics.[24,25,28,73–75]

Epidural morphine with or without bupivacaine has also been compared with intra-articular morphine with or without bupivacaine in dogs undergoing stifle surgery, showing that these techniques resulted in similar degrees of analgesia that were superior to placebo groups.[76,77] At this hospital, the author recommends the use of intra-articular and epidural injections in dogs undergoing stifle surgery by combining bupivacaine (0.5%, 0.1 mL/kg for intra-articular and 0.5%, 0.2 mL/kg for epidural) and morphine (0.1 mg/kg) for both techniques.

Cardiorespiratory Effects

The effects of epidural opioids on cardiorespiratory function depend on dose, as for systemic administration; therefore, it is more likely that lipophilic opioids result in changes related to higher epidural doses required for these opioids. Epidural fentanyl (4 μg/kg) in isoflurane-anesthetized cats decreased blood pressure and heart rate and increased $Paco_2$ for at least 2 hours.[78] In halothane-anesthetized dogs, epidural oxymorphone (0.1 mg/kg) combined with saline or bupivacaine (0.75% to a total volume of 0.2 mL/kg) induced a decrease in heart rate that coincided with lower cardiac and stroke volume index and a transient decrease in blood pressure.[64] In contrast, halothane-anesthetized dogs administered epidural morphine (0.1 mg/kg diluted in saline,

0.26 mL/kg) and maintained with 1.1% end-tidal pressure had better blood pressure and cardiac output than a control group maintained with an equipotent dose of halothane without epidural morphine (1.6% end-tidal pressure).[79]

One study reported the cardiorespiratory but not the analgesic effects of a combination of epidural morphine (0.1 mg/kg) and fentanyl (10 μg/kg) in sevoflurane-anesthetized dogs as a technique that could overcome the slow onset of morphine with the faster action of fentanyl. Systemic absorption of fentanyl resulted in decreases in blood pressure and vascular resistance and increases in $Pa{CO_2}$, which were not observed in dogs administered morphine alone.[80]

Other Beneficial Effects

The effects of epidural morphine on gut motility were recently investigated by assessing the appearance of the first interdigestive migrating complex (IMC) originating in the stomach and propagating to the distal intestine after abdominal surgery in dogs. Compared with epidural saline, epidural ropivacaine, and a low dose of continuous intravenous morphine, continuous epidural morphine (0.17 mg/kg administered every 24 hours) resulted in recovery of intestinal motility more rapidly than the other treatments. Intravenous morphine using the same dose was also superior to epidural saline and epidural ropivacaine.[81] Although morphine is known to delay gastric emptying and intestinal transit,[82] these effects are dose related and lower doses used systemically or administered by epidural injection can induce frequent high-amplitude contractions that lead to IMC.[81,83] Similar results have been seen after a combination of epidural morphine and bupivacaine in human patients who have ileus after major abdominal surgery.[84]

Adverse Side Effects

Pruritus, urinary retention, nausea, vomiting, and respiratory depression are the most common side effects mentioned in the human literature for epidural opioids. In the veterinary literature, these same side effects and delayed hair growth at the L-S intervertebral space have been reported with a low incidence (less than 11%).[28,85,86] Respiratory depression, assessed by a decrease in rate and an increase in end-tidal pressure or arterial carbon dioxide (CO_2) during surgery, was higher (26%) in dogs receiving epidural injections of morphine alone than in dogs receiving morphine and bupivacaine (7%), although the former group was maintained at a higher inhalational anesthetic concentration, which could have contributed to this adverse effect.[28] The respiratory depression associated with morphine is usually delayed and associated with rostral spread; therefore, it may take hours before it is noticed. In the study by Troncy and colleagues,[28] there is no mention as to whether the dose of morphine was related to respiratory depression, even though the range of doses used (0.1–0.4 mg/kg) exceeded the effective dose (0.1 mg/kg) used in the research setting.

In the human literature, doses of morphine per patient between 2 and 5 mg are recommended for the epidural route.[35,36] Although there is a dose-dependent effect for duration and quality of analgesia, a ceiling effect is observed at doses greater than 3.75 mg per patient;[35] conversely, the incidence of side effects depends on the dose at all doses. Therefore, the dose of morphine should probably not exceed 0.1 mg/kg in small animals.

Excessive doses of morphine can also cause myoclonus of pelvic limbs and the tail; this has been reported in a dog that received preservative-free morphine at an intrathecal dose of 0.15 mg/kg.[87] This effect has also been observed in rats overdosed with intrathecal morphine and may result from morphine's blocking action on glycine at the spinal cord level.[88]

Of the aforementioned side effects, urinary retention is probably the one that needs to be addressed in small animals to avoid discomfort and further complications. Manual compression is usually effective until normal function resumes. A urinary catheter may also be placed to facilitate continuous emptying. Urinary retention from opioids is the result of μ-agonistic actions on central (supraspinal) and spinal centers. Detrusor motor centers are centrally located in the brain stem reticular formation of the midbrain, pons, and medulla oblongata, and they are also spinally located in sacral parasympathetic segments in the dorsal horn. Agonistic actions of opioids on these centers inhibit bladder motility from detrusor relaxation and result in bladder filling.[89–91] Systemic opioids cause urinary retention by supraspinal actions, whereas intrathecal opioids cause it by spinal actions. Epidural opioids can induce urinary retention by supraspinal actions from systemic absorption of the opioid from the epidural space and also by spinal actions from absorption into the CSF and spinal cord. Inhibition of bladder function from systemic morphine can be reversed with systemic naloxone. In rats, morphine administered intravenously at a rate of 1 or 5 mg/kg induced central bladder relaxation, which was reversed with intravenously administered naloxone at a dose of only 0.1 mg/kg because of naloxone's higher degree of uptake in the brain.[91] Conversely, spinally induced bladder relaxation from intrathecal morphine injection of 5 μg was reversed with intrathecal naloxone at a rate of 10 to 20 μg but required a systemic naloxone intravenous dose of 1 mg/kg.[91] Because some of the urinary retention that results from epidural morphine is centrally mediated, it has been found that titration of naloxone (0.1–0.25 mL of 0.4 mg/mL diluted in saline [10 mL]; dose of 4–10-μg/bolus) while gently pressing on the abdomen may reverse urinary retention. This dose is unlikely to have any impact on the profound analgesia that results from morphine's spinal actions.

Local Anesthetics

Local anesthetics block voltage-gated sodium channels in nociceptive fibers at the nerve roots.[92] They can block A-δ and C nociceptive fibers; therefore, surgical pain is blocked effectively. B sympathetic fibers and A-β and A-α motor fibers are also affected, causing vasodilation, proprioceptive deficits, and motor blockade (see **Table 1**). Several factors determine which fibers are blocked more readily, including size and diffusion.[93,94] B sympathetic fibers are blocked at low concentrations. C fibers require higher concentrations of local anesthetics than A-δ fibers; however, because of their unmyelinated disposition, C fibers are blocked by differential diffusion before myelinated A-δ fibers. A-α motor fibers are more resistant. Therefore, the order of blockade seen clinically is: B, C, A-δ, and A-α.

Local anesthetics are also affected by the three routes of uptake from the epidural space. Higher concentrations than what is normally necessary within the nerve to cause blockade are required to counteract the routes of uptake from the epidural space. Local anesthetics are lipophilic drugs (lidocaine, O/B = 110; bupivacaine, O:B = 346–560; ropivacaine, O:B = 115) with similar permeability coefficients (lidocaine, 1.45 cm/min $\times$ 10^{-5}; bupivacaine = 1.60 cm/min $\times$ 10^{-5})[4] that can be readily absorbed systemically, and despite the fact that epidural doses are similar to systemic doses, it is less likely for them to produce supraspinal analgesia, except for lidocaine, because similar epidural doses used systemically are known to cause analgesia.[95] The predominant site of action after epidural administration is the nerve roots, which are bathed by the local anesthetic as it pools in the epidural space.

Among the commonly used local anesthetics in small animals, lidocaine and mepivacaine are faster in onset but of shorter duration and bupivacaine and ropivacaine are slower in onset but of longer duration (see **Table 2**). The lower protein binding of lidocaine (64%) and mepivacaine (75%) is responsible for their shorter action, and their more physiologic constant of dissociation (7.6–7.8) is responsible for their faster onset. Bupivacaine, because of its molecular size and lipophilicity, dissociates from the sodium channel at a slower rate than lidocaine.[92] Ropivacaine is also long acting, with a molecular size, pKa (8.1), and protein binding similar to bupivacaine (94%–96%), except that it has vasoconstrictive effects that contrast with the vasodilation produced by other local anesthetics.[96] In dogs, epidural bupivacaine 0.5% or 0.75% and ropivacaine 0.5% or 0.75% at 0.7 to 1.65 mg/kg resulted in similar times to onset and duration of blockade tested caudal to the thoracolumbar area and were associated with minimal cardiorespiratory changes.[97] Onset is of intermediate duration (<30 minutes), and the duration of analgesia for anatomic areas caudal to the diaphragm is approximately 2 hours for both drugs.[97] In other studies in which surgical procedures have been completed under epidural anesthesia with bupivacaine and sedation, doses of 1.0 to 1.5 mg/kg induced complete sensory blockade in 12 to 30 minutes and partial or complete sensory and motor blockade for 50 to 200 minutes.[20,46] Cardiovascular parameters, including cardiac index and blood pressure, are equally or better maintained than in dogs undergoing the procedure under general anesthesia.[20,98]

IQB-9302 [1-methylcyclopropyl-N-(2,6-dymethylphenyl)-2 piperidinecarboxamide] is a newer local anesthetic with properties similar to bupivacaine but more lipophilic and potent. Administered epidurally at 0.5, 1.0, or 1.5 mg/kg, it produced longer nociceptive complete blockade (243 versus 131 minutes for the high dose) and less motor blockade (4.7 versus 6.7 hours for the high dose) than bupivacaine.[46]

Excessive rostral epidural spread of local anesthetics to the thoracic area is associated with hypotension and potentially decreased cardiac output as a result of vasodilation and decreased vascular resistance.[99,100] These effects are more severe under conditions of compromised circulatory conditions and may result in decreased oxygen delivery (Do_2) at the splanchnic level[99] or, in more severe cases, cardiac arrest.[101] Conversely, the splanchnic circulation benefits from the vasodilation and increased microvascular hemoglobin oxygenation induced after epidural local anesthetics if physiologically stable conditions are present within the patient or if adequate measures are taken to re-establish compromised circulatory conditions with fluid resuscitation that preserves a positive correlation between Do_2 and microvascular hemoglobin oxygenation.[99]

Epidural anesthesia with local anesthetics shortens intestinal paralysis after colon anastomosis in dogs[26] by attenuating sympathetic efferent inhibitory pathways and by induced vasodilatation through sympathetic blockade.[102]

α_2-Agonists

Spinal α_2-receptors have presynaptic binding on primary afferents, block the release of substance P from C fibers, and have postsynaptic action on dorsal horn wide-dynamic-range neurons, which are all similar effects to opioids but are not antagonized by opioid antagonists.[55,61] Xylazine can also block A-δ fibers, inducing complete blockade of dermatomes, and has also been implicated in affecting A-α motor fibers, whereas other α_2-agonists are less likely to do so (see **Table 1**). B sympathetic fibers are not affected, but the systemic α-effects result in vasoconstriction.

The spinal effects of α_2-agonists also coexist with systemic effects from systemic vascular uptake, including sedation, analgesia (supraspinal), and less desirable effects (eg, bradycardia, increased vascular resistance, vomiting). Xylazine at doses of 0.1, 0.2, and 0.4 mg/kg decreases the MAC for isoflurane by 8%, 22%, and 33%, respectively, and associated with these doses, heart rate decreased and blood pressure increased compared with a placebo group that received epidural saline.[103] The high xylazine dose caused some degree of hind limb ataxia after recovery.[103] Dogs receiving epidural xylazine at a dose of 0.2 mg/kg and kept at a deeper level of isoflurane anesthesia (2%) had similar cardiovascular function as a placebo group, probably because of blunting elicited by the higher isoflurane concentration,[104] and similar findings were observed in dogs receiving epidural morphine (0.1 mg/kg) combined with a much lower dose of xylazine (0.02 mg/kg) while under 2% of isoflurane.[105]

Clonidine, more commonly used in human beings, has also been administered to dogs at constant rate infusions of 80, 200 and 320 μg/h at a rate of 4 mL every 24 hours for 28 days in a research study. These dogs exhibited a dose-dependent antinociceptive effect to thermally evoked skin twitch in the thoracic area and maximal effect in the lumbar area for all doses with development of tolerance over the 28-day period, and there were no effects on motor function or body temperature. Heart rate, blood pressure, and respiratory rate were decreased in a dose-dependent manner, but dogs showed progressive adaptation and returned to control values within days, except for respiratory rate, which remained decreased.[47]

Medetomidine (10 μg/kg) diluted in 1 mL of saline and injected at the L-S intervertebral space level in cats increased the pain threshold to electrical stimulation for the forelimb and hind limb within 20 minutes and lasted 245 minutes for the hind limb and 120 minutes for the forelimb.[66] Interestingly, in dogs administered 5 μg/kg, no analgesia was elicited to tail clamping; however, if combined with morphine (0.1 mg/kg), the analgesia was longer lasting (13 hours) than for morphine alone (6 hours).[106] Systemic effects observed in cats included mild sedation, vomiting in 12 of 15 cats within 7 minutes of injection, increases in blood pressure from increased vascular resistance, and decreases in heart rate and respiratory rate.[66,78] It is likely that a great component of the analgesic effects observed in this study is supraspinal. When the systemic effects of medetomidine tended to disappear, the combination of epidural morphine with medetomidine (0.1 mg/kg and 5 μg/kg, respectively) was not superior to epidural morphine (0.1 mg/kg) alone for dogs undergoing cranial cruciate ligament repair when evaluated in the postoperative period.[22] Using high doses of epidural medetomidine (30 μg/kg) in dogs, cardiovascular effects (bradycardia) persisted for longer than 2 hours and the MAC of isoflurane was decreased by 47%.[107]

Ketamine

Ketamine antagonizes *N*-methyl-D-aspartate receptors in the spinal cord and inhibits the excitatory actions of this glutamate receptor, reducing sensitization and nociception.[108] The use of epidural ketamine has resulted in variable degrees of analgesia or anesthesia and effects on motor function (see **Table 1**). Complete anesthesia of the perineal area for 5 to 10 minutes was observed in one study using 2.5 mg/kg.[109] The duration of analgesia is variable, being inadequate in a model of chemically induced synovitis,[110] adequate for 30 minutes for pinprick,[109] and adequate for 720 minutes using von Frey ligaments.[21] Systemic effects include hind limb incoordination or paralysis, salivation, and nystagmus, which are associated with the use of systemic doses (0.6–2.5 mg/kg) by the epidural route.[21,109–111]

The levogyral (S[+]) ketamine isomer has also been used epidurally (0.6 mg/kg); however, despite its twofold stronger potency, analgesic effects against von Frey ligament stimulation were less than 90 minutes, probably because the metabolism is faster for this isomer than for the racemic mixture.[21,112]

The use of epidural ketamine does not provide any advantage over opioids, local anesthetics, or α-agonists, and it is not recommended by this author.

Other Drugs

Epidural or intrathecal midazolam produces analgesia in rats and human beings that is mediated by means of the γ-aminobutyric acid $(GABA)_A$ receptor in the spinal cord.[113–115] Dogs administered a high dose of midazolam epidurally (1 mg/kg) to be able to demonstrate CSF concentrations achieved concentrations that were only 3% of those found in the systemic circulation;[116] however, it is expected that only low concentrations are necessary in the CSF to exert analgesic effects directly on the spinal cord. In fact, the analgesic epidural dose of midazolam in human studies is only 0.05 mg/kg.[115]

NSAIDs, including diclofenac, indomethacin, and ibuprofen, have been shown to provide analgesic effects by the epidural route and blocking spinal cyclooxygenase (COX)-2. This minimized the hyperalgesic mechanisms but not the acute noxious responses at the dorsal horn of the spinal cord in rats and people.[117,118] NSAIDs have intermediate lipophilicity, which facilitates their diffusion through the dural membranes, and a direct action on the spinal cord, but they also readily penetrate the blood-brain barrier because of systemic absorption by epidural vessels, and subsequently exert supraspinal action in addition to peripheral effects.[4,119] C-fiber stimulation induces prostanoid release in the spinal cord, which can be effectively blocked by COX-inhibitors, preventing the hyperalgesia induced by substance P and *N*-methyl-D-aspartate.[120] In an acute stifle synovitis model induced by sodium urate crystals injected into the joint of dogs, however, there was no advantage of injecting epidural deracoxib (1.5–3 mg/kg) over subcutaneous (3 mg/kg) administration, because both routes induced similar degrees of analgesia.[121]

Preservatives

Epidural injections are usually safe despite the use of drugs that may contain preservatives. Intrathecal injections should only be performed with preservative-free solutions to avoid direct toxic effects of the preservatives on the spinal cord.

Benzyl alcohol has also been shown to produce motor deficits that lasted 16 months in a woman injected with 0.9% sodium chloride (NaCl) with 1.5% benzyl alcohol epidurally.[122] Phenol and formaldehyde are the most toxic preservatives, whereas sodium metabisulfite and sodium edetate have not been shown to have neurotoxic effects when used for long-term intrathecal infusion in human beings.[123] Experimentally, preservative-containing preparations of morphine containing 0.1% sodium metabisulfite had no toxic or histopathologic effects in dogs administered this type of preparation epidurally.[124] Intrathecal administration using the higher epidural dose can produce prolonged sensory or motor deficits, however.[125] In rabbits administered intrathecal sodium bisulfite 0.2% at doses of 1.2 to 2.4 mg, neurotoxic effects, including irreversible hind limb paresis, were induced in 12 of 14 animals.[126] This concentration of sodium bisulfite (2 mg/mL) administered intrathecally to rabbits is 5 to 80 times higher than the intrathecal concentration (0.025–0.4 mg/mL) described by Sjoberg and colleagues[123] as being innocuous in human beings. Parabens are also considered safe for epidural and intrathecal injections.[127]

At the author's hospital, the Anesthesia Service uses morphine (15 mg/mL) containing 0.1% sodium metabisulfite for epidural injections, whereas patients in the ICU only receive preservative-free morphine. The recommended dose of morphine of 0.1 mg/kg results in a dose of sodium metabisulfite of 0.1 mg per 15 kg and reduces the risk for toxicity from accidental intrathecal injection. The lack of toxicity of metabisulfite by the epidural route is important to avoid complications; preservative-free solutions eliminate the risk completely. Therefore, it is advisable to use preservative-free solutions for intrathecal injections, whereas epidural injections can be performed with preservative-containing solutions as long as correct placement is verified using any of the different techniques already mentioned, the drug is diluted with preservative-free saline or preservative-free local anesthetic, and friendly preservatives are used. If an epidural injection is initially planned with preservative-containing drug and CSF is observed during puncture, indicating an intrathecal location, it is recommended to avoid the injection and, instead, to withdraw the needle to the epidural space, where the injection can be placed. If a preservative-free solution is used for the epidural injection and the injection is changed to an intrathecal injection because CSF is observed during puncture, it is recommended to decrease the dose at least 10 times to avoid the risk for side effects related to the higher bioavailability of the drug in the CSF.

SUMMARY

Current knowledge of drugs administered epidurally has allowed an effective way of providing analgesia for a wide variety of conditions in veterinary patients. Proper selection of drugs and dosages can result in analgesia of specific segments of the spinal cord with minimal side effects.

Epidural anesthesia is an alternative to general anesthesia with inhalation anesthetics, although the combination of both techniques is more common and allows for reduced doses of drugs used with each technique. Epidural anesthesia and intravenous anesthetics can also be used without inhalation anesthetics in surgical procedures caudal to the diaphragm.

Newer techniques are being incorporated in veterinary medicine, which include the use of epidural and spinal analgesia and anesthesia in addition to epidural or intrathecal injection in close proximity to spinal segments that innervate the desired specific dermatome, allowing for analgesia of those areas only. This area is promising, and further investigation is warranted to find practical techniques that can be applied in small animal species as they are currently applied in human medicine.

REFERENCES

1. Heylings DA. Supraspinous and interspinous ligaments in dog, cat and baboon. J Anat 1980;2:223–8.
2. Grau T, Leipold RW, Horter J, et al. The lumbar epidural space in pregnancy: visualization by ultrasonography. Br J Anaesth 2001;86:798–804.
3. Groen RJM, Ponssen H. Vascular anatomy of the spinal epidural space: considerations on the etiology of the spontaneous spinal epidural hematoma. Clin Anat 1991;4:413–20.
4. Bernards CM, Hill HF. Physical and chemical properties of drug molecules governing their diffusion through the spinal meninges. Anesthesiology 1992;77:750–6.
5. Fletcher TF. Spinal cord and meninges. In: Evans HE, Christensen GC, editors. Miller's anatomy of the dog. 2nd edition. Philadelphia: WB Saunders Co.; 1979. p. 945.
6. Hudson LC, Hamilton WP. Atlas of feline anatomy for veterinarians. Philadelphia: WB Saunders Co.; 1993. p. 198.
7. Geers C, Lecouvet FE, Behets C, et al. Polygonal deformation of the dural sac in lumbar epidural lipomatosis: anatomic explanation by the presence of meningovertebral ligaments. Am J Neuroradiol 2003;24:1276–82.

8. Ramsey HJ. Fat in the epidural space in young and adult cats. Am J Anat 1959; 104:345–79.
9. Ramsey HJ. Comparative morphology of fat in the epidural space. Am J Anat 1959;105:219–32.
10. Igarashi T, Hirabayashi Y, Shimizu R, et al. The fiberscopic findings of the epidural space in pregnant women. Anesthesiology 2000;92:1631–6.
11. Grundy EM, Zamora AM, Winnie AP. Comparison of spread of epidural anesthesia in pregnant and nonpregnant women. Anesth analg 1978;57:544–6.
12. Gorgi AA, Hofmeister EH, Higginbotham MJ, et al. Effect of body position on cranial migration of epidurally injected methylene blue in recumbent dogs. Am J Vet Res 2006;67:219–21.
13. Lee I, Yamagishi N, Oboshi K, et al. Distribution of new methylene blue injected into the lumbosacral epidural space in cats. Vet Anaesth Analg 2004; 31:190–4.
14. Brodbelt A, Stoodley M. CSF pathways: a review. Br J Neurosurg 2007;21: 510–20.
15. Rolbin SH, Cole AFD, Hew EM, et al. Effect of lateral position and volume on the spread of epidural anaesthesia in the parturient. Can Anaesth Soc J 1981;28: 431–5.
16. Norris MC, Leighton BL, DeSimone CA, et al. Lateral position and epidural anesthesia for cesarean section. Anesth Analg 1988;67:788–90.
17. Whalley DG, D'Amico JA, Rybicki LA, et al. The effect of posture on the induction of epidural anesthesia for peripheral vascular surgery. Reg Anesth 1995;20: 407–11.
18. Setayesh AR, Kholdebarin AR, Saber M, et al. The Trendelenburg position increases the spread and accelerates the onset of epidural anesthesia for cesarean section. Can J Anesth 2001;48:890–3.
19. Torske KE, Dyson DH. Epidural analgesia and anesthesia. Vet Clin North Am 2000;30:859–74.
20. Almeida TF, Fantoni DT, Mastrocinque S, et al. Epidural anesthesia with bupivacaine, bupivacaine and fentanyl, or bupivacaine and sufentanil during intravenous administration of propofol for ovariohysterectomy in dogs. J Am Vet Med Assoc 2007;230:45–51.
21. Duque JC, Valadão CAA, Farias A, et al. Pre-emptive epidural ketamine or S(+)-ketamine in post-incisional pain in dogs: a comparative study. Vet Surg 2004;33:361–7.
22. Pacharinsak C, Greene SA, Keegan RD, et al. Postoperative analgesia in dogs receiving epidural morphine plus medetomidine. J Vet Pharmacol Ther 2003; 26:71–7.
23. Valverde A, Dyson DH, McDonell WN. Epidural morphine reduces halothane MAC in the dog. Can J Anaesth 1989;36:629–32.
24. Kona-Boun JJ, Cuvelliez S, Troncy E. Evaluation of epidural administration of morphine or morphine and bupivacaine for postoperative analgesia after premedication with an opioid analgesic and orthopedic surgery in dogs. J Am Vet Med Assoc 2006;229:1103–12.
25. Fowler D, Isakow K, Caulkett N, et al. An evaluation of the analgesic effects of meloxicam in addition to epidural morphine/mepivacaine in dogs undergoing cranial cruciate ligament repair. Can Vet J 2003;44:643–8.
26. Jansen M, Jürgen F, Titel A, et al. Influence of postoperative epidural analgesia with bupivacaine on intestinal motility, transit time, and anastomotic healing. World J Surg 2002;26:303–6.

27. Klarica M, Rados M, Draganic P, et al. Effect of head position on cerebrospinal fluid pressure in cats: comparison with artificial model. Croat Med J 2006;47: 233–8.
28. Troncy E, Junot S, Keroack S, et al. Results of preemptive epidural administration of morphine with or without bupivacaine in dogs and cats undergoing surgery: 265 cases (1997–1999). J Am Vet Med Assoc 2002;221:666–71.
29. Stone JP, Tiwari VR, Shetty DY, et al. Injectate temperature and discomfort during epidural injection. Int J Obstet Anesth 2006;15:342–3.
30. Jones RS. Epidural analgesia in the dog and cat. Vet J 2001;161:123–31.
31. Bengis RG, Guyton AC. Some pressure and fluid dynamic characteristics of the canine epidural space. Am J Phys 1977;232:H255–259.
32. Rocco AG, Philip JH, Boas RA, et al. Epidural space as a Starling resistor and elevation of inflow resistance in a diseased epidural space. Reg Anesth 1997; 22:167–77.
33. Nordberg G, Hedner T, Mellstrand T, et al. Pharmacokinetics of epidural morphine in man. Eur J Clin Pharmacol 1984;26:233–7.
34. Palmer CM, Emerson S, Volgoropolous D, et al. Dose-response relationship of intrathecal morphine for postcesarean analgesia. Anesthesiology 1999;90: 437–44.
35. Palmer CM, Nogami WM, Van Maren G, et al. Postcesarean epidural morphine: a dose-response study. Anesth Analg 2000;90:887–91.
36. Dualé C, Frey C, Bolandard F, et al. Epidural versus intrathecal morphine for postoperative analgesia after Caesarean section. Br J Anaesth 2003;91:690–4.
37. Naganobu K, Hagio M. The effect of body position on the "hanging drop" method for identifying the extradural space in anaesthetized dogs. Vet Anaesth Analg 2007;34:59–62.
38. Iff I, Moens Y, Schatzmann U. Use of pressure waves to confirm the correct placement of epidural needles in dogs. Vet Rec 2007;161:22–5.
39. Tsui BCH, Gupta S, Finucane B. Confirmation of epidural catheter placement using nerve stimulation. Can J Anaesth 1998;45:640–4.
40. Tamai H, Sawamura S, Atarashi H, et al. The electrical properties of epidural catheters: what are the requirements for nerve stimulation guidance? Anesth Analg 2005;100:1704–7.
41. Read MR. Confirmation of epidural needle placement using nerve stimulation in dogs [abstract]. Fourth International Veterinary Academy of Pain Management (IVAPM) Annual Meeting 2007, Montreal (Canada).
42. Tsui BCH, Emery D, Uwiera RRE, et al. The use of electrical stimulation to monitor epidural needle advancement in a porcine model. Anesth Analg 2005;100: 1611–3.
43. de Medicis E, Tetrault JP, Martin R, et al. A prospective comparative study of two indirect methods for confirming the localization of an epidural catheter for postoperative analgesia. Anesth Analg 2005;101:1830–3.
44. Lim YJ, Bahk JH, Ahn WS, et al. Coiling of lumbar epidural catheters. Acta Anaesthesiol Scand 2002;46:603–36.
45. Hogan Q. Epidural catheter tip position and distribution of injectate evaluated by computed tomography. Anesthesiology 1999;90:964–70.
46. Gómez de Segura IA, Vazquez I, De Miguel E. Antinociceptive and motor-blocking action of epidurally administered IQB-9302 and bupivacaine in the dog. Reg Anesth Pain Med 2000;25:522–8.
47. Yaksh TL, Rathbun M, Jage J, et al. Pharmacology and toxicology of chronically infused epidural clonidine HCl in dogs. Fundam Appl Toxicol 1994;23:319–35.

48. Boikova NV, Volchkov VA, Strashnov VI, et al. Morphofunctional changes in spinal cord neurons after epidural lidocaine. Neurosci Behav Physiol 2004;34:597–601.
49. Swalander DB, Crowe DT, Hittenmiller DH, et al. Complications associated with the use of indwelling epidural catheters in dogs 81 cases (1996–1999). J Am Vet Med Assoc 2000;216:368–70.
50. Hansen BD. Epidural catheter analgesia in dogs and cats: technique and review of 182 cases (1991–1999). Journal of Veterinary Emergency and Critical Care 2001;11:95–103.
51. Cook TM. Combined spinal-epidural techniques. Anaesthesia 2000;55:42–64.
52. Novello L, Corletto F. Combined spinal-epidural anesthesia in a dog. Vet Surg 2006;35:191–7.
53. Gourlay GK, Cherry DA, Plummer JL, et al. The influence of drug polarity on the absorption of opioid drugs into CSF and subsequent cephalad migration following lumbar epidural administration: application to morphine and pethidine. Pain 1987;31:297–305.
54. Yaksh TL, Provencher JC, Rathbun ML, et al. Pharmacokinetics and efficacy of epidurally delivered sustained-release encapsulated morphine in dogs. Anesthesiology 1999;90:1402–12.
55. Sabbe MB, Grafe MR, Mjanger E, et al. Spinal delivery of sufentanil, alfentanil and morphine in dogs: physiologic and toxicologic investigations. Anesthesiology 1994;81:899–920.
56. Troncy E, Besner J-G, Charbonneau R, et al. Pharmacokinetics of epidural butorphanol in isoflurane-anesthetized dogs. J Vet Pharmacol Ther 1996;19:268–73.
57. Bernards CM, Shen DD, Sterling ES, et al. Epidural, cerebrospinal fluid, and plasma pharmacokinetics of epidural opioids (part I). Anesthesiology 2003;99:455–65.
58. Loper KA, Ready LB, Downey M, et al. Epidural and intravenous fentanyl infusions are clinically equivalent after knee surgery. Anesth Analg 1990;70:72–5.
59. George MJ. The site of action of epidurally administered opioids and its relevance to postoperative pain management. Anaesthesia 2006;61:659–64.
60. Valverde A, Conlon PD, Dyson DH, et al. Cisternal CSF and serum concentrations of morphine following epidural administration in the dog. J Vet Pharmacol Ther 1992;15:91–5.
61. Yaksh TL, Noueihed R. The physiology and pharmacology of spinal opiates. Annu Rev Pharmacol Toxicol 1985;25:433–62.
62. Mosing M, Leschnik M, Iff I. Specific gravity of cerebrospinal fluid in dogs and cats: comparison with different anaesthetic drug solutions (abstract). Veterinary Regional Anaesthesia and Pain Medicine 2006;4:28–9.
63. Yaksh TL. Multiple opiate receptor systems in brain and spinal cord. Part I. Eur J Anaesthesiol 1984;1:171–99.
64. Torske KE, Dyson DH, Conlon PD. Cardiovascular effects of epidurally administered oxymorphone and an oxymorphone-bupivacaine combination in halothane-anesthetized dogs. Am J Vet Res 1999;60:194–200.
65. Troncy E, Cuvelliez SG, Blais D. Evaluation of analgesia and cardiorespiratory effects of epidurally administered butorphanol in isoflurane-anesthetized dogs. Am J Vet Res 1996;57:1478–82.
66. Duke T, Cox AM, Remedios AM, et al. The analgesic effects of administering fentanyl or medetomidine in the lumbosacral epidural space of cats. Vet Surg 1994;23:143–8.

67. Ginosaur Y, Riley ET, Angst MS. The site of action of epidural fentanyl in humans. The difference between infusion and bolus administration. Anesth Analg 2003; 97:1428–38.
68. Leibetseder EN, Mosing M, Jones RS. A comparison of extradural and intravenous methadone on intraoperative isoflurane and postoperative analgesia requirements in dogs. Vet Anaesth Analg 2006;33:128–36.
69. Tusell JM, Andaluz A, Prandi D, et al. Effects of epidural anaesthesia-analgesia on intravenous anaesthesia with propofol. Vet J 2005;169:108–12.
70. Brose WG, Tanelian DL, Brodsky JB, et al. CSF and blood pharmacokinetics of hydromorphone and morphine following lumbar epidural administration. Pain 1991;45:11–5.
71. Pypendop BH, Pascoe PJ, Ilkiw JE. Effects of epidural administration of morphine and buprenorphine on the minimum alveolar concentration of isoflurane in cats. Am J Vet Res 2006;67:1471–5.
72. Golder FJ, Pascoe PJ, Bailey CS, et al. The effects of epidural morphine on the minimum alveolar concentration of isoflurane in cats. J Vet Anaesth 1998;25:52–6.
73. Torske KE, Dyson DH, Pettifer G. End tidal halothane concentration and postoperative analgesia requirements in dogs: a comparison between intravenous oxymorphone and epidural bupivacaine alone and in combination with oxymorphone. Can Vet J 1998;39:361–8.
74. Hendrix PK, Raffe MR, Robinson EP, et al. Epidural administration of bupivacaine, morphine or their combinations for post-operative analgesia in dogs. J Am Vet Med Assoc 1996;209:598–607.
75. Sibanda S, Hughes JML, Pawson PE, et al. The effects of preoperative extradural bupivacaine and morphine on the stress response in dogs undergoing femoro-tibial joint surgery. Vet Anaesth Analg 2006;33:246–57.
76. Day TK, Pepper WT, Tobias TA, et al. Comparison of intra-articular and epidural morphine for analgesia following stifle arthrotomy in dogs. Vet Surg 1995;24: 522–30.
77. Hoelzler MG, Harvey RC, Lidbetter DA, et al. Comparison of perioperative analgesic protocols for dogs undergoing tibial plateau leveling osteotomy. Vet Surg 2005;34:337–44.
78. Duke T, Cox AM, Remedios AM, et al. The cardiopulmonary effects of placing fentanyl or medetomidine in the lumbosacral epidural space of isoflurane-anesthetized cats. Vet Surg 1994;23:149–55.
79. Valverde A, Dyson DH, Cockshutt JR, et al. Comparison of the hemodynamic effects of halothane alone and halothane combined with epidurally administered morphine for anesthesia in ventilated dogs. Am J Vet Res 1991;52:505–9.
80. Naganobu K, Maeda N, Miyamoto T, et al. Cardiorespiratory effects of epidural administration of morphine and fentanyl in dogs anesthetized with sevoflurane. J Am Vet Med Assoc 2004;224:67–70.
81. Nakayoshi T, Kawasaki N, Suzuki Y, et al. Epidural administration of morphine facilitates time of appearance of first gastric interdigestive migrating complex in dogs with paralytic ileus after open abdominal surgery. J Gastrointest Surg 2007;11:648–54.
82. Wood JD, Galligan JJ. Function of opioids in the enteric nervous system. Neurogastroenterol Motil 2004;16:17–28.
83. Lewis TD. Morphine and gastroduodenal motility. Dig Dis Sci 1999;44:2178–86.
84. Barzoi G, Carluccio S, Bianchi B, et al. Morphine plus bupivacaine vs. morphine peridural analgesia in abdominal surgery: the effects on postoperative course in major hepatobiliary surgery. HPB Surg 2000;11:393–9.

85. Valverde A, Dyson DH, McDonell WN, et al. Use of epidural morphine in the dog for pain relief. Vet Comp Orth Traumatol 1989;2:55–8.
86. Herperger LJ. Postoperative urinary retention in a dog following morphine with bupivacaine epidural analgesia. Can Vet J 1998;39:650–2.
87. Kona-Boun JJ, Pibarot P, Quesnel A. Myoclonus and urinary retention following subarachnoid morphine injection in a dog. Vet Anaesth Analg 2003;30:257–64.
88. Tang AH, Schoenfeld MJ. Comparison of subcutaneous and spinal subarachnoid injections of morphine and naloxone in analgesic tests in the rat. Eur J Pharmacol 1978;52:215–23.
89. Rawal N, Möllefors K, Axelsson K, et al. An experimental study of urodynamic effects of epidural morphine and of naloxone reversal. Anesth Analg 1983;62: 641–7.
90. Dray A, Metsch R. Spinal opioid receptors and inhibition of urinary bladder motility in vivo. Neurosci Lett 1984;47:81–4.
91. Kontani H, Kawabata Y. A study of morphine-induced urinary retention in anesthetized rats capable of micturition. Jpn J Pharmacol 1988;48:31–6.
92. Butterworth JF IV, Strichartz GR. Molecular mechanisms of local anesthesia: a review. Anesthesiology 1990;72:711–34.
93. Huang JH, Thalhammer JG, Raymond SA, et al. Susceptibility to lidocaine of impulses in different somatosensory afferent fibers of rat sciatic nerve. J Pharmacol Exp Ther 1997;292:802–11.
94. Wildsmith JA, Gissen AJ, Takman B, et al. Differential nerve blockade: esters v. amides and the influence of pKa. Br J Anaesth 1987;59:379–84.
95. Valverde A, Doherty TJ, Hernandez J, et al. Effect of lidocaine on the minimum alveolar concentration of isoflurane in dogs. Vet Anaesth Analg 2004;31:264–71.
96. Hiroki I, Yukinaga W, Shuji D, et al. Direct effects of ropivacaine and bupivacaine on spinal pial vessels in canine: assessment with closed spinal window technique. Laboratory investigation. Anesthesiology 1997;87:75–81.
97. Duke T, Caulkett NA, Ball SD, et al. Comparative analgesic and cardiopulmonary effects of bupivacaine and ropivacaine in the epidural space of the conscious dog. Vet Anaesth Analg 2000;27:13–21.
98. Hewitt SA, Brisson BA, Sinclair MD, et al. Comparison of cardiopulmonary responses during sedation with epidural and local anesthesia for laparoscopic-assisted jejunostomy feeding tube placement with cardiopulmonary responses during general anesthesia for laparoscopic-assisted or open surgical jejunostomy feeding tube placement in healthy dogs. Am J Vet Res 2007;68:358–69.
99. Schwarte LA, Picker O, Höhne C, et al. Effects of thoracic epidural anesthesia on microvascular gastric mucosal oxygenation in physiological and compromised circulatory conditions in dogs. Br J Anaesth 2004;93:552–9.
100. Vagts DA, Iber T, Szabo B, et al. Effects of epidural anaesthesia on intestinal oxygenation in pigs. Br J Anaesth 2003;90:212–20.
101. Savvas I, Anagnostou T, Papazoglou LG, et al. Successful resuscitation from cardiac arrest associated with extradural lidocaine in a dog. Vet Anaesth Analg 2006;33:175–8.
102. Johansson K, Ahn H, Lindhagen J, et al. Effect of epidural anaesthesia on intestinal blood flow. Br J Surg 1988;75:73–6.
103. Soares JHN, Ascoli FO, Gremiao IDF, et al. Isoflurane sparing action of epidurally administered xylazine hydrochloride in anesthetized dogs. Am J Vet Res 2004;65:854–9.
104. Greene SA, Keegan RD, Weil AB. Cardiovascular effects after epidural injection of xylazine in isoflurane-anesthetized dogs. Vet Surg 1995;24:283–9.

105. Keegan RD, Greene SA, Weil AB. Cardiovascular effects of epidurally administered morphine and xylazine-morphine combination in isoflurane-anesthetized dogs. Am J Vet Res 1995;56:496–500.
106. Branson KR, Ko JC, Tranquilli WJ, et al. Duration of analgesia induced by epidurally administered morphine and medetomidine in dogs. J Vet Pharmacol Ther 1993;16:369–72.
107. Ewing KK, Mohammed HO, Scarlett JM, et al. Reduction of isoflurane anesthetic requirement by medetomidine and its restoration by atipamezole in dogs. Am J Vet Res 1993;54:294–9.
108. Lizarraga I, Chambers JP, Johnson CB. Depression of NMDA-receptor-mediated segmental transmission by ketamine and ketoprofen, but not L-NAME, on the in vitro neonatal rat spinal rat preparation. Brain Res 2006;1094:57–64.
109. Amarpal, Aithal HP, Kinjavdekar P, et al. Interaction between epidurally administered ketamine and pethidine in dogs. J Vet Med A Physiol Pathol Clin Med 2003;50:254–8.
110. Hamilton SM, Johnston SA, Broadstone RV. Evaluation of analgesia provided by the administration of epidural ketamine in dogs with a chemically induced synovitis. Vet Anaesth Analg 2005;32:30–9.
111. Acosta AD, Gomar C, Correa-Natalini C, et al. Analgesic effects of epidurally administered levogyral ketamine alone or in combination with morphine on intraoperative and postoperative pain in dogs undergoing ovariohysterectomy. Am J Vet Res 2005;66:54–61.
112. Geisslinger G, Hering W, Thomann P, et al. Pharmacokinetics and pharmacodynamics of ketamine enantiomers in surgical patients using a stereoselective analytical method. Br J Anaesth 1993;70:666–71.
113. Edwards M, Serrao JM, Gent JP, et al. On the mechanism by which midazolam causes spinally mediated analgesia. Anesthesiology 1990;73:273–7.
114. Nishiyama T, Hanoka K. The synergistic interaction between midazolam and clonidine in spinally-mediated analgesia in two different pain models of rats. Anesth Analg 2001;93:1025–31.
115. Nishiyama T. The post-operative analgesic action of midazolam following epidural administration. Eur J Anaesthesiol 1995;12:369–74.
116. Nishiyama T, Tamai H, Hanoka K. Serum and cerebrospinal fluid concentrations of midazolam after epidural administration in dogs. Anesth Analg 2003;96: 159–62.
117. Masue T, Dohi S, Asano T, et al. Spinal antinociceptive effect of epidural nonsteroidal antiinflammatory drugs on nitric oxide-induced hyperalgesia in rats. Anesthesiology 1999;91:198–206.
118. Lauretti GR, Reis MP, Mattos AL, et al. Epidural non-steroidal anti-inflammatory drugs for cancer pain. Anesth Analg 1998;86:117–8.
119. McCormack K. The spinal actions of nonsteroidal anti-inflammatory drugs and the dissociation between their anti-inflammatory and analgesic effects. Drugs 1994;5:28–45.
120. Malmberg AG, Yaksh TL. Hyperalgesia mediated by spinal glutamate or substance P receptor blockade by spinal cyclooxygenase inhibition. Science 1992;257:1276–9.
121. Karnik PS, Johnston S, Ward D, et al. The effects of epidural deracoxib on the ground reaction forces in an acute stifle synovitis model. Vet Surg 2006;35: 34–42.
122. Craig DB, Habib GG. Flaccid paraparesis following obstetrical epidural analgesia: possible role of benzyl alcohol. Anesth Analg 1977;56:219–21.

123. Sjoberg M, Karlsson PA, Nordborg C, et al. Neuropathological findings after long-term intrathecal infusion of morphine and bupivacaine for pain treatment in cancer patients. Anesthesiology 1992;76:173–86.
124. King FG, Baxter AD, Mathieson G. Tissue reaction of morphine applied to the epidural space of dogs. Can Anaesth Soc J 1984;31:268–71.
125. Covino BG, Marx GF, Finster M, et al. Prolonged sensory/motor deficits following inadvertent spinal anesthesia. Anesth Analg 1980;59:399–400.
126. Wang BC, Hillman DE, Spielholz NI, et al. Chronic neurological deficits and nesacaine-CE. An effect of the anesthetic 2-chloroprocaine, or the antioxidant, sodium bisulfite? Anesth Analg 1984;63:445–7.
127. Hodgson PS, Neal JN, Pollock JE, et al. The neurotoxicity of drugs given intrathecally (spinal). Anesth Analg 1999;88:797–809.

Paravertebral Blockade of the Brachial Plexus in Dogs

Kip A. Lemke, DVM, MS*, Catherine M. Creighton, DVM

KEYWORDS

- Paravertebral blockade • Brachial plexus • Dogs
- Local anesthesia • Regional anesthesia • Lidocaine
- Bupivacaine • Electrical nerve location
- Electrical nerve stimulation • Percutaneous electrode
- Guidance

Local anesthetic techniques are often used perioperatively in combination with other analgesic drugs as an integral part of multimodal strategies to manage pain in small animals.[1,2] Surgical trauma and inflammation produce sensitization of peripheral sensory fibers, and the subsequent barrage of nociceptive input produces sensitization of projection neurons in the dorsal horn of the spinal cord. Local anesthetics are the only class of analgesic drugs that can produce complete blockade of peripheral nociceptive input and prevent sensitization of central nociceptive pathways and the development of pathologic pain. Preoperative use of local anesthetic techniques reduces inhalant requirements and autonomic responses to noxious surgical stimuli. These reductions improve cardiopulmonary function during surgery and promote a rapid smooth recovery from anesthesia after surgery. Perioperative use of local anesthetic techniques also attenuates the neuroendocrine or stress response to surgical trauma and inflammation and reduces the incidence of postoperative complications dramatically.[3]

Neural blockade of the brachial plexus is used during the period around the time of surgery to manage pain in dogs undergoing surgical procedures of the forelimb. The block has traditionally been performed by injecting local anesthetic into the axillary space at the level of the shoulder.[4,5] Although the axillary technique is relatively easy to perform, a large volume of local anesthetic is required, onset time is slow (20–30 minutes), structures proximal to the elbow are not anesthetized, and incomplete blockade of the brachial plexus is relatively common. Further, neural blockade of the elbow and antebrachium is easier to achieve by selectively blocking the radial,

Department of Companion Animals, Atlantic Veterinary College, University of Prince Edward Island, 550 University Avenue, Charlottetown, Prince Edward Island, Canada, C1A 4P3
* Corresponding author.
E-mail address: klemke@upei.ca (K.A. Lemke).

Vet Clin Small Anim 38 (2008) 1231–1241
doi:10.1016/j.cvsm.2008.06.003 vetsmall.theclinics.com
0195-5616/08/$ – see front matter

ulnar, median, and musculocutaneous nerves above the humeral epicondyles. Given these drawbacks, the traditional axillary technique has limited clinical utility.

Paravertebral blockade of the brachial plexus was developed at the Atlantic Veterinary College and was first described by Lemke and Dawson[1] in 2000. Recently, the anatomic landmarks, technical merits, and reliability of the paravertebral technique were confirmed independently in an anatomic study by Hofmeister and colleagues.[6] A modified paravertebral technique, which was also developed at the Atlantic Veterinary College, is described for the first time in this article. Both paravertebral techniques have several advantages over the traditional axillary technique. Key anatomic landmarks are easier to identify, smaller amounts of local anesthetic are required, the entire forelimb (including the shoulder) is anesthetized, and complete blockade of the brachial plexus is easier to achieve. Unilateral blockade of the phrenic nerve and hemidiaphragmatic paresis are likely complications with both paravertebral techniques. Inadvertent intravascular injection and pneumothorax are potential complications with the paravertebral techniques and with the axillary technique. All three techniques are unreliable in obese or heavily muscled dogs, because anatomic landmarks are obscured. With both paravertebral techniques, a clear understanding of the anatomy of the brachial plexus and surrounding structures is required to use these techniques safely and effectively.

CLINICAL ANATOMY

The canine brachial plexus is formed by ventral branches of the sixth (C_6), seventh (C_7), and eighth (C_8) cervical spinal nerves, and the first thoracic (T_1) spinal nerve (**Figs. 1** and **2**).[7–9] Contributions from the fifth cervical (C_5) and the second thoracic (T_2) spinal nerves are small (<1 mm) or absent.[7,9] The phrenic nerve originates from ventral branches of C_5, C_6, and C_7, and runs medial to the brachial plexus before entering the thoracic inlet ventral to the subclavian artery.

Several major vessels are close to the cervical spinal nerves that form the brachial plexus (**Figs. 3** and **4**). The vertebral artery runs medial to the ventral branches of C_6, C_7, and C_8 as they emerge from their respective intervertebral foramina. The costocervical artery runs next to the ventral branch of T_1 as it emerges from the intervertebral foramen and wraps around the medial surface of the first rib. The vertebral ganglion is located within the thoracic inlet near the origin of the vertebral artery and provides most, if not all, of the postganglionic sympathetic innervation to the heart.[10]

Innervation to the shoulder and brachium is supplied by C_6, C_7, and C_8, and innervation to the elbow and antebrachium is supplied by C_7, C_8, and T_1. Consequently, neural blockade of the ventral branches of C_6, C_7, and C_8 is sufficient for surgical procedures of the shoulder and brachium. The suprascapular nerve arises primarily from C_6 and provides sensory innervation to the lateral aspect of the shoulder joint capsule and motor innervation to the supraspinatus and infraspinatus muscles. The subscapular nerve arises from C_6 and C_7 and provides motor innervation to the subscapular muscle. The musculocutaneous nerve arises primarily from C_7 and provides sensory innervation to the craniomedial aspect of the antebrachium (medial cutaneous antebrachial nerve) and motor innervation to the coracobrachialis, biceps brachii, and brachialis muscles. The axillary nerve arises from C_7 and C_8, and provides sensory innervation to the caudal aspect of the shoulder joint capsule and the lateral aspect of the brachium (lateral cutaneous brachial nerve). The axillary nerve also provides motor innervation to the subscapularis, teres major, teres minor, and deltoideus muscles. The radial nerve arises from C_7, C_8, and T_1 and provides sensory innervation to the lateral aspect of the elbow joint capsule and the craniolateral aspect of the

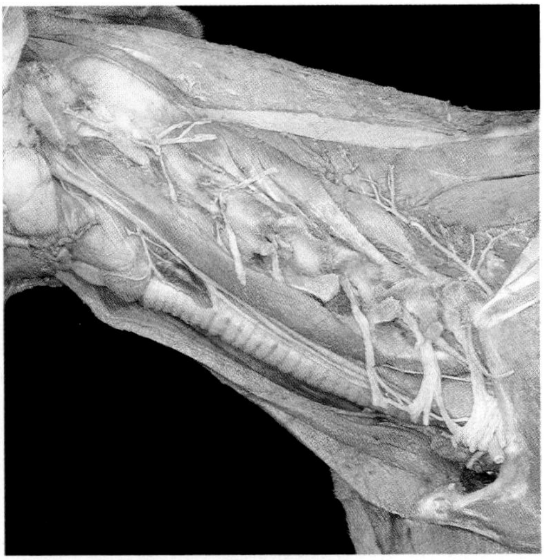

Fig. 1. Superficial dissection of the nerves of the canine brachial plexus (*lateral view*). Note the location of the large ventral wing of the transverse process of the sixth cervical vertebra, the head and costochondral junction of the first rib, and the axillary artery and vein. Ventral branches of the sixth and seventh cervical nerves can be blocked as they cross the cranial and caudal margins of the transverse process, respectively. Ventral branches of the eighth cervical nerve and the first thoracic nerve can be blocked as they cross the cranial and caudal margins of the head of the first rib, respectively. Alternately, ventral branches of the eighth cervical and first thoracic nerves can be blocked where they converge above the axillary artery along the cranial margin of the first rib. (*From* Done SH, Goody PC, Evans SA, et al. Color atlas of veterinary anatomy, the dog and cat. Vol 3. London: Elsevier; 1996. p. 3.14; with permission.)

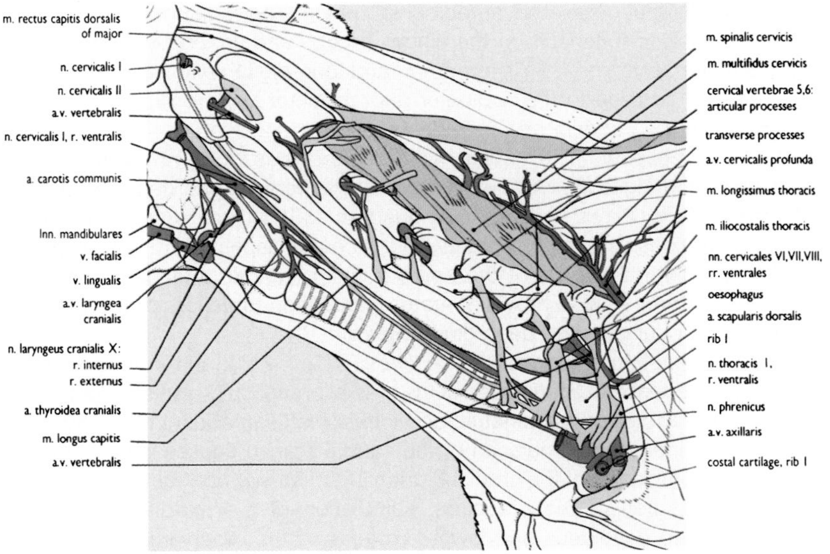

Fig. 2. Detailed legend for the superficial dissection of the nerves of the canine brachial plexus (*lateral view*). (*From* Done SH, Goody PC, Evans SA, et al. Color atlas of veterinary anatomy, the dog and cat. Vol 3. London: Elsevier; 1996. p. 3.14; with permission.)

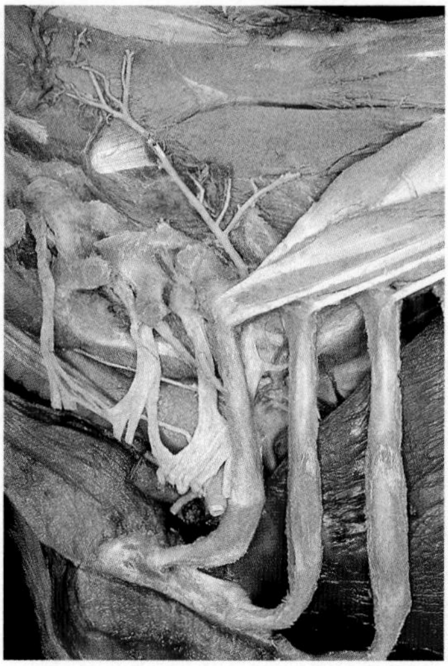

Fig. 3. Deep dissection of the nerves of the canine brachial plexus (*lateral view*). Note the location of the large ventral wing of the transverse process of the sixth cervical vertebra, the head and costochondral junction of the first rib, and the axillary artery and vein. Ventral branches of the sixth and seventh cervical nerves can be blocked as they cross the cranial and caudal margins of the transverse process, respectively. Ventral branches of the eighth cervical nerve and the first thoracic nerve can be blocked as they cross the cranial and caudal margins of the head of the first rib, respectively. Alternately, ventral branches of the eighth cervical and first thoracic nerves can be blocked where they converge above the axillary artery along the cranial margin of the first rib. (*From* Done SH, Goody PC, Evans SA, et al. Color atlas of veterinary anatomy, the dog and cat. Vol 3. London: Elsevier; 1996. p. 3.15; with permission.)

antebrachium (lateral cutaneous antebrachial nerve). The radial nerve also provides motor innervation to extensors of the elbow (triceps and anconeus) and the carpus and digits (extensor carpi radialis, common and long digital extensors, and extensor carpi ulnaris) in addition to the supinator and abductor pollicis longus. The median nerve arises from C_8 and T_1 and provides sensory innervation to the medial aspect of the elbow joint capsule. The median nerve also provides motor innervation to flexors of the carpus and digits (flexor carpi radialis and superficial and deep digital flexors) and to the pronator teres and pronator quadratus. The ulnar nerve arises from C_8 and T_1 and provides sensory innervation to the caudal aspect of the elbow joint capsule and caudolateral aspect of the antebrachium (caudal cutaneous antebrachial nerve). The ulnar nerve also provides motor innervation to flexors of the carpus and digits (flexor carpi ulnaris and deep digital flexor).

Electrical stimulation of the ventral branches of C_6, C_7, C_8, and T_1 induces characteristic motor responses.[7] Stimulation of the cranial branch of C_6 causes contraction of the brachiocephalicus, supraspinatus, and infraspinatus in addition to outward rotation of the shoulder, and stimulation of the caudal branch causes inward rotation of the shoulder. Stimulation of the cranial branch of C_7 causes contraction of the biceps and outward rotation of the brachium, stimulation of the middle branch causes contraction of the deltoideus and inward rotation of the brachium, and stimulation of the caudal branch causes contraction of the triceps and extension of the carpus. Stimulation of C_8 causes contraction of the triceps and extension of the elbow, carpus, and digits, and stimulation of T_1 causes flexion of the carpus and digits.

Fig. 4. Detailed legend for the deep dissection of the nerves of the canine brachial plexus (*lateral view*). (*From* Done SH, Goody PC, Evans SA, et al. Color atlas of veterinary anatomy, the dog and cat. Vol 3. London: Elsevier; 1996. p. 3.15; with permission.)

Electrical stimulation of more distal nerves of the brachial plexus also induces characteristic motor responses.[8] Stimulation of the suprascapular nerve (C_6) causes extension of the shoulder, and stimulation of the subscapular nerve (C_6 and C_7) causes inward rotation of the shoulder and abduction of the limb. Stimulation of the musculocutaneous nerve (C_7) causes flexion of the shoulder, elbow, and carpus. Stimulation of the axillary nerve (C_7 and C_8) causes flexion of the shoulder, abduction of the elbow, and inward rotation of the carpus. Stimulation of the radial nerve (C_7, C_8, and T_1) causes extension of the elbow, carpus, and digits in addition to splaying of the toes. Stimulation of the combined median-ulnar nerve trunk (C_8 and T_1) causes flexion of the elbow, carpus, and digits.

PARAVERTEBRAL TECHNIQUE

Indications

The paravertebral technique is used during the period around the time of surgery to provide analgesia and muscle relaxation for surgical procedures of the shoulder and brachium. The technique is relatively easy to perform provided that the anatomy of the brachial plexus is reviewed and that key anatomic landmarks are accurately identified. The technique is difficult to perform in obese dogs and in dogs with heavy cervical musculature, and it should not be performed if the transverse process of the sixth cervical vertebra and the head of the first rib cannot be identified.

Clinical Technique

The nerves of the brachial plexus can be successfully blocked in most patients by injecting 1–3 mL of 2% lidocaine or 0.5% bupivacaine using a 22-gauge (0.7-mm), 1-inch (25-mm), or 1.5-inch (38-mm) needle at each of the four sites (C_6, C_7, C_8,

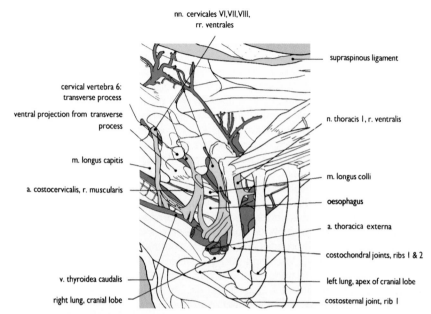

and T_1). Particular attention should be paid to the location of the jugular groove, thoracic inlet, and major vessels that are close to the nerves of the brachial plexus. Syringes should be aspirated before each injection to avoid inadvertent intravascular administration. Doses of local anesthetics should be calculated carefully for small patients, and the total dose (based on lean body weight) should not exceed 8 mg/kg of 2% lidocaine or 2 mg/kg of 0.5% bupivacaine. For dogs weighing less than 10 kg, the maximum total dose is divided by four to obtain the dose for injection at each site.

After clipping and aseptic preparation of the site, the scapula is shifted caudally to expose the transverse process of the sixth cervical vertebra and the head of the first rib (see **Figs. 1** and **2**). An index finger is placed on the large ventral wing of the transverse process, and the cranial and caudal margins of the process are isolated. Ventral branches of C_6 and C_7 are relatively superficial at this site (<2–3 cm under the skin) and are just dorsal to the cranial and caudal margins of the transverse process, respectively. Placement of an index finger on this key anatomic landmark also covers the jugular groove and prevents inadvertent injection of local anesthetic near the jugular vein, carotid artery, and vagosympathetic trunk. The needle is inserted dorsal to the cranial and caudal margins of the process and is directed medially. Local anesthetic (1–3 mL or less for dogs weighing less than 10 kg) is injected along the nerve above the dorsolateral surface of the transverse process at each site. Ventral branches of C_8 and T_1 are located dorsal to the cranial and caudal margins of the head of the first rib, respectively (see **Figs. 3** and **4**). Next, with the scapula still shifted caudally, the first rib is palpated medial to the cranial margin of the scapula. An index finger is placed just ventral to the head of the rib, and the cranial and caudal margins are isolated. Placement of an index finger on this key anatomic landmark also covers the thoracic inlet and prevents inadvertent injection of local anesthetic near major vessels and the vertebral ganglion or within the pleural space. The needle is inserted dorsal to the cranial and caudal margins and is directed medially. Local anesthetic (1–3 mL or less for dogs weighing less than 10 kg) is injected dorsal to the head of the rib at each site. Care should be taken to avoid intravascular injection.

Potential Complications

The phrenic nerve originates from ventral branches of C_5, C_6, and C_7, and runs medial to the brachial plexus (see **Figs. 1** and **2**). Blockade of the ventral branches of C_6 and C_7 or direct blockade of the phrenic nerve with local anesthetics can produce hemidiaphragmatic paresis. In human patients, a similar technique (interscalene block) consistently produces paralysis of the phrenic nerve and hemidiaphragmatic paresis, but adequate pulmonary function is maintained.[11,12] Similarly, unilateral or bilateral blockade of the phrenic nerve does not seem to compromise pulmonary function in conscious or anesthetized dogs.[13–16] Unilateral blockade of the brachial plexus should be avoided in patients that have compromised pulmonary function, however, and blockade of the brachial plexus should not be performed bilaterally. Accidental epidural or intrathecal administration is an unlikely but potential complication, and needles should be directed caudally to avoid insertion into intervertebral foramina. Inadvertent intravascular injection and direct nerve injury are also potential complications.

MODIFIED PARAVERTEBRAL TECHNIQUE

Indications

The modified paravertebral technique was also developed at the Atlantic Veterinary College and is used during the period around the time of surgery to provide analgesia and muscle relaxation for surgical procedures of the shoulder and brachium. The modified technique is easier to perform than the standard technique because the ventral branches of C_8 and T_1 are blocked at their junction on the cranial border of the first rib rather than dorsal to the head of the rib. This technique is also difficult to perform in obese dogs and in dogs with heavy cervical musculature and should not be performed if the transverse process of the sixth cervical vertebra and the first rib cannot be identified.

Clinical Technique

After clipping and aseptic preparation of the site, the scapula is shifted caudally and the transverse process of the sixth cervical vertebra is identified (see **Figs. 1** and **2**). The index finger is place on the transverse process, and the cranial and caudal margins of the process are identified. The ventral branches of C_6 and C_7 are blocked using the same approach as the standard technique. Next, with the scapula still shifted caudally, the axillary artery and the costochondral junction of the first rib are identified (see **Figs. 3** and **4**). The ventral branches of C_8 and T_1 converge 1 to 2 cm dorsal to the axillary artery and costochondral junction along the cranial margin of the first rib. Local anesthetic (1–3 mL or less in dogs weighing less than 10 kg) is injected along the cranial margin of the rib at one or two sites. Care should be taken to avoid intravascular injection and insertion of the needle into the thoracic inlet and pleural space.

Potential Complications

As with the standard technique, blockade of the phrenic nerve is a likely complication. Accidental epidural or intrathecal administration is an unlikely but potential complication, and needles should be directed caudally when blocking the ventral branches of C_6 and C_7 to avoid insertion into intervertebral foramina. Blockade of the ventral branches of C_8 and T_1 should be performed above the axillary artery along the cranial margin of the first rib. Needle placement within the thoracic inlet could result in pneumothorax, inadvertent intravascular injection, or blockade of the vertebral ganglion. Direct nerve injury is also a potential complication.

RADIAL, ULNAR, MEDIAN, AND MUSCULOCUTANEOUS NERVES TECHNIQUE

Indications

Complete neural blockade for surgical procedures of the elbow and antebrachium can be produced by blocking the radial, ulnar, median, and musculocutaneous (RUMM) nerves above the humeral epicondyles.[1] This technique is easier to perform than the axillary and paravertebral techniques, and the potential for complications is lower. The radial nerve is blocked above the lateral epicondyle of the humerus between the lateral head of the triceps and brachialis. The ulnar, median, and musculocutaneous nerves are blocked above the medial epicondyle of the humerus next to the brachial artery. The musculocutaneous nerve lies cranial to the brachial artery, and the median and ulnar nerves lie caudal to the artery.

Clinical Technique

The RUMM nerves can be successfully blocked in most patients by injecting 1–2 mL of 2% lidocaine or 0.5% bupivacaine using a 22-gauge (0.7-mm) 1-inch (25-mm) needle at each of the three sites (radial, ulnar-median, and musculocutaneous). Particular attention should be paid to the location of the brachial artery and vein along the medial surface of the humeral shaft. Aseptic technique should be used, and syringes should be aspirated before each injection to avoid inadvertent intravascular administration. Doses of local anesthetics should be calculated carefully for small patients, and the total dose (based on lean body weight) should not exceed 8 mg/kg of 2% lidocaine or 2 mg/kg of 0.5% bupivacaine. For dogs weighing less than 10 kg, the maximum total dose is divided by three to obtain the dose for injection at each site.

The radial nerve can be palpated above the lateral epicondyle of the humerus between the brachialis and lateral head of the triceps. The needle is inserted proximal to the lateral epicondyle, and local anesthetic (1–2 mL) is injected along the nerve. The musculocutaneous nerve is cranial to the brachial artery, and the median and ulnar nerves are caudal to the artery. The needle is inserted proximal to the medial epicondyle over the brachial artery, and local anesthetic (1–2 mL) is injected along the cranial and caudal margins of the artery. Care should be taken to avoid intravascular injection.

Potential Complications

This technique is easier to perform than the standard and modified paravertebral techniques, and the potential for complications is lower. Inadvertent intravascular injection and direct nerve injury are potential complications.

ELECTRICAL NERVE LOCATORS

Successful neural blockade of the forelimb depends on precise localization of the ventral branches of C_6, C_7, C_8, and T_1 or more distal nerves of the brachial plexus. The location of superficial nerves can be determined by direct palpation, whereas deeper nerves require identification of distinct landmarks and an intimate knowledge of regional anatomy. Electrical nerve locators (ENLs) are used routinely to facilitate neural blockade of the brachial plexus in human patients.[17–19] These devices can also be used to facilitate neural blockade of the brachial plexus in dogs using the standard or modified paravertebral technique, and they can also be used to localize and block more distal nerves of the brachial plexus (RUMM technique). Anatomic landmarks are often obscured in obese and heavily muscled dogs, and ENLs can be used in these patients to localize the nerves of the brachial plexus. Clinical use of ENLs facilitates correct needle placement and may shorten onset time, prolong duration of action, and reduce the risk for nerve injury. These devices are also excellent educational tools for professional students and for practicing veterinarians.

Most ENLs consist of a constant-current generator that is connected to an insulated needle and a remote electrode that is attached to the skin (**Fig. 5**). A 22-gauge (0.7-mm), 1.5-inch (38-mm) pinpoint-tip insulated needle is appropriate for neural blockade of the forelimb in most dogs (**Fig. 6**). When the insulated needle penetrates the skin, the circuit is closed and a constant current stimulus is delivered at a frequency of 1 or 2 Hz and for a duration of 0.1 to 0.2 milliseconds. Resistance varies with tissue impedance and the position of the remote electrode and ranges from 0.5 to 3.0 kΩ. Consequently, the current generator must vary the voltage according to Ohm's law ($I = V/R$; I, current; V, voltage; R, resistance) to maintain a constant stimulus strength. Some models include a percutaneous electrode that allows transcutaneous stimulation and localization of nerves before needle placement (**Fig. 7**). The resistance between the percutaneous electrode and the remote electrode is approximately 25 kΩ, and a proportionally higher current (10 mA) and stimulus duration (0.5 ms) are required to depolarize adjacent nerve fibers.

The current required to depolarize motor nerve fibers varies with the distance of the needle tip from the fiber (r) according to Coulomb's law [$E = K(Q/r^2)$; E, threshold current required; K, constant; Q, minimal current]. As the needle tip approaches the nerve, less current is required to depolarize the nerve fibers and produce a motor response. Clinical use of ENLs can be divided into a search phase, an approach phase,

An Update on Nonsteroidal Anti-Inflammatory Drugs (NSAIDs) in Small Animals

Mark G. Papich, DVM, MS

KEYWORDS

- NSAIDs • Anti-inflammatory drugs • Analgesic drugs
- Dogs • Cats • Pain • Arthritis • COX-1

There are several nonsteroidal anti-inflammatory drugs (NSAIDs) to choose from (**Box 1**). The pharmacologic activity of the NSAIDs has been reviewed in other articles, textbooks, popular journals, and promotional material distributed by drug sponsors. It is not necessary to review in-depth information on chemistry, mechanism of action, history, discovery, or pharmacokinetics of these drugs, because that information has been described previously. The clinical use and dosages of these drugs are provided in a recent book by the author,[1] and this topic was last reviewed by this author in 2000.[1,2] A description of the chemistry, mechanism of action, and clinical use of the cyclooxygenase-2 inhibiting (COXIB) class of NSAIDs was provided in a thorough review.[3] Pharmacokinetics and pharmacodynamics of NSAIDs were reviewed extensively by Lees and colleagues.[4] Guidelines for clinical use in dogs[5] and cats[6] was recently provided in excellent reviews. This article primarily reviews developments that were not available at the time of this author's previous review in 2000 and discusses issues for which updates are necessary.

MECHANISM OF ACTION

The review articles by experts in this area are sufficient to describe the basic pharmacology and mechanism of action of these drugs.[7,8] The most significant development in our understanding of NSAIDs occurred in the early 1990s with a revision in the understanding of the targets of these drugs. At that time, it was discovered that there are two isoenzymes (isoforms) of cyclooxygenase (prostaglandin synthase) that are responsible for synthesis of prostaglandins. Prostaglandin synthase-1 (COX-1) is

Department of Molecular Biomedical Sciences, North Carolina State University College of Veterinary Medicine, 4700 Hillsborough Street, Raleigh, NC 27606, USA
E-mail address: mark_papich@ncsu.edu

Vet Clin Small Anim 38 (2008) 1243–1266
doi:10.1016/j.cvsm.2008.09.002 **vetsmall.theclinics.com**
0195-5616/08/$ – see front matter

Box 1
Currently available nonsteroidal anti-inflammatory drugs for dogs

Aspirin[a]

Phenylbutazone[b]

Carprofen (Rimadyl, and generic)[f]

Etodolac (EtoGesic)

Meloxicam (Metacam)[c,f,1]

Ketoprofen (Anafen)[d,4]

Deracoxib (Deramaxx)

Firocoxib (Previcox)

Meclofenamic acid (Arquel)[e,11]

Tepoxalin (Zubrin)

Tolfenamic acid (Tolfedine)[d,f]

[a] Aspirin is not US Food and Drug Administration (FDA)–registered for dogs, but some forms are marketed for dogs as if there were FDA approval. There is an approved combination with methylprednisolone (Cortaba tablets, 0.5 mg of methylprednisolone and 300 mg of aspirin).
[b] Registered for dogs but not actively marketed.
[c] Registered for cats also as a single dose.
[d] Registered in Canada only.
[e] Registered but not marketed.
[f] Also available as an injectable and oral; the others are all available in oral forms.

usually a constitutive enzyme expressed in tissues.[9] Prostaglandins, prostacyclin, and thromboxane synthesized by this enzyme are responsible for normal physiologic functions. Prostaglandin synthase-2 (COX-2), on the other hand, is inducible and synthesized by macrophages and inflammatory cells after stimulation by cytokines and other mediators of inflammation. In some tissues, COX-2 may be constitutive. For example, COX-2 production of prostaglandins was found to be constitutive in canine pyloric and duodenal mucosa,[10] even though it previously was believed to be induced only in the presence of injury or inflammation. COX-2 may be up-regulated in these tissues, responding to inflammatory stimuli to produce a protective and healing role.[11] There is evidence, confirmed in two independent studies,[10,12] that prostaglandin synthesis is inherently higher in gastric mucosa than duodenal mucosa. This suggests that, in the duodenum, there may be a greater requirement for induction of COX-2, and that there is a protective mechanism to emerge in the duodenum rather than in the stomach. The perception that COX-2 is a bad enzyme and COX-1 is a good enzyme is probably overly simplistic because we now understand that there is some overlap in the functions of these isoforms.[13] Nevertheless, the target of most of the most recently developed NSAIDs has been COX-2—or to spare COX-1 as much as possible—with the goal of producing analgesia and suppressing inflammation without inhibiting physiologically important prostanoids.

Selectivity of COX-2 versus COX-1 is often expressed as the COX-1/COX-2 inhibitory ratio. This ratio is derived from an in vivo study in which the inhibitory effect, usually expressed as the inhibitory concentration to inhibit 50% of activity (IC_{50}), is measured from stimulating cells that are capable of expressing products of these enzymes. In the whole blood assay, the source for COX-1 products (thromboxane or TXA_2) is platelets, and the source of COX-2 products (PGE_2) is leukocytes. The ratio is expressed as COX-1 [IC_{50}]/COX-2 [IC_{50}], or simply COX-1/COX-2. The higher the value above 1.0, the more specific the drug is for COX-2 compared with COX-1. There is subjective value placed on the magnitude of the ratio to consider the drug as "COX-1 sparing," "COX-2 specific," "COX-2 preferential," or "COX-2 selective." These terms have been used by many authors without any true definition of the magnitude of the ratio used to determine the criteria for each term.

Is there a COX-3?

After the discovery of COX-1 and -2, interest emerged of the presence of yet another isozyme, the COX-3 enzyme. Interest in COX-3 began after a discovery, in dog tissues, that there was a central cyclooxygenase that was inhibited by acetaminophen.[14] This substance was called COX-3. It is believed now that COX-3 is a variant of COX-1, rather than a distinct isomer.[15,16] The term "COX-3" has even been rejected by some authors.[17] This variant of the COX enzyme was selectively inhibited by acetaminophen in dogs[15] and this inhibition may represent a target for a central mechanism for some NSAIDs, including acetaminophen and dipyrone. As proposed by Chandrasekharan and colleagues,[15] other NSAIDs that produce analgesia, but are not selective for COX-2, perhaps have a central mechanism of action targeting COX-3. Despite the initial interest in COX-3, this enzyme may be more prominent in dogs than in people or laboratory rodents.[17] Subsequently, there has been little focus on inhibition of this enzyme in the human literature and some of the initial enthusiasm about COX-3 has waned. (See the review by Kis and colleagues[18] for a more in-depth treatment of this topic.) Nevertheless, there is evidence to suggest that an enzyme exists centrally in dogs, at levels that are distinct from humans and laboratory animals, that may be a central target for some NSAIDs. It may be worthwhile to consider this method of treatment in dogs for some types of pain (see later discussion).

Inconsistencies Among the Studies

When one examines the drugs registered for veterinary medicine, there is disagreement in the literature with respect to the selectivity for the COX-1 versus COX-2 enzyme (**Table 1**). For example, deracoxib is considered a highly selective COX-2

Table 1
COX-1/COX-2 inhibitory ratios based on IC_{50} values in dogs

Drug	Streppa et al 2002[a]	Ricketts et al 1998[21,a]	Kay-Mugford et al 2000[22,a]	Cryer et al 1998[b]	Brideau et al 2001[b]	Wilson et al 2004[23,b]	Gierse et al 2002[19,c]
Ketoprofen	0.17	0.23	0.36	0.125	0.6	0.5	—
Aspirin	0.39	<0.3	—	0.32	—	0.37	—
Etodolac	0.53	0.52	—	7.92	—	6.3	3.4
Ibuprofen	0.74	—	—	0.6	—	—	—
Piroxicam	2	—	—	1.27	—	1.75	—
Meloxicam	2.72	2.9	12.3	—	10	—	—
Meclofenamic acid	5	15.4	—	12.1	—	5	—
Phenylbutazone	9.7	>2.6	—	—	0.6	—	—
Carprofen	16.8	129	1.75	—	6.5	5.3	65
Deracoxib	—	—	—	—	—	—	1275

[a] Assay with canine cell lines.
[b] Assay with human cell lines.
[c] Assay with purified enzymes.

inhibitor based on an assay performed in purified enzymes.[19] In this study, the COX-1/COX-2 ratio was 1275, much higher than other drugs tested. But when tested in canine whole blood and compared with other NSAIDs, deracoxib had a ratio of only 12. In this study, carprofen had a ratio of 6 to 7, and firocoxib (the newest NSAID for dogs) had a ratio of 384 to 427.[20]

Some of the confusion regarding understanding the action of the veterinary NSAIDs is that in vitro studies to examine their relative effects on COX-1 versus COX-2 have varied in their techniques and the cell system used. For example, in a study using canine enzyme systems, carprofen had a COX-1/COX-2 ratio of 129.[21] In another study, using cell lines of another species (sheep and rodent) the ratio was 1.0,[7] and in a study using canine macrophages, the ratio was 1.75.[22] Yet another study on carprofen showed a ratio of 5.3 and that it was 1000 times less potent in whole blood than in cell culture.[23] This emphasizes the effect of protein binding on in vitro assays (see later discussion). An in vivo study with carprofen in dogs did not demonstrate that it was capable of inhibiting prostaglandins systemically in dogs.[24]

Carprofen is not the only drug for which conflicting results have been reported. The ratios for etodolac, another NSAID approved for dogs, has a COX-1/COX-2 ratio of 8.1 in humans, but 0.52 to 0.53 in dogs. Another study with etodolac showed that the selectivity for COX-2 was 10 times greater in people than dogs.[19,25] Dr. Vane, a preeminent expert on COX inhibition, concludes that the inhibitory activity of a drug for COX-1 to its inhibitory activity for COX-2 can vary according to whether tests are done on pure enzymes, cell homogenates, or intact cells, or with the types of cells used.[7] According to Dr. Lees, one of the leading investigators of NSAIDs in veterinary medicine, there are several unexplored questions to be answered for veterinary drugs.[26]

What is the Best Assay?

In view of the discrepancies among studies and techniques, it is now generally accepted that the whole-blood assay should be the gold standard for determining COX-1/COX-2 specificity. The first evidence of this technique was published in 1992[27] and it is now used in most of the veterinary drug studies. The advantage of the whole-blood assay is that it incorporates the components into the assay that normally occur in circulating blood: proteins, cells, platelets, and circulating enzymes. These components are not present in isolated cells or enzyme systems used for some earlier assays.

Because the NSAIDs are highly protein bound, this is particularly important because only a small fraction—the unbound fraction—is biologically active in the blood. The whole-blood assay measures COX-2 products (PGE_2) from stimulated leukocytes, and COX-1 products (TXA_2) from stimulated platelets.

Taking the whole-blood assay one step further is to perform an ex vivo assay in which blood samples are collected after administration of the NSAID. This assay is perhaps more clinically relevant than the in vitro assay because it accounts for differences in metabolism among the drugs, pharmacokinetic variations, and the potential presence of active metabolites.[28,29] The ex vivo assay allows the investigator to study the time course of prostaglandin inhibition (duration of effect) and may be more relevant to predict clinical and adverse effects of NSAIDs.[29]

Pharmacokinetic-pharmacodynamic modeling

There has been tremendous interest in combining the pharmacodynamic studies that measure COX-1 and COX-2 inhibitory concentrations with the pharmacokinetics of the drug to derive the clinically optimal and safe doses for animals. Pharmacokinetics and pharmacodynamics (PK-PD) can be useful for preclinical evaluation to select the most appropriate dose to use in further studies. These approaches were described in an excellent review by Lees and colleagues,[4,30] and demonstrated for specific drugs in studies by Giraudel and colleagues.[31,32] The approach by these investigators is to use a blood concentration corresponding to 80% inhibition of COX-2 (IC_{80}) to produce a therapeutic effect, and only 20% inhibition of COX-1 (IC_{20}) to avoid adverse effects. As reviewed by Hinz and Brune[29] 80% COX-2 inhibition to predict clinical effects also has been supported by other studies. A drug concentration producing 50% inhibition may not be enough to produce a therapeutic effect and an inhibitory concentration of 80% may be more realistic.

Using these inhibitory concentration values as targets, PK-PD mathematical modeling can be performed by taking into consideration the corresponding pharmacokinetics of the drug (plasma clearance). Safe and effective doses can be derived to attain these blood concentration targets. The calculations and descriptions of the model are beyond this article but are well described in the citations above. In a PK-PD modeling approach using these techniques, the investigators determined a dose of meloxicam of 0.17 mg/kg every 24 hours in cats.[32] At this dose inhibition of COX-1 actually exceeded 20%.[32] This dose is below the US Food and Drug Administration (FDA)–registered single dose for cats, but higher than the chronic dose registered in Europe (doses of meloxicam are discussed later in the section on cats). The PK-PD approach suggested that meloxicam is safe for a single dose of 0.3 mg/kg, despite high COX-1 inhibition, but for chronic treatment lower doses are necessary to minimally inhibit COX-1. This agrees with the clinical experience with meloxicam in cats.

Rather than using an in vitro assay, such as the whole-blood assay, to measure cyclooxygenase inhibition as the pharmacodynamic surrogate marker for efficacy, another approach is to use an in vivo measure. An in vivo measure is more likely to reflect physiologic and pathologic conditions and predict clinical outcome. Several in vivo models have been used to test NSAIDs in animals. These are described in more detail by Lees and colleagues.[30] An in vivo model may involve inducing inflammation in a tissue cage and measuring the inhibition of inflammation in response to the drug concentration. It may use an injection of an irritant in a joint and observing the response by measuring the degree of lameness produced, heat, and pain. Injections of an irritant (kaolin) have been administered to cats to measure inflammatory pain and heat. Values such as 50% inhibitory concentration (IC_{50}) can be calculated from the in vivo model, as for the in vitro model.

Using this approach, induced inflammation in cats was used for PK-PD modeling of meloxicam.[31] These investigators calculated a single dose of 0.25 to 0.3 mg/kg of meloxicam to produce optimum analgesic, anti-inflammatory, and antipyretic effects. This dose agrees with the dose derived from clinical trials that led to the current FDA-registered dose for cats.

Do in vitro Tests Predict in vivo Performance?

Whether or not in vitro measurements of COX-1 versus COX-2 inhibition predict in vivo response and safety has been debated. PK-PD approaches to dose determination may not always agree with results from clinical trials. Deviations from clinically-derived doses are attributed to effects of NSAIDs that may not directly correlate with blood concentrations. As the authors of the studies cited above explained,[4,30–32] participation of other mechanisms of action in the anti-inflammatory effects of NSAIDs may explain deviations from these models, along with the accumulation of the active compound in the target cells or biotransformation leading to active metabolites. These effects cannot be measured with in vitro whole-blood assays alone. For example, although carprofen etodolac and meloxicam all have been shown to inhibit COX-2 with different magnitudes of COX-1/COX-2 ratios and meloxicam generally being more selective, carprofen and etodolac were equally effective for reducing pain scores in experimentally treated dogs[33] but were more effective than meloxicam. Likewise, according to safety studies available from the drug sponsor, firocoxib, carprofen, and etodolac all were similar with respect to incidence of gastrointestinal adverse effects in dogs, even though they vary widely in the COX1/COX-2 ratios, with deracoxib being the most COX-2 specific.

Many in vitro studies have agreed qualitatively with results from in vivo assays. When effects of meloxicam were compared with aspirin in dogs, meloxicam, which is a somewhat selective COX-2 inhibitor using a whole-blood assay, also had a sparing effect on gastrointestinal prostaglandins (COX-1 mediated) compared with aspirin.[34] Meloxicam also was a potent inhibitor of lipopolysaccharide-induced prostaglandin synthesis (COX-2 mediated). These findings are consistent with COX-2 inhibition and COX-1–sparing effects of meloxicam, but demonstrate the lack of such specificity for aspirin. In a follow-up study by the same laboratory they compared carprofen, deracoxib, and etodolac.[35] All three drugs failed to inhibit prostaglandins in the stomach mucosa, and thromboxane in platelets, consistent with a COX-1–sparing effect. All three drugs produced the same degree of COX-1 sparing, despite a wide range in COX-1/COX-2 inhibitory ratios among these drugs. In the same study, etodolac did not suppress the COX-2–mediated product, PGE_2, in a blood assay compared with carprofen and deracoxib on days 3 and 10 of treatment. Carprofen and deracoxib did not differ in their in vivo effects on either COX-1 or COX-2 inhibition, despite large differences for in vitro COX-1/COX-2 ratios. In a more recent study, the same laboratory showed that firocoxib and meloxicam, both of which have a preference for COX-2 but have widely different COX-1/COX-2 ratios, were similar in their ability to suppress COX-2–mediated prostaglandins in whole blood and sparing COX-1–mediated prostaglandins in gastric mucosa.[12] These results suggest that the in vitro assays may be helpful for demonstrating qualitative differences among the NSAIDs, but do not provide a quantitative measure of difference in efficacy or safety.

Is Prostaglandin Inhibition all there is?

Although we assume that prostaglandin inhibition is the most important mechanism of action for most NSAIDs, there may be other mechanisms, some not fully understood, that also may explain the actions of these drugs. For example, some NSAIDs, including salicylates, may inhibit nuclear factor kappa-B (NF-κB). NF-κB is an important promoter for inflammatory mediators.

Carprofen seems to be a COX-1–sparing drug,[25] but there is not agreement among investigators on whether it also inhibits COX-2 in vivo. Although there is evidence for inhibitory effects on the enzyme cyclooxygenase in some models, carprofen did not show an in vivo anti-prostaglandin effect in dogs,[24] which may explain the low rate of gastrointestinal adverse effects at approved doses. In one study, the investigators were unable to show that carprofen inhibited either COX-1 or COX-2,[36] suggesting either a central mechanism of action or activity on other pathways.

IS THERE REALLY AN ADVANTAGE FOR COX-2 INHIBITORS?

After the discovery of two isoenzymes, COX-1 and -2, there was a focus in drug development toward developing highly selective COX-2 inhibitors. Drugs that emerged from this work were celecoxib (Celebrex), valdecoxib (Bextra, now discontinued), and rofecoxib (Vioxx, now discontinued).[37] These are often referred to as the

COXIBs and they were among the top-selling prescription drugs of any category in human medicine. The removal of rofecoxib and valdecoxib from the human market has been well chronicled in the human literature and is discussed later. The background and pharmacology of the COXIBs was reviewed thoroughly by Bergh and Budsberg.[3]

Deracoxib was the first veterinary drug in this group; the next one approved was firocoxib (Previcox). Both are licensed for dogs to treat pain associated with osteoarthritis. Other COX-2–specific drugs may follow in veterinary medicine. Based on in vitro tests in one study, firocoxib is more specific for COX-2 than deracoxib, with a COX-1/COX-2 ratio of 384 to 427 compared with deracoxib with a ratio of 12.[38] In efficacy studies, firocoxib was compared with etodolac and carprofen and was shown in some measurements to have better improvement in lameness scores. Although studies that have performed safety assessment comparisons among drugs have been scarce and of low statistical power, firocoxib, carprofen, and etodolac all were similar with respect to incidence of vomiting and anorexia in dogs. There was a lower incidence of diarrhea with firocoxib compared with carprofen and etodolac and less melena compared with etodolac (data available from drug sponsor).

Evaluations of the COXIBs in people have shown that they are not necessarily more effective than older drugs, but they may be safer for the gastrointestinal tract[39] during short-term evaluations. In veterinary studies, there is no convincing evidence that drugs with higher COX-1/COX-2 ratios produce fewer gastrointestinal or renal adverse effects than drugs with low ratios. One of the veterinary drugs with selective COX-2 inhibitory action, deracoxib, was shown to be safe in studies performed by the manufacturer.[3] In 2005, however, investigators from North Carolina State University reported on 29 cases of gastrointestinal perforation and bleeding in association with deracoxib use in dogs.[40] Most occurred in the duodenum near the pyloric junction. Some of these animals may have had predisposing factors that contributed to the gastrointestinal perforations (for example, high dose or concurrent corticosteroid administration).

The adverse reactions from the COXIBs in people have resulted in removal of some from the market. Thousands of lawsuits against the drug sponsor are still being settled in the courts. The studies that originally demonstrated safety and led to initial FDA approval in people have been criticized.[41–43] Some reviews have pointed out that these selective COX-2 inhibitors may have been no better for long-term therapy than older established drugs, many with mixed COX-1/COX-2 inhibition in gastrointestinal safety and efficacy.[44,45] Some skeptics have proposed that selective COX-2 inhibitors may not be appropriate for all patients because COX-2 enzyme products may be involved in actions other than inflammation. For example, COX-2 products may be biologically important for angiogenesis, renal function, regulation of bone resorption, reproductive function, and healing of gastroduodenal ulcers.[46]

The safety concern in people from COX-2 selective drugs is a higher risk for cardiovascular problems because they preserve COX-1, which may promote platelet aggregation and vasoconstriction.[47] This cardiovascular risk is why the popular drug rofecoxib (Vioxx) was voluntarily taken off the market, soon followed by valdecoxib (Bextra). Some experts believe that the high COX-2 selectivity of this drug led to this increased risk.[48,49] There have been serious concerns expressed about the events that led up this withdrawal and whether or not the public was aware of the safety concerns. Editorials in major journals[41,43] suggested that the drug review process was inadequate for these drugs and we anticipate closer scrutiny of highly selective COX-2 human drugs in the future.[50,51]

DUAL INHIBITORS

There have been older drugs promoted to be dual inhibitors of arachidonic acid metabolites, but none were commercially successful. Dual inhibitor drugs effectively inhibit both cyclooxygenase (COX) and lipoxygenase (LOX). Therefore, they inhibit synthesis of inflammatory prostaglandins (PG) and leukotrienes (LT). Interest in a dual inhibitor has focused on the potential benefits in inhibiting LOX, which may include higher gastrointestinal safety and greater analgesic efficacy.[52] Lipoxygenase metabolites are involved in hyperalgesia and inflammatory responses.[13] Older drugs believed to have dual inhibitor capability were benoxaprofen and ketoprofen. Benoxaprofen was taken off the market, and the evidence for ketoprofen acting as a dual inhibitor is weak. A new drug being evaluated in people and dogs is licofelone, which is a true dual inhibitor, but it is not yet on the market. Licofelone may have greater gastrointestinal safety than other NSAIDs.[53]

Corticosteroids have been shown to be dual inhibitors in some studies because they inhibit phospholipase A_2, the enzyme that forms arachidonic acid from cell membranes. Corticosteroid inhibition of both LT and PG by way of this mechanism may not be clinically relevant, however. There is evidence that corticosteroids block COX-2 gene expression resulting in inhibition of synthesis of COX-2, which may be responsible for some anti-inflammatory effects. By inhibition of COX-2 in the gastrointestinal tract during conditions in which COX-2 products are needed for healing and repair, corticosteroids may exacerbate or produce injury to the gastrointestinal mucosa.[11,54,55]

The only drug approved in Europe and the United States that acts as a dual inhibitor in animals is tepoxalin (Zubrin). The metabolite is active, but only acts as a COX inhibitor. The COX inhibitor functions are more specific for COX-1 than COX-2, although this was not a canine-specific assay (data from Schering-Plough). In vivo and in vitro studies in dogs administered tepoxalin showed that it inhibited COX-1– and COX-2–mediated prostaglandins in blood and gastroduodenal mucosa, but it also inhibited LOX activity, consistent with its proposed mechanism of action.[12,56]

Despite being a nonselective COX inhibitor (primarily COX-1 using in vitro assays), tepoxalin has a gastrointestinal safety profile that matches other more selective COX-2 inhibitors. Tepoxalin has been effective in dogs that have osteoarthritis and showed gastrointestinal safety at several times the label dose. A question remaining about tepoxalin is the duration of the LOX inhibitory effect. The half-life for the LOX inhibitor parent drug is much shorter than the metabolite, which has little LOX inhibition (**Table 2**). The other question remaining to be answered for tepoxalin is the contribution of anti-LOX action on the overall therapeutic effect. Studies in osteoarthritis in dogs (the registered indication for tepoxalin) have not revealed whether it is the COX or the LOX inhibition (or possibly some other mechanism) that is responsible for a favorable clinical effect. Whether the dual inhibition action of tepoxalin will be effective for other inflammatory diseases (eg, respiratory disease, dermatitis) has not been reported.

IS IT TIME TO RECONSIDER ACETAMINOPHEN?

Veterinarians have been reluctant to consider acetaminophen treatment in animals because of its well-known toxicity in cats.[57] It should not be prescribed to cats under any circumstances—but what about dogs? Acetaminophen has been safe in dogs, even when administered at high doses. Although it produces analgesic effects, it does not produce anti-inflammatory effects at clinically relevant doses.[58–60] A study in a canine surgery model that demonstrated anti-inflammatory effects used doses that are higher than recommended clinically.[59] Acetaminophen has not produced

Table 2
Pharmacokinetic data for nonsteroidal anti-inflammatory drugs at the dosages tested in dogs

Drug	Half-Life in Dogs	Test Dose
Aspirin	8 h	10–20 mg/kg q8–12 h, oral
Carprofen	8 h (range 4.5–10)	4.4 mg/kg q24 h, or 2.2 mg/kg q12 h, oral
Deracoxib	3 h at 2–3 mg/kg;19 h at 20 mg/kg	3–4 mg/kg q24 h, oral
Etodolac	7.7 h fasted; 12 h nonfasted	10–15 mg/kg q24 h, oral
Flunixin	3.7 h	1 g/kg, oral or IM, once
Meloxicam	12–36 h	0.2 mg/kg initial, then 0.1 mg/kg q24 h, oral
Naproxen	74 h	5 mg/kg initial, then 2 mg/kg q48 h, oral
Phenylbutazone	6 h	15–22 mg/kg q12 h, oral
Piroxicam	40 h	0.3 mg/kg, q24 h, or q48 h, oral
Tepoxalin	1.6 h parent drug; 13 h for active metabolite	20 mg/kg initial; then 10 mg/kg q24 h, oral
Firocoxib	7.8 h	5 mg/kg q24 h, oral

renal or gastric injury in dogs when prescribed at commonly recommended doses for dogs (15 mg/kg orally, every 8 to 12 hours). Evidence of toxicity was not observed in dogs until doses of 100 mg/kg were exceeded.[61] It has been administered to dogs anecdotally, when other alternatives either are contraindicated or have caused adverse effects. It has been administered to dogs in combination with codeine, oxycodone (Percocet), and hydrocodone (Vicodin), despite a lack of clinical studies on the effectiveness of these preparations. Clinical-effectiveness seems to be mostly anecdotal.

More recent investigations reveal that acetaminophen actually is a COX inhibitor, but acts in cells in which low concentrations of arachidonic acid are present.[17] There is evidence that the site of acetaminophen action is the peroxidase enzyme component of prostaglandin H_2 synthase.[17] (Prostaglandin H_2 synthase consists of the peroxidase and cyclooxygenase portions, but it has collectively been referred to as "COX" in most recent studies.) The target for traditional NSAIDs is the cyclooxygenase portion of prostaglandin H_2 synthase. As reviewed by Davies and colleagues,[16] the COX inhibition probably occurs at site-specific tissues, sparing the gastrointestinal mucosa, platelets, and kidneys, but acting centrally. There also is evidence that it is a selective COX-2 inhibitor in selected tissues.[62]

Other supporting evidence for acetaminophen is that it seems to inhibit the COX-1 variant that was referred to as COX-3 earlier in this article.[15] The action is more prominent in dogs than in any other species and acts centrally, without affecting prostaglandin synthesis at other sites in the body that could potentially lead to adverse effects (for example, kidney and gastrointestinal mucosa). Other selected NSAIDs (dipyrone, phenacetin) also seem to inhibit COX-3. Because COX-3 may have a centrally mediated effect to produce analgesia and pyrexia, particularly dogs in which it was first discovered, perhaps acetaminophen has a role in treatment of some types of pain when other traditional NSAIDs are not appropriate.

In review articles, other authors have not supported this mechanism for the action of acetaminophen.[18,19,29] Other proposed mechanisms of action for acetaminophen involve pathways that may also be affected by other drug categories. Descending inhibitory pain pathways are mediated by serotonin (5-HT_3). Acetaminophen can stimulate the inhibitory pain pathway mediated by serotonin, and this can be blocked by serotonin antagonists.[63] This evidence suggests that acetaminophen may directly activate serotonin receptors. Other drugs that have been used to treat pain in animals—tricyclic antidepressants (eg, amitriptyline) and selective serotonin reuptake inhibitors (eg, fluoxetine)—modulate serotonin activity by inhibiting the reuptake of serotonin at the synapse. These drugs also have been used in some pain syndromes. One of the enantiomers of tramadol, a widely used analgesic in people and animals, also affects serotonin systems. Although it is appealing to consider studies in which acetaminophen could be combined with these agents to treat pain in animals, there are no such reports available in animals. Clearly, there is a risk of combining drugs that act on the serotonergic system without understanding the implications. Other drugs used in veterinary medicine that affect serotonin systems include serotonin-reuptake inhibitors, tricyclic antidepressants, and selegiline. On the other hand, some antiemetic drugs (eg, ondansetron) compete with serotonin receptors. The benefits and risks of adding another drug to a patient already receiving any of these other drugs would have to be weighed.

PHARMACOKINETIC FEATURES

For most of the NSAIDs there are adequate pharmacokinetic data for dogs, and some for cats, available in the reviews cited previously. Most of the traditional drugs in this group are weak acids that are highly protein bound and most of them have a small volume of distribution (some new drugs are an exception to this standard). These drugs are excreted at varying rates, depending on the metabolic pathway and extent of enterohepatic circulation. There are tremendous species differences in drug elimination among the NSAIDs. For some drugs the enterohepatic cycling may increase the risk for toxicosis because the local effects of the drug may be focused on the intestinal mucosa through repeated cycling in the biliary system.

Although the drug distribution, half-life, and clearance have been characterized for most NSAIDs used in animals, this information has not always been of use for predicting safe and effective dosage regimens. For example, NSAIDs such as ibuprofen and indomethacin easily cause toxicity in dogs even though they have short half-lives. On the other hand, naproxen and piroxicam have long half-lives of 74 hours and 40 hours, respectively, but have been used safely when dosed carefully. Among the small animal NSAIDs, half-lives do not correlate with the frequency of administration. Most currently used NSAIDs are given once a day, but half-lives vary widely (see **Table 2**).

As reviewed by Lees and colleagues,[4] an important feature of the NSAID pharmacokinetics is that anti-inflammatory and analgesic effects persist longer than the plasma half-lives would predict. In dogs, several NSAIDs have half-lives of 24 hours or less, (aspirin and carprofen, 8 hours; phenylbutazone, 6 hours; flunixin, 3.7 hours; meloxicam, 10–24 hours; etodolac, 8–12 hours), but have been administered once every 24 hours with effective results.[64] One explanation for the long duration of effect is the high protein binding. The tissue protein binding (for example the protein in an inflamed site) may serve as a reservoir for the drug after it has been eliminated from the plasma. The NSAID may thus persist in inflamed sites longer than the plasma.

IS A WASHOUT TIME NECESSARY?

As cited above, the pharmacologic effects may persist for longer than predicted by the half-life. Does this warrant a washout period between treatments? The washout time is the period between administrations of an NSAID when switching from one drug to another. Some promotional material published by veterinary pharmaceutical companies has advocated such a washout period when switching from one NSAID to another in animals. That is, when switching from one NSAID to another—which may be necessary because it is recognized that animals may respond to individual drugs differently, despite a shared mechanism of action—some unsupported citations have advocated an unspecified time to wash out the effects of one NSAID before another is administered. In one of the studies investigating this effect it was stated that, "In general, veterinarians are advised to discontinue an NSAID for 24 hours to 7 days before initiating administration of a second NSAID."[65] The intended purpose of a washout is to allow any residual effect from previous administration to wane before introducing another drug. Despite the well-meaning intentions, there is little scientific support for this practice. We do not know how much residual effect remains after a dose, and how long the period should be. Most NSAIDs used chronically are administered once per day (see **Table 2**), even some that have long half-lives. Piroxicam, a human drug that has a half-life of 35 to 40 hours in dogs, has been safely administered once daily.[66–68] The concept of assigning a washout time has gained support primarily through discussions on Internet sites and NSAID promotions by sponsors without any convincing scientific evidence for support. A remaining question is: should the patient be without treatment for 2 to 7 days before another NSAID is administered while waiting for the washout? This is indeed an important consideration because it may be common to switch NSAIDs between immediate postoperative care (with an injectable NSAID) to be followed by at-home treatment with another drug administered orally.

The Role of Aspirin-Triggered Lipoxin

The FDA-approved labels for these drugs give no guidance on prescribing that indicates that a washout period is needed, or how long it should be. A case can be made for caution when switching between treatment with aspirin and a COX-2 inhibitor. Aspirin is a nonselective COX inhibitor, and at low doses is more COX-1 selective. (Aspirin is not an FDA-approved drug for dogs.) As reviewed by Brune,[69] and Wallace and Fiorucci,[70] during treatment with aspirin a pathway is induced to produce lipoxin (lipoxin A4), also known as aspirin-triggered lipoxin (ATL). ATL is generated by COX-2 and has a protective role, reducing inflammation. Over time, gastrointestinal adaptation occurs, which is believed to be mediated by ATL, and induces the gastrointestinal mucosa to become more tolerant of potential injury caused by NSAIDs.[71,72]

COX-2 inhibitors inhibit the synthesis of ATL. If aspirin is administered simultaneously with a COX-2 inhibitor, or if a COX-2 inhibitor is administered before aspirin, it may prevent the process of adaptation, making the gastrointestinal mucosa more vulnerable to injury from NSAIDs.

There is evidence that gastric adaptation also involves other factors. As discussed by Brzozowski and colleagues,[73] who showed attenuation of gastric mucosal injury after repeated exposure to aspirin, gastric adaptation may rely on enhanced production of growth factors, increased cell proliferation, and mucosal regeneration. In this article the authors also argued that gastric adaptation is a long-lasting effect that produces increased resistance of the adapted mucosa to subsequent damage by ulcerogenic agents.

What is the evidence that NSAID adaptation and ATL synthesis is important in our patients? Most of the studies and review papers deal primarily with laboratory rodent studies. But studies in dogs from many years ago (Hurley and Crandal, 1964; Phillips 1973)[74] demonstrated that adaptation to administration of aspirin is possible in dogs. These reports showed that lesions were observed initially after aspirin treatment. After 1 to 2 weeks of aspirin treatment, the lesions resolved in the face of continued administration. The adaptation to aspirin in the dogs of this study was accompanied by an increase in gastric blood flow, reduction in inflammatory cell infiltration, and an increase in mucosal cell regeneration and mucosal content of epidermal growth factor. These observations are consistent with the role of ATL. There is reason to suspect that ATL is synthesized after aspirin treatment in dogs and this can potentially be inhibited by COX-2 inhibitors. Additional evidence for up-regulation of COX-2 after mucosal injury was demonstrated by Wooten and colleagues,[10] in which COX-2 was increased in the duodenum of dogs after administration of aspirin after 3 days. It is plausible that treatment with a COX-2 inhibitor would suppress this induction, and possibly the protection derived from COX-2. A washout time of several days between switching from a COX-2 inhibitor to aspirin therefore seems appropriate. Additionally, caution should be exercised when administering aspirin simultaneously with a COX-2 inhibitor. The phenomenon of adaptation from chronic administration is not without controversy, because other studies have failed to demonstrate gastric adaptation after aspirin administration to dogs. When dogs received aspirin at a high dose of 25 mg/kg every 8 hours, there was no evidence of adaptation; the lesions were as severe or worse on day 28 compared with earlier in the study.[75]

Does adaptation occur with other nonsteroidal anti-inflammatory drugs?
There are insufficient data to resolve this question and some conflicting evidence. The study cited earlier by Dowers and colleagues[65] suggests that some adaptation may occur after repeated administration of NSAIDs other than aspirin. In their study the observed gastrointestinal lesions from administration of deracoxib and carprofen were worse early in the course of treatment to day 2, but improving by day 5. There was also conflicting evidence in that study that indicated that residual effects of NSAID treatment to these experimental dogs may have occurred. On day 1 of the crossover study, lesions were observed, despite a 16-day washout time to allow recovery of the previous crossover in the preceding weeks of the study. The investigators of this study suggested that sequential NSAID administration may exert long-term effects and requires further study. On the other hand, evidence for long-term effects after 2 months of treatment was not observed by Raekallio and colleagues,[76] but there is evidence that adaptation occurred in these dogs. Dogs that had arthritis were treated every day for two months with carprofen. Plasma proteins were lower at 4 weeks, but recovered to pretreatment levels by 8 weeks. The protein loss may have been from changes in permeability of the gastrointestinal mucosa, but recovered by two months.

Is a Washout Period Needed Between Nonsteroidal Anti-Inflammatory Drugs Other than Aspirin?

A washout time when switching between NSAIDS other than aspirin is not supported by evidence. Although ATL can be synthesized independently of aspirin, there has not been conclusive evidence that ATL is induced by drugs other than aspirin, despite investigations to identify other potential candidates.[70,77] A precaution to avoid switching between NSAIDs without a washout period because it decreases ATL and increases risk for adverse reactions seems to apply only to aspirin treatment in combination with other drugs.

In a clinical trial the COX-2 inhibitor firocoxib was administered to dogs after a washout period ranging from 1 to 5 days. After analysis of 1000 patients, there was no increased risk from switching from another NSAID to firocoxib within 7 days compared with a longer washout period.[78] The washout time within the 7-day period varied from 0 days to 7 days. Most common washout time within the 7-day period was 2 days or longer. Furthermore, there was no observed risk when switching from one NSAID to another within 1 week, compared with administration of an NSAID without any previous treatment. The study only examined administering firocoxib after another NSAID and the results cannot necessarily be extended to other drugs. Furthermore, the study did not include aspirin, which would have induced ATL.

When dogs were administered sequential NSAIDs (deracoxib and carprofen), there was no evidence that following one NSAID treatment (injectable carprofen) with another (oral deracoxib) in sequential treatment produced treatment-related lesions in the gastrointestinal tract.[65] A clinical report described gastrointestinal lesions in dogs associated with administration of deracoxib.[40] Many of the dogs in that report had severe ulceration and had received either a high dose, concurrent treatment with a corticosteroid, or another NSAID in close temporal association with deracoxib. It has already been established in other studies that concurrent treatment with an NSAID and a corticosteroid exacerbates the gastroduodenal lesions.[11,54,55] The NSAID therapy reported by Lascelles and colleagues[40] was variable and consisted of different drugs and doses, making it difficult to determine whether these dogs were predisposed to NSAID-induced injury or if the NSAID therapy compounded the toxicity from deracoxib. COX-2 is important for healing to occur when gastrointestinal injury has occurred. By administering a COX-2 inhibitor to the dogs described in the clinical report,[40] the ability for mucosal recovery, regeneration, and healing may have been compromised. This evidence supports a recommendation that if gastrointestinal injury or compromise is observed, or even suspected, administration of another NSAID, particularly a COX-2 inhibitor, before allowing for healing to occur could produce additional injury.

ADVERSE EFFECTS OF NONSTEROIDAL ANTI-INFLAMMATORY DRUGS

Gastrointestinal Toxicity

Among the adverse reactions caused by NSAIDs, gastrointestinal problems are the most frequent reason to discontinue NSAID therapy or consider alternative treatment. The FDA's Freedom of Information (FOI) Summary for all the approved veterinary drugs provides the documentation of safety tests conducted prior to a drug's registration. The FOI summaries also provide the adverse events reported from clinical trials that led to FDA approval. For all drugs, adverse events that can be attributed to the gastrointestinal tract (vomiting, anorexia, diarrhea), but not necessarily to ulceration, are the most common. In animals, gastrointestinal effects can potentially range from mild gastritis and vomiting to severe gastrointestinal ulceration, bleeding, and even death. Gastrointestinal adverse events also have been documented for the past 3 decades in the veterinary literature. Gastrointestinal toxicity is caused by two mechanisms: direct irritation of the drug on the gastrointestinal mucosa and prostaglandin inhibition.[11,46,79] Direct irritation occurs because the acidic NSAIDs become more lipophilic in the acid milieu of the stomach and diffuse into the gastric mucosa where they cause injury. Prostaglandins have a cytoprotective effect on the gastrointestinal mucosa and inhibition of these compounds results in decreased cytoprotection, diminished blood flow, decreased synthesis of protective mucus, and inhibition of mucosal cell turnover and repair. In the gastrointestinal tract of healthy dogs, COX-1 is the primary COX enzyme that produces prostaglandins (primarily PGE_2),[23] but COX-2 may also be present and up-regulated after exposure to an irritant.[10] Two independent reports have confirmed a higher level of prostaglandin synthesis in the canine stomach compared with the mucosa.[10,12] A pattern is emerging to suggest that in the stomach there is an endogenous high level of COX-1–synthesized prostaglandins because of the requirement to protect the stomach from high shear forces and gastric acid and produce mucosal bicarbonate. Consistent with published studies, inhibition of COX-1 in the stomach increases the risk for gastric erosions and ulcers. In the duodenum the prostaglandin requirement is lower because there is less acid, less requirement for mucosal bicarbonate (bicarbonate is secreted by the pancreas), and less shear force because of the trituration of food that has already occurred in the stomach. Injury or insult to the duodenum induces COX-2 to produce protective and healing prostaglandins. If the COX-2–mediated prostaglandins are inhibited by NSAIDs, it may increase the risk for duodenal ulceration.

An examination of published reports of gastrointestinal toxicity from administration of NSAIDs in animals indicates that the most serious problems are caused from doses that are higher than recommended, but toxicity also has been observed from relatively mild doses in susceptible individuals. Some factors may increase the risk for gastrointestinal toxicosis, including concurrent corticosteroids and other gastrointestinal diseases. In people, there is now evidence that genetic variation may determine one's susceptibility to NSAIDs.[80]

The most recently-approved NSAIDs in the United States for dogs are carprofen, etodolac, meloxicam, deracoxib, firocoxib, and tepoxalin (see **Box 1**). A few other drugs are approved in Canada and Europe (eg, tolfenamic acid and ketoprofen). For the newer veterinary-registered NSAIDs, the gastrointestinal safety profile compared with older drugs has contributed to their popularity in veterinary medicine. There is no evidence in the published literature using controlled clinical trials to show that one is noticeably safer or more effective than another, however. For example, in a study in which carprofen, meloxicam, and ketoprofen were compared in dogs after endoscopic evaluation after 7 and 28 days of administration, there was no statistical difference among the drugs with respect to development of gastroduodenal lesions.[81] In another study that compared the gastrointestinal effects of recommended doses of carprofen, etodolac, and aspirin on the canine stomach and duodenum for 28 days, etodolac and carprofen produced significantly fewer lesions than aspirin, but lesion scores in the carprofen- and etodolac-treated groups were no different than administration of placebo.[82]

The putative explanation for the safety of carprofen, etodolac, deracoxib, firocoxib, and meloxicam is that these drugs have preferential inhibitory action for COX-2 over COX-1 (high COX-1/COX-2 ratio). Perhaps a more accurate description of these drugs is that they have a COX-1–sparing effect.[39] COX-1/COX-2 ratios many not necessarily correlate with gastrointestinal safety, however, and the calculated ratios may vary from study to study and from species to species. Some drugs may lose their COX-2 selectivity at high doses.[46] The dose dependence was shown for etodolac. At the label dose it was safe, but at higher doses (2.7 × dose) it produced gastrointestinal lesions, and at the high dose (5.3 × dose) it caused death. At high doses, meloxicam—a drug ordinarily associated with good gastrointestinal safety[34,83]—also has produced some gastrointestinal toxicity.[84] According to one report, the sponsors of this drug in Europe recommended reducing the original approved dose from 0.2 mg/kg to 0.1 mg/kg because of some initial gastrointestinal problems.[81]

Renal Injury from Nonsteroidal Anti-Inflammatory Drugs

In the kidney, prostaglandins play an important role in modulating the tone of blood vessels and regulating salt and water balance. Renal injury caused by NSAIDs has been described in people and horses, but has not been as well documented in small animals. Reported cases of toxicity occurred when high doses were used or when there were other complicating factors. Renal injury occurs as a result of inhibition of renal prostaglandin synthesis. In animals that have decreased renal perfusion caused by dehydration, anesthesia, shock, or pre-existing renal disease, this leads to renal ischemia.[64,85]

Healthy animals are somewhat immune from adverse effects from NSAIDs,[86] but if there is renal compromise (eg, dehydration, tubular dysfunction, electrolyte depletion, or anesthesia), the kidney depends on COX-1 and COX-2 for prostaglandin synthesis to autoregulate water metabolism, tubular function, and renal blood flow.[87] Animals that have renal disease are more at risk for dehydration, which can increase the likelihood of NSAID-induced nephropathy.

Renal toxicity associated with NSAIDs is characterized by decreased renal perfusion, sodium and fluid retention, and decreased tubular function. In people, pain in the kidney area has been recorded. One should not assume that NSAIDs that are more specific for the COX-2 enzyme are safer for the kidneys. Both COX-1 and COX-2 enzymes are involved in renal blood flow regulation and tubular function. Some of the prostaglandins that play an important role in salt and water regulation and hemodynamics in the kidney are synthesized by COX-2 enzymes.[88] Constitutive COX-2 is found in various sections of the kidney and administration of drugs that are selective for COX-2 may adversely affect the kidney during conditions in which the kidney is stressed because of dehydration, decreased perfusion, or disease. Administration of a specific COX-2 inhibitor to salt-depleted people decreased renal blood flow, glomerular filtration rate, and electrolyte excretion.[88] Corticosteroids may also increase the risk for injury because it was shown that administration of prednisolone to dogs in combination with either meloxicam or ketoprofen has a potential for serious adverse effects on the kidneys and the gastrointestinal tract.[55]

Of the currently available NSAIDs, the effect of carprofen and meloxicam on renal function has been the most extensively studied. Because these drugs are used in perioperative situations in an injectable formulation, investigations were performed to determine if there was any evidence of renal toxicity, particularly during conditions of anesthesia. In one study, carprofen, ketorolac, and ketoprofen were examined in healthy dogs undergoing surgery, but without intravenous fluid administration. There were minor increases in renal tubular epithelial cells on urine sediment, but carprofen had no adverse effects on renal function.[86] Some ketorolac- and ketoprofen-treated dogs had transient azotemia. In other studies, administration of carprofen to anesthetized healthy dogs had no adverse effects on renal function (Bergmann and colleagues, 2005).[89–93]

Meloxicam did not produce adverse renal effects in healthy dogs after short-term administration, with and without pimobendan.[94] In healthy dogs anesthetized and treated with acepromazine to produce hypotension, preanesthetic administration of meloxicam did not produce any altered renal function.[95] Healthy dogs administered meloxicam before anesthesia and electrical nociceptive stimulus did not have decreased renal function associated with treatment.[90] Tepoxalin was evaluated in anesthetized, healthy, normotensive, normovolemic dogs at a dose of 10 mg/kg (currently registered dose) using renal scintigraphy.[96] There were no adverse effects on renal function detected. In another study with tepoxalin on renal function, there were no adverse effects when it was administered to dogs in combination with an angiotensin-converting enzyme (ACE) inhibitor.[96]

The common design in the studies cited above was that dogs were healthy, generally young, and NSAID doses were from a single dose and within the recommended range. Deviations from this design, use of higher doses, longer treatment, or administration to clinical patients with other problems could produce different results.

Renal effects following deracoxib administration to dogs were reported by the manufacturer. At high doses, there is a dose-dependent effect on renal tubules. It is well tolerated in most dogs up to 10 mg/kg for 6 months, but there is a potential for a dose-dependent renal tubular degeneration/regeneration at doses of 6 mg/kg or higher. (Clinically approved dose for long-term treatment is 1–2 mg/kg per day.) Long-term administration of carprofen, etodolac, flunixin, ketoprofen, or meloxicam to dogs did not induce any evidence of renal injury as measured by urinalysis and serum biochemistry.[97]

There is another form of analgesic nephritis, usually caused by chronic use of acetaminophen (eg, Tylenol) in people.[98] This syndrome has not been described in domestic animals.

Are there increased effects with angiotensin-converting enzyme inhibitors and nonsteroidal anti-inflammatory drugs?

Because ACE inhibitors carry a risk for decreased renal perfusion, administration of ACE inhibitors and NSAIDs has been suggested to increase the risk.[99] The review by Lefebvre and Toutain[100] examines the role of ACE inhibitors on the kidney and the potential for complications from coadministration of NSAIDs. For example, in humans there is concern that in some patients the combination of an ACE inhibitor and an NSAID may increase the risk for renal injury.[99] Only one study examining this combination has been published for dogs.[96] It was concluded in that study that tepoxalin did not alter renal function in healthy beagle dogs receiving an ACE inhibitor. Such an effect of other NSAID combinations has not been adequately studied in veterinary medicine to make adequate conclusions.

Sensitivity of Nonsteroidal Anti-Inflammatory Drugs in Cats

A complete and in-depth review of NSAIDs in cats was published by Lascelles and colleagues.[6] The toxic effects of salicylates in cats are well documented. Cats are susceptible because of slow clearance and dose-dependent elimination. Affected cats may have hyperthermia, respiratory alkalosis, metabolic acidosis, methemoglobinemia, hemorrhagic gastritis, and kidney and liver injury. Cats also are prone to acetaminophen toxicosis because of their deficiency in drug-metabolizing enzymes. Cases of acetaminophen toxicity in cats also have been well documented. Treatment of acetaminophen toxicity consists of measures to replenish compounds that can conjugate the metabolites of acetaminophen and increase clearance, such as acetylcysteine[57] or S-adenosyl methionine. Despite the sensitivity in cats to some of the NSAIDs, there are still drugs in this group have been used safely. Aspirin has been used at doses of 10 mg/kg every other day.[1] There are also reports of the safe use of ketoprofen (registered in Canada) at a dose of 1 mg/kg/day for 4 days and flunixin meglumine (1 mg/kg once) in cats for short-term treatment.

In the United States meloxicam is registered for single use at 0.3 mg/kg and also is used in Canada and Europe. The label instructions carefully warn not to administer more than one dose. When cats were administered high doses (5 $\times$ dose) vomiting and other gastrointestinal problems were reported. With repeated doses (9 days) of 0.3 mg/kg per day to cats, inflamed gastrointestinal mucosa and ulceration was observed. (Earlier in this article the PK-PD analysis of meloxicam indicated that this dose would be high for repeated doses.) On the other hand, many veterinarians have administered meloxicam to cats for multiple doses at lower doses. Some regimens recommend meloxicam in cats at 0.1 mg/kg initially, followed by decreased doses. If a favorable response is seen in the first few days, increase the dose interval to once every 48 to 72 hours, at a lower dose of 0.05 mg/kg and as low as 0.025 mg/kg. In Europe the approved dose for cats is 0.05 mg/kg per day for chronic use. There are safety data from the sponsor to support this claim. Long-term safety of meloxicam in cats was published at a lower dose of 0.01 to 0.03 mg/kg, which is lower than the approved European dose.[101]

Use of carprofen in cats has been discouraged because of reports of gastroduodenal toxicosis when it was administered according to canine dose rates. Carprofen is approved for single-dose administration in Europe. Tepoxalin has not been tested clinically in cats, even though pharmacokinetic studies showed that both the parent drug and metabolite would allow for safe dosing at 10 mg/kg. At high doses, however, it has produced adverse effects and a safe dose for routine therapeutic use has not been identified. There is one report of use of firocoxib in cats.[102] In this report, cats were given doses of 0.75 to 3 mg/kg (single dose), which was effective for attenuating experimentally induced fever. Other selections of NSAIDs in cats should be guided by the review cited earlier.[6]

Hepatic Safety

As pointed out in a recent review, any NSAID has the potential for causing hepatic injury.[103] The author states that NSAIDs as a class have been associated with considerable hepatotoxicity. Hepatotoxicity caused by NSAIDs can be either idiosyncratic (unpredictable, non–dose related) or intrinsic (predictable and dose related).[104,105] Toxicity to acetaminophen and aspirin are intrinsic; reactions to other drugs tend to be idiosyncratic and unpredictable. Administration of NSAIDs to animals that have hepatic disease has been questioned because of the role of the liver in metabolizing these drugs, but there is no evidence that prior hepatic disease predisposes a patient to NSAID-induced liver injury. Drug enzyme systems are remarkably preserved in hepatic disease and pre-existing hepatic disease is not necessarily a contraindication for administration of an NSAID. Patients that have liver disease may be more prone to gastrointestinal ulceration, and there is concern that administration of NSAIDs could increase the risk for this complication.

Carprofen was approved by FDA in October 1996 for relief of pain and inflammation in dogs. Before this approval, it was registered for treatment of dogs in Europe (Zenecarp) and was evaluated in clinical trials. In studies in dogs that had arthritis, it was effective and had a low incidence of adverse effects.[106] In long-term studies in which carprofen was administered from 2 weeks to 5 years, the incidence of adverse reactions was only 1.3%. Vomiting, diarrhea, anorexia, and lethargy were the most common adverse reactions documented. Attention has focused on the hepatotoxicity caused by carprofen because of a report in the published literature.[107] Hepatic injury signs are also among the most common adverse events reported for carprofen to the FDA adverse events reporting site. In this report, 21 dogs were described in which carprofen was associated with acute, idiosyncratic hepatotoxicosis. Affected dogs had diminished appetites, vomited, and were icteric, with elevations in hepatic enzymes and bilirubin. Dogs received the usual recommended dose and developed signs an average of 19 days after therapy was initiated. No predisposing conditions were identified. Most dogs recovered without further consequences. Many of the dogs in that report were Labrador retrievers, but there is no follow-up evidence to show that this breed of dogs has increased risk for carprofen hepatotoxicity.[108] Among the other drugs, the newest drug, firocoxib, caused fatty liver changes in young dogs when administered at high doses (manufacturer's data). Other NSAIDs used in veterinary medicine also have potential for causing liver injury, but they are uncommon. In a study of long-term administration for 90 days, there were only minor and clinically unimportant changes in serum biochemical variables in dogs after administration of carprofen, etdolac, flunixin, ketoprofen, and meloxicam.[97] Idiosyncratic reactions are rare (1/1000 to 1/10,000 patients). Any unexplained increase in hepatic enzymes or bilirubin 7 to 90 days after initiating NSAID administration should be investigated.

CLINICAL DRUG SELECTION

When selecting a drug for treatment in animals, there are several choices (see **Box 1**). Veterinarians should not allow unsubstantiated claims to affect the selection of one drug over another. Over the past several years we have learned some important information about these drugs that should guide treatment (**Box 2**), and one of the most significant of these is that we really do not know which NSAID drug is best. Each has advantages and disadvantages. There are different dosage forms that include injectable, oral liquid, rapidly dissolving tablets, regular tablets, and chewable tablets. The preference for each of these depends on the clinical situation and the pet owner. There are veterinary generic formulations of popular drugs and there are still some human-labeled drugs used off- label (eg, piroxicam).

For acute pain, such as perioperative use, there is good evidence of efficacy from oral and injectable formulations that has been published in previous reports and reviews. For these and other indications, NSAIDs have been used for short-term durations of 1 or 2 days to decrease fever and decrease pain from surgery or trauma. Preoperative injections of carprofen to dogs were shown to be beneficial to decrease postoperative pain in dogs after ovariohysterectomy.[109] Meloxicam effects for surgical pain have been reported and were shown to be superior to butorphanol in some of the pain assessments that were measured.[110–112]

Oral NSAIDs also may be used for acute treatment of myositis, arthritis, and postoperative pain, or they may be administered chronically for osteoarthritis. Drugs that have been administered in the United States to small animals are listed in **Box 1**, and some veterinarians also have used human-label drugs, such as aspirin, piroxicam, and naproxen. If these human-label drugs are considered, consult appropriate references for accurate dosing because it may differ from the human dose schedule. The most recently approved drugs are carprofen, etodolac, meloxicam, firocoxib, tepoxalin, and deracoxib. Doses are listed in **Table 2**. For long-term use there are no controlled studies that compare which is the most effective. When drugs are compared with one another it is difficult, using subjective measurements, to demonstrate differences between these drugs for reducing pain in animals. Without a very large number of patients, the statistical power to detect differences among drugs in clinical veterinary studies is difficult.

In summary, there are several choices of NSAIDs for treating dogs that have osteoarthritis. Like people, there may be greater differences among individuals in their

Box 2
What have we learned about nonsteroidal anti-inflammatory drugs?

All NSAIDs, regardless of COX-1/COX-2 specificity, are capable of producing gastrointestinal lesions, particularly at high doses.

All NSAIDs (selective or nonselective) can produce other gastrointestinal signs, including vomiting, diarrhea, and decreased appetite, without producing ulceration.

All NSAIDs have potential for producing hepatic injury. Susceptibility seems to be idiosyncratic and unpredictable.

All NSAIDs have the potential for producing renal injury. Previous renal disease, salt depletion, and dehydration increase the risk.

No NSAID is consistently more clinically effective than another.

response than there are differences among the drugs. In past practice, veterinarians often selected aspirin or phenylbutazone as an initial drug, and then progressed to off-label human drugs (eg, piroxicam) or other agents as an alternative. Now we have the advantage of several approved NSAIDs for which there are excellent published studies and FDA or foreign approval to guide clinical use and safe dosages. Among the drugs available (see **Box 1**) there may be variations among animals with respect to tolerance of adverse effects and clinical response. It is a rational approach to consider a rotating schedule of two or more drugs to identify which drug is better tolerated, more effective, and easier to administer in each patient. When considering a switch from one NSAID to another, the necessity of a washout period should be considered.

REFERENCES

1. Papich MG. Saunders handbook of veterinary drugs. 2nd edition. St. Louis (MO): Elsevier-Saunders Co.; 2007.
2. Papich MG. Pharmacologic considerations for opiate analgesic and nonsteroidal anti-inflammatory drugs. Vet Clin North Am Small Anim Pract 2000;30:815–37.
3. Bergh MS, Budsgerg SC. The COXIB NSAIDs: potential clinical and pharmacologic importance in veterinary medicine. J Vet Intern Med 2005;19:633–43.
4. Lees P, Landoni MF, Giraudel J, et al. Pharmacodynamics and pharmacokinetics of nonsteroidal anti-inflammatory drugs in species of veterinary interest. J Vet Pharmacol Ther 2004b;27(6):479–90.
5. Lascelles BDX, McFarland JM, Swann H. Guidelines for safe and effective use of NSAIDs in dogs. Vet Ther 2005;6(3):237–50.
6. Lascelles BDX, Court MH, Hardie EM, et al. Nonsteroidal anti-inflammatory drugs in cats: a review. Vet Anaesth Analg 2007;34:228–50.
7. Vane JR, Botting RM. New insights into the mode of action of anti-inflammatory drugs. Inflamm Res 1995;44:1–10.
8. Laneuville O, Breuer DK, DeWitt DL, et al. Differential inhibition of human prostaglandin endoperoxide synthases-1 and -2 by nonsteroidal anti-inflammatory drugs. J Pharmacol Exp Ther 1994;271:927–34.
9. Meade EA, Smith WL, DeWitt DL. Pharmacology of prostaglandin endoperoxide synthase isozymes-1 and -2. Ann N Y Acad Sci 1994;714:136–42.
10. Wooten JG, Blikslager AT, Ryan KA, et al. Cyclooxygenase expression and prostanoid production in pyloric and duodenal mucosae in dogs after administration of nonsteroidal anti-inflammatory drugs. Am J Vet Res 2008;69(4):457–64.
11. Konturek SJ, Konturek PC, Brzozowski T. Prostaglandins and ulcer healing. J Physiol Pharmacol 2005;56(Suppl 5):5–31.
12. Punke JP, Speas AL, Reynolds LR, et al. Effects of firocoxib, meloxicam, and tepoxalin on prostanoid and leukotriene production by duodenal mucosa and other tissues of osteoarthritic dogs. Am J Vet Res 2008;69(9):1203–9.
13. Bertolini A, Ottani A, Sandrini M. Dual acting anti-inflammatory drugs: a reappraisal. Pharmacol Res 2001;44:437–50.
14. Flower RJ, Vane JR. Inhibition of prostaglandin synthetase in brain explains the antipyretic activity of paracetamol (4-acetamidophenol). Nature 1972;240(5381): 410–1.
15. Chandrasekharan NV, Dai H, Roos KL, et al. A cyclooxygenase-1 variant inhibited by acetaminophen and other analgesic/antipyretic drugs: cloning, structure, and expression. Proc Natl Acad Sci U S A 2002;99(21):13926–31 (with commentary in Proc Natl Acad Sci U S A. 99(21):13371–13373, 2002).

16. Davies NM, Good RL, Roupe KA, et al. Cyclooxygenase-3: axiom, dogma, anomaly, enigma or splice error?—not as easy as 1, 2, 3. J Pharm Pharm Sci 2004;7(2):217–26.
17. Aronoff DM, Oates JA, Boutaud O. New insights into the mechanism of action of acetaminophen: its clinical pharmacologic characteristics reflect its inhibition of the two prostaglandin H2 synthases. Clin Pharmacol Ther 2005;79:9–19.
18. Kis B, Snipes JA, Busija DW. Acetaminophen and the cyclooxygenase-3 puzzle: sorting out facts, fictions, and uncertainties. J Pharmacol Exp Ther 2005;315(1): 1–7.
19. Gierse JK, Staten NR, Casperson GF, et al. Cloning, expression, and selective inhibition of canine cyclooxygenase-1 and cyclooxygenase-2. Vet Ther 2002;3: 270–80.
20. McCann ME, Andersen DR, Zhang D, et al. In vitro effects and in vivo efficacy of a novel cyclo-oxygenase-2 inhibitor in dogs with experimentally induced synovitis. Am J Vet Res 2004;65:503–12.
21. Ricketts AP, Lundy KM, Seibel SB. Evaluation of selective inhibition of canine cyclooxygenase 1 and 2 by carprofen and other nonsteroidal anti-inflammatory drugs. Am J Vet Res 1998;59:1441–6.
22. Kay-Mugford P, Benn SJ, LaMarre J, et al. In vitro effects of nonsteroidal anti-inflammatory drugs on cyclooxygenase activity in dogs. Am J Vet Res 2000; 61:802–10.
23. Wilson JE, Chandrasekharan NV, Westover KD, et al. Determination of expression of cyclooxygenase-1 and -2 isozymes in canine tissues and their differential sensitivity to nonsteroidal anti-inflammatory drugs. Am J Vet Res 2004;65:810–8.
24. McKellar QA, Delatour P, Lees P. Stereospecific pharmacodynamics and pharmacokinetics of carprofen in the dog. J Vet Pharmacol Ther 1994;17:447–54.
25. Glaser KB. Cyclooxygenase selectivity and NSAIDs: cyclooxygenase-2 selectivity of etodolac (lodine). Inflammopharmacology 1995;3:335–45.
26. Lees P. Pharmacology of drugs used to treat osteoarthritis in veterinary practice. Inflammopharmacology 2003;11:385–99.
27. Patrignani P, Panara MR, Greco A, et al. Biochemical and pharmacological characterization of the cyclooxygenase activity of human blood prostaglandin endoperoxide synthases. J Pharmacol Exp Ther 1994;271(3):1705–12.
28. Blain H, Boileau C, Lapicque F, et al. Limitation of the in vitro whole blood assay for predicting the COX selectivity of NSAIDs in clinical use. Br J Clin Pharmacol 2002;53(3):255–65.
29. Hinz B, Brune K. Can drug removals involving cyclooxygenase-2 inhibitors be avoided? A plea for human pharmacology. Trends Pharmacol Sci 2008;29(8): 391–7.
30. Lees P, Giraudel J, Landoni MF, et al. PK-PD integration and PK-PD modelling of nonsteroidal anti-inflammatory drugs: principles and applications in veterinary pharmacology. J Vet Pharmacol Ther 2004a;27(6):491–502.
31. Giraudel JM, Diquelou A, Laroute V, et al. Pharmacokinetic/pharmacodynamic modelling of NSAIDs in a model of reversible inflammation in the cat. Br J Pharmacol 2005a;146(5):642–53.
32. Giraudel JM, Diquelou A, Lees P, et al. Development and validation of a new model of inflammation in the cat and selection of surrogate endpoints for testing anti-inflammatory drugs. J Vet Pharmacol Ther 2005b;28(3):275–85.
33. Borer LR, Peel JE, Seewald W, et al. Effect of carprofen, etodolac, meloxicam, or butorphanol in dogs with induced acute synovitis. Am J Vet Res 2003;64: 1429–37.

34. Jones CJ, Streppa HK, Harmon BG, et al. In vivo effects of meloxicam and aspirin on blood, gastric mucosal, and synovial fluid prostanoid synthesis in dogs. Am J Vet Res 2002;63:1527–31.
35. Sessions JK, Reynolds LR, Budsberg SC. In vivo effects of carprofen, deracoxib, and etodolac on prostanoids production in blood, gastric mucosa, and synovial fluid in dogs with chronic osteoarthritis. Am J Vet Res 2005;66:812–7.
36. Bryant CE, Farnfield BA, Janicke HJ. Evaluation of the ability of carprofen and flunixin meglumine to inhibit activation of nuclear factor kappa B. Am J Vet Res 2003;64:211–5.
37. FitzGerald GA, Patrono C. The Coxibs, selective inhibitors of cyclooxygenase-2. N Engl J Med 2001;345:433–42.
38. McCann ME, Rickes EL, Hora DF, et al. In vitro effects and in vivo efficacy of a novel cyclooxygenase-2 inhibitor in cats with lipopolysaccharide-induced pyrexia. Am J Vet Res 2005;66:1278–84.
39. Peterson WL, Cryer B. COX-1-sparing NSAIDs—is the enthusiasm justified? J Am Med Assoc 1999;282:1961–3 [see also pages 1921 and 1929 of this issue.].
40. Lascelles BDX, Blikslager AT, Fox SM, et al. Gastrointestinal tract perforation in dogs treated with a selective cyclooxygenase-2 inhibitor: 29 cases (2002–2003). J Am Vet Med Assoc 2005;227:1112–7.
41. Drazen JM. COX-2 inhibitors – a lesson in unexpected problems. N Engl J Med 2005;352:1131–2.
42. Malhotra S, Shafiq N, Pandhi P. COX-2 inhibitors: a CLASS act, or just VIGORously promoted. MedGenMed 2004;6(1). Available at: www.medscape.com.
43. Psaty BM, Furberg CD. COX-2 inhibitors—lessons in drug safety. N Engl J Med 2005;352:1133–5.
44. Jüni P, Rutjes AWS, Dieppe PA. Are selective COX 2 inhibitors superior to traditional non steroidal anti-inflammatory drugs? Br Med J 2002;324:1287–8.
45. Rainsford KD. The ever-emerging anti-inflammatories. Have there been any real advances? J Physiol 2001;95:11–9.
46. Wolfe MM, Lichtenstein DR, Singh G. Gastrointestinal toxicity of nonsteroidal antiinflammatory drugs. N Engl J Med 1999;340:1888–99.
47. Mukherjee D, Nissen SE, Topol EJ. Risk of cardiovascular events associated with selective COX-2 inhibitors. JAMA 2001;286:954–9.
48. FitzGerald GA. Coxibs and cardiovascular disease. N Engl J Med 2004;351:1709–11.
49. Topol EJ. Failing the public health—rofecoxib, Merck and the FDA. N Engl J Med 2004;351:1707–9.
50. Eisenberg RS. Learning the value of drugs—is rofecoxib a regulatory success story? N Engl J Med 2005;352:1285–7.
51. Okie S. Raising the safety bar—the FDA's Coxib meeting. N Engl J Med 2005;345:1283–5.
52. Trang T, McNaull B, Quirion R, et al. Involvement of spinal lipoxygenase metabolites in hyperalgesia and opiate tolerance. European Journal of Pharmacology 2004;491:21–30.
53. Moreau M, Daminet S, Martel-Pelletier J, et al. Superiority of the gastrointestinal safety profile of licofelone over rofecoxib, a COX-2 selective inhibitor in dogs. J Vet Pharmacol Ther 2005;28:81–6.
54. Boston SE, Moens NM, Kruth SA, et al. Endoscopic evaluation of the gastroduodenal mucosa to determine the safety of short-term concurrent administration of meloxicam and dexamethasone in healthy dogs. Am J Vet Res 2003;64(11):1369–75.

55. Narita T, Sato R, Motoishi K, et al. The interaction between orally administered non-steroidal anti-inflammatory drugs and prednisolone in healthy dogs. J Vet Med Sci 2007;69(4):353–63.
56. Agnello KA, Reynolds LR, Budsberg SC. In vivo effects of tepoxalin, an inhibitor of cyclooxygenase and lipoxygenase, on prostanoid and leukotriene production in dogs with chronic osteoarthritis. Am J Vet Res 2005;66(6):966–72.
57. Hjelle JJ, Grauer GF. Acetaminophen-induced toxicosis in dogs and cats. J Am Vet Med Assoc 1986;188:742–6.
58. Bradley JD, Brandt KD, Katz BP, et al. Comparison of an anti-inflammatory dose of ibuprofen, an analgesic dose of ibuprofen, and acetaminophen in the treatment of patients with osteoarthritis of the knee. N Engl J Med 1991;325:87–91.
59. Mburu DN, Mbugua LA, Skoglund LA, et al. Effects of paracetamol (acetaminophen) and acetylsalicylic acid on the post-operative course after experimental orthopaedic surgery in dogs. J Vet Pharmacol Ther 1988;11:163–71.
60. Mburu DN. Evaluation of the anti-inflammatory effects of a low-dose of acetaminophen following surgery in dogs. J Vet Pharmacol Ther 1991;14:109–11.
61. Savides MC, Oehme FW, Nash SL, et al. The toxicity and biotransformation of single doses of acetaminophen in dogs and cats. Toxicol Appl Pharmacol 1984;74:26–34.
62. Hinz B, Cheremina O, Brune K. Acetaminophen (paracetamol) is a selective cyclooxygenase-2 inhibitor in man. FASEB J 2007;22(2):383–90.
63. Pickering G, Esteve V, Loriot M-A, et al. Acetaminophen reinforces descending inhibitory pain pathways. Clin Pharmacol Ther 2008;84(1):47–51.
64. Mathews KA. Nonsteroidal anti-inflammatory analgesics in pain management in dogs and cats. Can Vet J 1996;37:539–45.
65. Dowers KL, Uhrig SR, Mama KR, et al. Effect of short-term sequential administration of nonsteroidal anti-inflammatory drugs on the stomach and proximal portion of the duodenum in healthy dogs. Am J Vet Res 2006;67(10):1794–801.
66. Galbraith EA, McKellar QA. Pharmacokinetics and pharmacodynamics of piroxicam in dogs. Vet Rec 1991;128:561–5.
67. Knapp DW, Richardson RC, Chan TCK, et al. Piroxicam therapy in 34 dogs with transitional cell carcinoma of the urinary bladder. J Vet Intern Med 1994;8(4):273–8.
68. Schmidt BR, Glickman NW, DeNicola DB, et al. Evaluation of piroxicam for the treatment of oral squamous cell carcinoma in dogs. J Am Vet Med Assoc 2001;218:1783–6.
69. Brune K. Safety of anti-inflammatory treatment—new ways of thinking. Rheumatology 2004;43(Suppl 1):i16–20.
70. Wallace JL, Fiorucci S. A magic bullet for mucosal protection.and aspirin is the trigger!. Trends Pharmacol Sci 2003;24(7):323–6.
71. Fiorucci S, de Lima OM Jr, Mencarelli A, et al. Cyclooxygenase-2-derived lipoxin A4 increases gastric resistance to aspirin-induced damage. Gastroenterology 2002;123(5):1598–606.
72. Souza MH, de Lima OM Jr, Zamuner SR, et al. Gastritis increases resistance to aspirin-induced mucosal injury via COX-2-mediated lipoxin synthesis. Am J Physiol Gastrointest Liver Physiol 2003;285(1):G54–61.
73. Brzozowski T, Konturek PC, Konturek SJ, et al. Role of prostaglandins in gastroprotection and gastric adaptation. J Physiol Pharmacol 2005;56(Suppl 5):33–55.
74. Taylor LA, Crawford LM. Aspirin-induced gastrointestinal lesions in dogs. J Am Vet Med Assoc 1968;152(6):617–9.
75. Sennello KA, Leib MS. Effects of deracoxib or buffered aspirin on the gastric mucosa of healthy dogs. J Vet Intern Med 2006;20:1291–6.

76. Raekallio MR, Hielm-Björkman AK, Kejonen J, et al. Evaluation of adverse effects of long-term orally administered carprofen in dogs. J Am Vet Med Assoc 2006; 228(6):876–80.
77. Wallace JL, Wallace JL, Zamuner SR, et al. Aspirin, but not NO-releasing aspirin (NCX-4016), interacts with selective COX-2 inhibitors to aggravate gastric damage and inflammation. Am J Physiol Gastrointest Liver Physiol 2004;286(1):G76–81.
78. Ryan WG, Moldave K, Carithers D. Switching NSAIDs in practice: insights from the Previcox (firocoxib) experience trial. Vet Ther 2007;8(4):263–71.
79. Whittle BJ. Mechanisms underlying intestinal injury induced by anti-inflammatory COX inhibitors. Eur J Pharmacol 2004;500(1–3):427–39.
80. Lee YS, Kim H, Wu TX, et al. Genetically mediated interindividual variation in analgesic responses to cyclooxygenase inhibitory drugs. Clin Pharmacol Ther 2006;79(5):407–18.
81. Forsyth SF, Guilford WG, Haslett SJ, et al. Endoscopy of the gastroduodenal mucosa after carprofen, meloxicam and ketoprofen administration in dogs. J Small Anim Pract 1998;39:421–4.
82. Reimer ME, Johnston SA, Leib MS, et al. The gastrointestinal effects of buffered aspirin, carprofen, and etodolac in healthy dogs. J Vet Intern Med 1999;13:472–7.
83. Doig PA, Purbrick KA, Hare JE, et al. Clinical efficacy and tolerance of meloxicam in dogs with chronic osteoarthritis. Can Vet J 2000;41(4):296–300.
84. Enberg TB, Braun LD, Kuzma AB. Gastrointestinal perforation in five dogs associated with the administration of meloxicam. Journal of Veterinary Emergency and Critical Care 2006;16:34–43.
85. Mathews KA, Doherty T, Dyson DH, et al. Nephrotoxicity in dogs associated with methoxyflurane anesthesia and flunixin meglumine analgesia. Can Vet J 1990; 31:766–71.
86. Lobetti RG, Joubert KE. Effect of administration of nonsteroidal anti-inflammatory drugs before surgery on renal function in clinically normal dogs. Am J Vet Res 2000;61:1501–6.
87. Gambaro G, Perazella MA. Adverse renal effects of anti-inflammatory agents: evaluation of selective and nonselective cyclo-oxygenase inhibitors. J Intern Med 2003;253:643–52.
88. Rossat J, Maillard M, Nussberger JU, et al. Renal effects of selective cyclooxygenase-2 inhibition in normotensive salt-depleted subjects. Clin Pharmacol Ther 1999;66:76–84.
89. Boström IM, Nyman GC, Lord PF, et al. Effects of carprofen on renal function and results of serum biochemical and hematologic analyses in anesthetized dogs that had low blood pressure during anesthesia. Am J Vet Res 2002;63:712–21.
90. Crandell DE, Mathews KA, Dyson DH. Effect of meloxicam and carprofen on renal function when administered to healthy dogs prior to anesthesia and painful stimulation. Am J Vet Res 2004;65(10):1384–90.
91. Frendin JH, Boström IM, Kampa N, et al. Effects of carprofen on renal function during medetomidine-propofol-isoflurane anesthesia in dogs. Am J Vet Res 2006;67(12):1967–73.
92. Ko JCH, Miyabiyashi T, Mandsager RE, et al. Renal effects of carprofen administered to healthy dogs anesthetized with propofol and isoflurane. J Am Vet Med Assoc 2000;217:346–9.
93. Bergmann HML, Nolte IJA, Kramer S. Effects of preoperative administration of carprofen on renal function and hemostasis in dogs undergoing surgery for fracture repair. Am J Vet Res 2005;66:1356–63.

94. Fusellier M, Desfontis J-C, LeRoux A, et al. Effect of short-term treatment with meloxicam and pimobendan on the renal function in healthy beagle dogs. Journal of Veterinary Pharmacology and Therapeutics 2008;31:150–5.
95. Boström IM, Nyman G, Hoppe A, et al. Effects of meloxicam on renal function in dogs with hypotension during anaesthesia. Vet Anaesth Analg 2006;33(1):62–9.
96. Kay-Mugford PA, Grimm KA, Weingarten AJ, et al. Effect of preoperative administration of tepoxalin on hemostasis and hepatic and renal function in dogs. Vet Ther 2004;5:120–7.
97. Luna SP, Basílio AC, Steagall PV, et al. Evaluation of adverse effects of long-term oral administration of carprofen, etodolac, flunixin meglumine, ketoprofen, and meloxicam in dogs. Am J Vet Res 2007;68(3):258–64.
98. de Broe ME, Elseviers MM. Analgesic nephropathy. N Engl J Med 1998;338: 446–52.
99. Loboz KK, Shenfield GM. Drug combinations and impaired renal function—the triple whammy. Br J Clin Pharmacol 2005;59:239–43.
100. Lefebvre HP, Toutain PL. Angiotensin-converting enzyme inhibitors in the therapy of renal diseases. J Vet Pharmacol Ther 2004;27(5):265–81.
101. Gunew MN, Menrath VH, Marshall RD. Long-term safety, efficacy and palatability of oral meloxicam at 0.01-0.03 mg/kg for treatment of osteoarthritic pain in cats. J Feline Med Surg 2008;10(3):235–41.
102. McCann ME, Rickes EL, Hora DF, et al. In vitro effects and in vivo efficacy of a novel cyclooxygenase-2 inhibitor in cats with lipopolysaccharide-induced pyrexia. Am J Vet Res 2005;66:01278–84.
103. Lee WM. Drug induced hepatotoxicity. N Engl J Med 2003;349:474–85.
104. Bjorkman D. Nonsteroidal anti-inflammatory drug-associated toxicity of the liver, lower gastrointestinal tract, and esophagus. Am J Med 1998;105(Suppl 5A): 17S–21S.
105. Tolman KG. Hepatotoxicity of non-narcotic analgesics. Am J Med 1998; 105(Suppl 1B). 13S–7S.
106. Vasseur PB, Johnson AL, Budsberg SC, et al. Randomized, controlled trial of the efficacy of carprofen, a nonsteroidal antiinflammatory drug, in the treatment of osteoarthritis in dogs. J Am Vet Med Assoc 1995;206:807–11.
107. MacPhail CM, Lappin MR, Meyer DJ, et al. Hepatocellular toxicosis associated with administration of carprofen in 21 dogs. J Am Vet Med Assoc 1998;212:1895–901.
108. Hickford FH, Barr SC, Erb HN. Effect of carprofen on hemostatic variables in dogs. Am J Vet Res 2001;62(10):1642–6.
109. Lascelles BDX, Cripps PJ, Jones A, et al. Efficacy and kinetics of carprofen, administered preoperatively or postoperatively, for the prevention of pain in dogs undergoing ovariohysterectomy. Vet Surg 1998;27:568–82.
110. Budsberg SC, Cross AR, Quandt JE, et al. Evaluation of intravenous administration of meloxicam for perioperative pain management following stifle joint surgery in dogs. Am J Vet Res 2002;63(11):1557–63.
111. Caulkett N, Read M, Fowler D, et al. A comparison of the analgesic effects of butorphanol with those of meloxicam after effective ovariohysterectomy in dogs. Can Vet J 2003;44(7):565–70.
112. Mathews KA, Pettifer G, Foster R, et al. Safety and efficacy of preoperative administration of meloxicam, compared with that of ketoprofen and butorphanol in dogs undergoing abdominal surgery. AM J Ver Res 2001;62(6):882–8.

Managing Pain in Feline Patients

Sheilah A. Robertson, BVMS, PhD, MRCVS

KEYWORDS

- Diagnosis • Behavior • Psychopharmacology
- Cognitive Dysfunction • Pheromone

It is estimated that there are 200 million pet cats worldwide, with 76 million in the United States alone. In many European countries, the United States, and China, cats now outnumber dogs.[1] The need for perioperative pain management is great, because most pet cats are spayed or castrated and, in the United States, many are also declawed. Over a 5-year period, the use of specific analgesics in cats undergoing surgical procedures in South Africa increased from 13% in 2000 to 56% in 2005, and 94% now receive a perioperative drug with analgesic properties.[2] A similar trend in increased use of analgesics in cats was recently reported among Canadian veterinarians.[3] In 2005, 50% of cats in New Zealand were estimated to receive perioperative pain relief for castration.[4] These improvements are thought to be a result of continuing education and review articles.[2,3] Despite these encouraging numbers, there is still room for improvement; some animals are receiving no analgesics; "strong" (pure μ-agonist) opioids, local anesthetics, and α_2-agonists are still underused,[3] and as many as 42% of veterinarians[4] and 96% of nurses thought that their ability to assess and treat pain was inadequate and could be improved.[5] The goals of the newly published American Animal Hospital Association and American Association of Feline Practitioners pain management guidelines are to demonstrate to practitioners the wide range of situations in which pain management should be instituted, to encourage them to embrace alleviation of pain as central to good medicine, and to demonstrate the many resources at their disposal to help them in this mission.[6] The incidence of chronic pain in cats is not well documented, but feline osteoarthritis (OA) is a disease that is beginning to be addressed and occurs in many cats older than the age of 10 years.[7–9] Other methods for improving pain management include client education and developing validated methods of pain assessment.[10] Challenges that still face the feline practitioner are the cat's unique metabolism, which has an impact on the choice of drugs, especially for long-term use, and the lack of analgesic agents with market authorization. This article aims to review the current knowledge of pain assessment in cats and the most effective methods for its alleviation.

Department of Large Animal Clinical Sciences, College of Veterinary Medicine, University of Florida, PO Box 100136, Gainesville, FL 32610-0136, USA
E-mail address: robertsons@vetmed.ufl.edu

Vet Clin Small Anim 38 (2008) 1267–1290
doi:10.1016/j.cvsm.2008.06.008 vetsmall.theclinics.com
0195-5616/08/$ – see front matter

PAIN ASSESSMENT

The benefits of pain management are numerous; however, to treat pain, we must first recognize it. Assessment of pain in animals is not an easy task but is essential for successful pain management. Pain is a complex multidimensional experience involving sensory and affective (emotional) components. It is now accepted that animals do experience pain, even if they cannot communicate it in the same way that people do.[11] Pain is a subjective and individual experience. Human beings show large interindividual differences in quality, intensity, and response to intervention that are genetically determined,[12] and recent antinociceptive studies suggest that this is also true in cats;[13,14] therefore, the importance of assessing pain in each feline patient cannot be overemphasized. In animals, pain is what the observer says it is, and because all judgments are subjective, if we "get it wrong," animals suffer.

Currently, there is no robustly tested or validated pain scoring system for cats. In a recent survey, only 8.1% of practices were using a pain scoring system, yet 80.3% of veterinary nurses agreed that they are useful clinical tools. It is clear that pain assessments must be based on behavior rather than on objective measures, such as heart rate, blood pressure, plasma cortisol, or β-endorphin values[15–17]; however, pressure platform gait analysis can be used in cats for studying acute musculoskeletal pain and the effect of analgesic intervention, and this does seem to be a reliable objective measure.[18–20] There is no question that as more studies focus on analyzing pain behaviors in cats, our ability to recognize pain is going to improve; we must accept that it is currently a subjective and inaccurate science, but ignoring pain simply because it is difficult to measure is not an option.

Any pain scoring system that is adopted for use must be reliable, sensitive, and also simple and quick to perform in a busy clinical setting. There are many to choose from, including simple descriptive scales, numeric rating scales, and visual analog scales (VASs). It is now accepted that systems that include behavior assessments and observation and interaction with the animal are most reliable. Knowledge of normal behavior for the individual being evaluated is essential; often, owners and animal technicians who spend a lot of time with the animal are the best judges. Deviations from normal behavior suggest pain, anxiety, fear, or some combination of stressors. In acute pain states, wound sensitivity has correlated well with visual analog pain scores in cats,[21] suggesting that this simple clinically applicable technique is a valuable tool and should be incorporated into an overall assessment protocol.

Signs that have been suggested as indicative of pain in cats include a hunched posture with the head held low, squinted eyes, sitting quietly and seeking no attention, trying to hide, or resentment at being handled. Waran and colleagues[22] have analyzed the behavior of cats before and after ovariohysterectomy using a detailed ethogram. In that study, the display of "half-tucked-up" and "crouching" postures was correlated with abdominal pain. Excessive licking or biting at a surgical incision should initiate a prompt reassessment for pain. A cat sitting quietly in the back of the cage after surgery may be painful and ignored by caretakers if it is believed that signs of pain are always overt. Interacting with the cat to assess its interest in its surroundings and caregivers and gentle wound palpation or palpation of the suspected source of pain (eg, the abdomen in cases of pancreatitis or cystitis) to make a final decision is a good approach. A simple descriptive score (SDS) based on the cat's response to an observer approaching, its back being stroked, and its response to wound palpation (VASs) and dynamic interactive visual analog scales (DIVASs) can be used by a trained observer to differentiate between control (no surgery), cats that did have surgery, and treated and untreated cats.[15,21] Although interaction is ideal, this is impossible in some cats because of their socialization status (eg, feral cats) or because they are too painful. In these situations, analgesics should still be given if an injury or surgery has occurred; in most cases, there is an improvement in their overall behavior and they often become less hostile. Monitoring the response to a "test" dose of analgesic is also recommended when one is not sure if a cat is in pain.

Once the effects of anesthesia have worn off, cats should perform normal tasks, such as grooming and climbing into a litter box, if they are comfortable. Some cats dislike bandages, especially if they are restrictive, and respond by shaking their legs, biting at the bandage, or throwing themselves around. These reactions could indicate pain or dislike of the bandage; thus, it is important to differentiate between the two by palpation. Pain assessment after surgery should be an integral part of care just as temperature, pulse, and respiration are. In general, the more frequent the observations, the more likely it is that subtle signs of pain may be detected, but this must be weighed against what is practical.

Cats may experience chronic pain associated with dental and gum disease, cancer, interstitial cystitis, chronic wounds, dermatitis, and OA; of these, the latter has received the most attention. The behavioral changes that accompany OA may be insidious and easily missed or assumed to be inevitable with advancing age. Lameness in cats is not a common owner complaint or a common clinical sign related to OA in cats, but changes in behavior, including decreased grooming, reluctance to jump up on favorite places, and soiling outside the litter box, should prompt the veterinarian to look for sources of chronic pain. Other changes that owners may report in some cats are altered sleeping habits (an increase or decrease), less activity, withdrawing from human interaction, hiding, and dislike of being stroked or brushed.

In a prospective clinical trial, alterations in the cat's ability to jump and the height of the jump were the most frequent signs of feline OA (seen in 67%–71% of cats), but stiffness and lower activity levels were also noted by owners.[9] Lascelles and colleagues[23,24] hypothesized that cats with OA would have lower activity levels and used a validated accelerometer-based activity monitor to test this theory. After treatment with a nonsteroidal anti-inflammatory drug (NSAID), activity levels did increase and this was reflected in a client-specific questionnaire. A small activity monitor can be mounted on the cat's collar and is a valuable tool for assessing treatment outcomes.

DRUG METABOLISM

Cats have a low capacity to handle drugs that require hepatic glucuronidation, which has been explained by molecular genetic studies.[25–27] Domestic cats have fewer hepatic UDP-glucuroninosyltransferase (UGT) isoforms, which represent major phase II drug-metabolizing enzymes, as a result of mutations of UGT and the presence of pseudogenes. It is suggested that because cats are carnivores, they had no evolutionary need to develop systems that metabolized the phytoalexins, a group of compounds found in cruciferous plants. The clinical consequence of this is twofold: toxic side effects may occur if doses and dosing intervals are not adjusted, or, alternatively, if the parent compound is metabolized to an active component by way of this pathway, the drug may be less effective. The cat's susceptibility to toxic side effects of phenolic drugs, such as acetaminophen (paracetamol), and the long half-life of aspirin can be explained by the deficient glucuronidation pathway. A goal of future feline research should be to focus on identifying analgesic drugs that do not depend on the glucuronidation pathway.

ANALGESIC DRUGS

The "classic" analgesic drug categories include the opioids, NSAIDs, and local anesthetics. α_2-Agonists provide analgesia in addition to sedation and muscle relaxation. Other drugs with potential as analgesic agents in cats include ketamine and other *N*-methyl-D-aspartate (NMDA) inhibitors, such as amantadine, and the tricyclic antidepressants amitriptyline and clomipramine, the anticonvulsant agent gabapentin, and tramadol.

OPIOIDS

This section discusses some general features of opioids unique to cats and also covers individual drugs and different routes of administration.

There are many causes of acute pain in cats, including surgery, trauma, procedural pain, and several medical conditions, such as pancreatitis, peritonitis, and cystitis. Because of their efficacy, good safety margin, and versatility, opioids comprise the backbone of acute pain management in most species, including human beings.

The lethal dose of individual opioids is not well documented in the cat, but in the rat, the median lethal dose of morphine is 64 mg/kg and it is 234 mg/kg for buprenorphine,[28] which are 32 times and greater than 4000 times the recommended analgesic dose, respectively. The safety of opioids is also enhanced by their reversibility with specific antagonists, such as naloxone or naltrexone.

EVALUATION OF OPIOIDS IN THE CAT

In the laboratory setting, opioids have been studied in cats using various noxious stimulus models and measuring changes in the threshold to the stimulus before and after drug administration. Although this is a measure of antinociception and these stimuli are not the same as clinical pain, these studies have been useful for measuring onset time and intensity and duration of antinociception produced by opioids, and they have also been used to study the influence of various routes of drug administration. The models used include thermal,[29] mechanical,[30] electrical,[31] and visceral[32] stimulation. Another method has been the measurement of the minimum alveolar concentration (MAC) of inhalant anesthetic agents. This is an indirect method based on the assumption that because the technique involves a noxious stimulus (electrical or mechanical) applied to the anesthetized animal, a reduction in MAC after administering a putative analgesic supports its efficacy. Many opioids with clear analgesic properties in conscious cats are not MAC sparing, and these studies should no longer be used to evaluate analgesics,[33] at least in this species.

SIDE EFFECTS OF OPIOIDS

It is a misconception that all opioids cause excitement or so-called "morphine mania" in cats. Unfortunately, this fear of excitement has been one of the reasons why practitioners have historically been hesitant to use opioids in cats. Such reports were based on early literature when excessive doses, far in excess of those required to provide analgesia, were administered.[34] With appropriate dosing, the behavioral effects usually include euphoria, with purring, rolling, and kneading with the front paws.

The practitioner should be aware of opioid-related hyperthermia in cats. At doses of morphine greater than 1.0 mg/kg, cats may become hyperthermic,[35] and pethidine (meperidine) at three times clinically recommended doses resulted in temperatures as high as 41.7°C (107°F).[36] Alfentanil infusions in anesthetized cats resulted in significantly elevated rectal temperatures,[37] and in a clinical study of cats undergoing onychectomy, those treated with a transdermal fentanyl (TDF) patch had higher rectal temperatures than those given butorphanol.[38] In a retrospective clinical study,[39] there was a strong association between the use of hydromorphone (at 0.05–0.1 mg/kg administered intravenously, intramuscularly, or subcutaneously on one or more occasions) and hyperthermia (defined as a rectal temperature >40°C [104°F]). Rectal temperatures higher than 40°C (104°F) were recorded in 75% of the cats that received hydromorphone, and a peak temperature of 42.5°C (108.5°F) occurred in one cat. In a research setting, hydromorphone at a dose of 0.1 mg/kg administered intravenously was associated with a significant increase in skin temperature, whereas doses of 0.025 and 0.05 mg/kg were not.[40] In a prospective clinical study, hydromorphone was implicated in perianesthetic hyperthermia in feline patients, although it may occur with other drugs.[41]

Opioids cause marked mydriasis in cats; this may cause them to bump into objects, and they may not see a handler approaching. For these reasons, approach slowly while talking to the cat so that it is not startled. Also, keep them out of bright light while their pupils are dilated.

Vomiting and salivation (which suggest nausea) are seen after morphine and hydromorphone injection but are uncommon after administration of butorphanol, buprenorphine, fentanyl, meperidine, or methadone. The incidence of nausea and vomiting is also related to the route of administration; subcutaneous hydromorphone results in a higher incidence of vomiting than the intravenous or intramuscular route.[42] When administered to painful cats or in combination with acepromazine, the incidence of opioid-induced vomiting is considerably less.

The effects on bowel function of pain itself and of analgesics and sedatives used clinically must be considered. Pain can cause bowel stasis, abdominal distention, discomfort, and vomiting, all of which add to a patient's overall misery. Analgesic intervention often results in a dramatic improvement, but opioids are known to decrease bowel motility, especially with long-term use. Intramuscular acepromazine (0.1 mg/kg) combined with buprenorphine (0.01 mg/kg) or medetomidine (50 μg/kg) alone provided good restraint without altering orocecal transit time in cats, whereas ketamine (5 mg/kg) and midazolam (0.1 mg/kg) did decrease gastrointestinal motility.[43] The effects of opioids on bowel function may be opioid-specific and related to dose and duration, but there are few scientific data available for cats. In this author's experience, constipation associated with opioid use is uncommon in cats. Cats receiving opioids should be well hydrated to counteract any potential constipating effects.

INDIVIDUAL VARIATION

Individual variability in the pharmacokinetics and pharmacodynamics effects of opioids has been demonstrated in many species, and this variability seems to be multifactorial, with gender, genotype, and type of noxious stimulus affecting an individual's response. It is now apparent that individuals are unique with respect to number, morphology, and distribution of opioid receptors and that these differences are genetically determined.[44] Klepstad and colleagues[45] discussed that even for one drug (morphine), genetic variability in patient response is multifactorial and involves genes that code for the enzymes that metabolize morphine, the μ-opioid receptors, and blood-brain barrier transporters. Pharmacogenetics is an increasingly important emerging area of research related to analgesia.

The morphology and sequencing of feline opioid receptors have not been extensively studied compared with other species,[46] but in controlled research environments, marked variation in analgesic response to opioids has been reported, suggesting that cats also express genetic variability. In two independent studies of butorphanol in cats using a thermal antinociceptive model, investigators demonstrated significant intercat differences in intensity and duration of effect.[13,14] Individual variability in response to butorphanol was also noted in a visceral nociception model, wherein the duration of effect varied from 0 to at least 360 minutes in individual cats.[47] As stated previously, this underscores the importance of carefully assessing pain in cats, because one analgesic at a set dose is unlikely to be equally effective in all patients.

DOSE-RELATED EFFECTS

In the literature, wide ranges of doses of opioids are often suggested with little foundation. The effect of dose on onset, duration, and intensity of effect is difficult to compare among studies because of the individual variation among cats. Two randomized crossover dose-response studies using a thermal threshold model have been published. In both, the intravenous route of administration was used to avoid any differences in absorption, uptake, distribution, or metabolism among cats. The first study examined doses of 0.1, 0.2, 0.4, and 0.8 mg/kg of butorphanol.[13] Results indicated that the duration of the antinociceptive action of butorphanol was 90 minutes and that there was no dose-response relation in cats, supporting the assumption that butorphanol is an agonist-antagonist opioid and rapidly reaches a ceiling effect. Wegner and Robertson[40] concluded that doses of hydromorphone less than 0.1 mg/kg have a minimal effect and that perhaps a critical number of opioid receptors must be occupied before a response is measurable. More studies are needed with other opioids to determine the relation between dose and intensity and duration of effect.

ROUTES OF ADMINISTRATION

In a hospital setting, the intravenous, intramuscular, and subcutaneous routes of administration are most commonly used. Studies comparing opioids given by the intravenous and intramuscular routes show that the route of administration does influence pharmacokinetic variables.[48] What we are most interested in, however, is the pharmacodynamic effect of opioids, and, with respect to the route of administration, this has not been extensively studied in cats. The subcutaneous route is attractive in cats because it is simpler than an intravenous injection and less painful than an intramuscular injection. The route of administration of hydromorphone affects the onset time, intensity of effect, and duration of antinociceptive effects, with the subcutaneous route being the least effective.[42]

Oral Administration

Administering pills orally to cats is notoriously difficult, and in most species, oral administration of opioids results in greatly reduced plasma levels because of "first-pass" hepatic metabolism. For these reasons, the oral route of administration of opioids has not received much attention. One exception is tramadol, which has some opioid effects and good oral bioavailability.

Transdermal Delivery Systems

There has been great interest in transdermal delivery of drugs because this may offer a "hands-off" approach to pain management and could provide a constant delivery of drug, thereby avoiding the peaks and troughs seen with intermittent bolus administration. These systems are also attractive for cats that are difficult to handle. Fentanyl and buprenorphine are available in a transdermal patch formulation and are discussed elsewhere in this article. Despite their widespread use and promotion by compounding pharmacies, the claims of efficacy of transdermal formulations of creams containing opioids designed to be rubbed into the skin of cats have not been scientifically supported.[49]

Transmucosal Uptake

Based on reports of the efficacy of transmucosal uptake of buprenorphine in human beings, studies in cats were conducted and showed almost 100% bioavailability of the injectable formulation when placed on oral mucus membranes.[50,51] It was also found to be well tolerated and as effective as the intravenous route when assessed using a thermal threshold model.[51]

Epidural Administration

Morphine, buprenorphine, fentanyl, meperidine (pethidine), and methadone have been administered by means of the epidural route in cats. In a laboratory-based study, fentanyl only resulted in an increase in pain threshold at the 20-minute test point.[31] Epidural buprenorphine and morphine did not decrease the MAC of isoflurane-anesthetized cats,[52] whereas epidural morphine decreased the MAC of halothane by up to 42% in dogs.[53] In conscious cats, however, epidural morphine (100 μg/kg) had significant antinociceptive effects lasting up to 16 hours.[54] The effects of buprenorphine are dose related, with 12.5 μg/kg lasting 10 hours in one study[54] and 20 μg/kg lasting up to 24 hours in another (P.V. Steagall, personal communication, 2007).

In a clinical setting, morphine seems to be the most clinically useful epidural opioid in terms of analgesia achieved and duration of action, although in a clinical review, 2 of 23 cats that received epidural morphine had urinary retention.[55]

SPECIFIC OPIOIDS

Butorphanol

Butorphanol is a μ-antagonist that produces analgesia through its κ-agonist activity. It is commonly used in cats in North America and is generally given at doses from 0.1 to 0.4 mg/kg,[56] but its analgesic properties have been questioned in dogs and cats.[57] Butorphanol exhibits a "ceiling" effect after which increasing the dose does not produce any further analgesia[13]; after intravenous administration, there were no significant differences in thermal antinociception produced with 0.1, 0.2, 0.4, or 0.8 mg/kg. In an experimental visceral pain model (rectal distention with a balloon),[47] the most effective intravenous dose of butorphanol was 0.1 mg/kg, which produced analgesia for 350 ± 10 minutes, and the most effective subcutaneous dose was 0.4 mg/kg, which resulted in 298 ± 45 minutes of analgesia. The same investigators could only demonstrate somatic antinociception after high doses of intravenous butorphanol.

Clinical impressions and experimental investigations indicate that butorphanol is short acting (<90 minutes)[13,57,58] and requires frequent dosing to be effective. Butorphanol seems to be a poor analgesic choice in the face of somatic and visceral pain but would be a reasonable choice for acute visceral pain, such as that associated with acute cystitis or enteritis; however, if pain relief is not achieved, giving additional doses may be of no value.

Buprenorphine

Buprenorphine is the most popular opioid used in small animal practices in the United Kingdom,[59] where it now has market authorization for use in cats, and it is also widely used in the rest of Europe, Australia, and South Africa.[60,61] Intramuscular doses of

0.01 mg/kg resulted in a slow onset (2 hours) of analgesia with a variable duration ranging from 4 to 12 hours.[58] At a dose of 0.02 mg/kg administered intramuscularly, the thermal threshold was significantly increased from 35 minutes to 5 hours after treatment.[14] Systemic uptake of buprenorphine after oral transmucosal (OTM) dosing is almost 100% complete.[50,51] The pH of the cat's mouth is between 8 and 9, which would enhance absorption, and this may explain the effectiveness of this route in cats compared with other species with a neutral oral pH. There was no difference in the onset of analgesia (within 30 minutes), time to peak effect (90 minutes), or duration of action (6 hours) when 0.02 mg/kg was administered by the intravenous or OTM route in research cats.[51]

In clinical studies, buprenorphine produced better analgesia than morphine in cats undergoing a variety of soft tissue and orthopedic procedures,[62] was superior to oxymorphone for sterilization (with or without onychectomy),[63] and provided longer pain relief than meperidine (pethidine) after ovariohysterectomy.[64] Buprenorphine rarely causes vomiting or dysphoria and has not been associated with hyperthermia.[39]

A transdermal (matrix patch) delivery system for buprenorphine (Transtec; Napp Pharmaceuticals, Cambridge, United Kingdom) is now available for use in human beings. In cats, there was systemic uptake after application of a 35-μg/h patch, but plasma concentrations were quite variable, and over a 4-day period, no effective analgesia was demonstrated.[65] These investigators concluded that, similar to constant rate infusions (CRIs), a "loading dose" of buprenorphine may be required at the time of patch application to achieve a steady-state plasma concentration and to create a gradient between plasma and the central nervous system or that a patch with a greater delivery rate may be required.

Fentanyl

Fentanyl is a potent short-acting pure μ-agonist that is commonly used clinically as a CRI,[66] although there are no published data on the pharmacokinetic profile of fentanyl over time when administered in this fashion to cats. In a cat-specific study, 10 μg/kg (administered intravenously) provided rapid onset (peak action <5 minutes) of significant analgesia that lasted 110 minutes, with no excitement, salivation, or vomiting.[49] In that study, plasma fentanyl concentrations and analgesia were closely correlated, and it was concluded that at a plasma value of greater than 1.07 ng/mL, fentanyl provides analgesia similar to that reported for dogs.[67] Fentanyl is an excellent choice in many critical care or postsurgery situations, because the infusion rate can be quickly adjusted up or down to meet the individual needs of the patient. In addition, the use of fentanyl alone rarely causes dysphoria; the usual response is a cat that is calm, comfortable, and kneading and purring.

TDF patches have been used for acute perioperative pain in cats.[38,68,69] Plasma fentanyl concentrations are variable in cats after patch placement,[38,68] and in one study,[70] two of six cats never achieved plasma fentanyl concentrations greater than 1 ng/mL. Factors affecting plasma levels include the size of the patch compared with the weight of the cat, skin permeability, and body temperature. In critical care patients, hypothermia, hypovolemia, and diminished skin perfusion decrease absorption. Because intravenous access is available in these patients, instituting a CRI of fentanyl is a much better choice for the reasons outlined previously. In normothermic (38°C) cats, mean serum levels were 1.83 ± 0.63 ng/mL compared with 0.59 ± 0.30 ng/mL in hypothermic (35°C) animals.[71] In cats weighing less than 4 kg, placement of a 25-μg/h patch with full exposure of the adhesive layer resulted in a steady-state plasma concentration of 1.78 ± 0.92 ng/mL compared with 1.14 ± 0.86 ng/mL when only one half of the adhesive was exposed.[72] For extremely small cats or kittens, a 12.5-μg/h patch can be used. In general, cats achieve a steady-state plasma concentration within 6 to 12 hours after patch placement,[73] and this persists for up to 18 to 20 hours[70] after removal. During the uptake phase, other opioids must be administered to provide analgesia, and all except butorphanol, which may antagonize fentanyl, could be used. The TDF patches have proved useful in cats undergoing onychectomy or ovariohysterectomy.[38,68,69] In dogs, the use of fentanyl patches did not provide better analgesia and increased the cost to the client compared with a systemically administered opioid;[74] a similar comparison has not been made for cats.

Hydromorphone

Hydromorphone has become popular in veterinary medicine and has, to a great extent, replaced oxymorphone because it is less expensive.[75] The relation between dose and thermal antinociception after intravenous hydromorphone administration has been studied in cats; at doses of 0.025 and 0.05 mg/kg, there was a small increase in thermal antinociception of short duration,[40] whereas an intravenous dose of 0.1 mg/kg produced a substantial increase in thermal antinociception for up to 7 hours.[40,76] The route of administration has a significant effect on quality and duration of analgesia and on side effects. When the analgesic and side effects of 0.1 mg/kg given by the intravenous, intramuscular, or subcutaneous route were compared, the intravenous route produced the greatest intensity and duration of antinociceptive effect with the least incidence of vomiting and salivation.[42] The incidence of hyperthermia associated with the use of hydromorphone in cats,[39,41] as discussed previously in this article, has limited its use by some veterinarians in clinical practice.

Meperidine (Pethidine)

Meperidine (pethidine) is only given by the intramuscular or subcutaneous route because of reports of excitement after intravenous dosing. In clinical studies (3.3–10 mg/kg administered intramuscularly), it seems to be effective and has a fast onset but short duration of action.[77,78] Research studies suggest that at 5 mg/kg, its duration of action is less than 1 hour.[29]

Methadone

Methadone is a synthetic opioid agonist but also has activity as an NMDA antagonist. It is widely used to manage cancer pain and neuropathic-type pain with considerable success in human patients. In people, this opioid is unusual in that it has good oral bioavailability and a long elimination half-life, making it convenient for "at-home" use. In dogs, the pharmacokinetic profile of methadone was quite different from that of people, with low oral bioavailability, rapid clearance, and a short elimination half-life.[79] The pharmacokinetic profile of this drug has not been reported in cats.

Racemic methadone has been evaluated in cats in a research setting,[80] and it and levo-methadone have been assessed around the time of surgery in clinical cases.[81,82] In one study, 0.2 mg/kg of methadone given subcutaneously increased the thermal threshold at 1 to 3 hours and the mechanical threshold from 45 to 60 minutes after administration.[80]

Racemic methadone (0.6 mg/kg administered intramuscularly) and levo-methadone (0.3 mg/kg administered intramuscularly) given before surgery provided effective analgesia as judged by assessment of behavior and palpation of the wound in cats after ovariectomy and without adverse behavioral, respiratory, or cardiovascular side effects.[81] Levo-methadone (0.3 mg/kg administered every 8 hours for 5 days, beginning at extubation) was not as effective as carprofen or buprenorphine in cats after major orthopedic surgery and was associated with excitement in some cats.[82]

Morphine

Morphine has been widely used in cats, and doses of 0.1 to 0.2 mg/kg are effective in clinical cases and do not cause excitement.[83] Clinically[83] and in research models,[58] onset of action is slow. Morphine seems to be less effective in cats compared with dogs, and this may be related to cats' limited production of the active morphine metabolite morphine-6-glucuronide (M-6-G),[48] which may contribute significantly to morphine's overall analgesic effect in human beings. M-6-G could only be detected in three of six cats after intravenous administration and was not measurable after intramuscular dosing.[48] It may be that higher doses of morphine would be more beneficial in cats because of the primary dependence on the parent compound to produce analgesia.

Nalbuphine

Nalbuphine is classified as an opioid agonist-antagonist, and although it was popular in the past, it is not as widely used in cats today. Using an electrical stimulus to evaluate somatic antinociception, Sawyer and Rech[47] could not demonstrate any effects at doses ranging from 0.75 to 1.5 mg/kg administered intravenously. They were able to demonstrate a dose-related effect on visceral pain thresholds: 3.0 mg/kg administered intravenously had a duration of effect of 180 ± 39 minutes.

Oxymorphone

Oxymorphone has been a popular analgesic for many years in the United States.[84] Clinically, oxymorphone does not seem to be associated with hyperthermia, vomiting and nausea, or adverse behavioral effects, but it was not as effective as buprenorphine for postoperative pain control after onychectomy with or without castration or ovariohysterectomy.[63]

COMBINATIONS OF OPIOIDS

The combinations of oxymorphone and butorphanol,[32] hydromorphone and butorphanol,[85] and buprenorphine and butorphanol[14] have been reported in cats. The rationale behind these studies is to combine the attributes of each drug in the combination and to minimize the side effects of each. Multiple combinations are possible, given the dose range of each drug. The results of these combinations were quite different, however, and may be a result of actual drug effects or the doses of each used. Low doses of oxymorphone and butorphanol in combination produced greater levels of antinociception than when used individually.[32] The addition of butorphanol (0.4 mg/kg administered intramuscularly) to hydromorphone (0.1 mg/kg administered intramuscularly) decreased the intensity of antinociception during the first 2 hours but extended the duration of observable antinociception from 5.75 to 9 hours.[85] A combination of 0.2 mg/kg of butorphanol administered intramuscularly and 0.02 mg/kg of buprenorphine administered intramuscularly had no demonstrable advantages over either drug used alone.[14] In this author's opinion, mixing of opioids in a clinical situation often results in unpredictable effects.

CONSTANT RATE INFUSION OF OPIOIDS

Fentanyl, alfentanil, sufentanil, and remifentanil are used as infusions in human beings and several domestic species. CRIs are used as part of a balanced anesthetic protocol, with other injectable agents, such as propofol, or with inhalant agents. They can also be used in conscious cats to provide continuous analgesia and avoid the peaks and troughs and break-through pain associated with intermittent bolus administration. Ideally, target-controlled infusion rates based on pharmacokinetic data and a plasma concentration-effect relation should be used.

Fentanyl is the drug used most often in a clinical setting, yet there are no data on the influence of inhalant anesthetics or propofol on its metabolism in cats. In a prospective randomized study of injured cats requiring surgery, it was concluded that fentanyl (CRI of 20 μg/kg/h) and propofol (12 mg/kg/h) provided better cardiovascular stability than isoflurane and fentanyl but required intermittent positive-pressure ventilation to maintain end-tidal carbon dioxide (CO_2) values less than 50 mm Hg.[86] In conscious cats, fentanyl CRI (2–4 μg/kg/h, increased to 10 μg/kg/h when needed) is a versatile and effective way to manage pain. Target-controlled infusions of alfentanil have been studied in isoflurane-anesthetized research cats [37] and were associated with an increase in rectal temperature, metabolic acidosis, decrease in PaO_2, and excitement during recovery if the cats were handled. Combinations of propofol with fentanyl, alfentanil, or sufentanil provided satisfactory anesthesia in a research setting using a noxious stimulus to evaluate depth of anesthesia.[87] Although it is not possible to compare infusion rates of alfentanil between the studies by Ilkiw and colleagues[37] and Mendes and Selmi[87] because of different methodologies, the latter investigators reported hypothermia and not hyperthermia.

The pharmacokinetics and analgesic effects of remifentanil have recently been reported in cats.[33,88] Elimination is rapid, but isoflurane does alter its disposition;[88] therefore, different infusion rates may be required in conscious versus anesthetized cats. At an infusion rate of 1.6 μg/kg/min, significant analgesia was achieved in awake cats without excitement, but infusion rates as high as 16 μg/kg/min did not change the MAC of isoflurane.[33] Correa and colleagues[89] were able to perform ovariohysterectomies in cats using propofol (0.3 mg/kg/min) combined with remifentanil (0.2 μg/kg/min), but recovery was prolonged, taking up to 140 minutes for some cats to stand.

LONG-TERM USE OF OPIOIDS

Little is known about long-term use of opioids in cats, including the issue of dependency. Side effects, such as euphoria, dilated pupils, and inappetence, can be problematic. The use of opioid antagonists that work only at peripheral sites to antagonize undesirable systemic effects but not centrally mediated analgesia shows great promise in human beings[90] but has not been widely explored in veterinary medicine.

TRAMADOL

Although not classified as an opioid, tramadol has weak binding affinity at μ-receptors and is also thought to interact with noradrenergic and serotonergic systems. Tramadol does produce opioid-like behavior in cats, and mydriasis occurs. It is available as injectable and oral formulations and is also sold in combination with acetaminophen (paracetamol), which must not be used in cats. Until recently, the use of tramadol in cats has been empiric, but new pharmacokinetic data[91] should lay the foundation for selecting doses for clinical evaluation. A dose of 1 mg/kg administered subcutaneously failed to provide thermal antinociception in research cats,[92] but compared with postoperative tolfenamic acid alone, premedication with tramadol (4 mg/kg administered subcutaneously) improved the comfort level of cats for the first 8 hours after ovariohysterectomy.[93] Oral tramadol is 62% bioavailable, and peak plasma concentration is reached at 45 minutes; however, compared with its use in dogs,[94] it is slowly eliminated in cats.[91] These features make it a good candidate for long-term treatment of cats in their home environment, and the pharmacokinetic data suggest that the dose should be lower and the dosing interval longer than those used in dogs. There are no published studies on the use of tramadol for chronic pain in cats, but anecdotal reports suggest it is worth pursuing.

EPIDURAL ADMINISTRATION OF OPIOIDS

Opioids exert their major analgesic effect in the dorsal horn of the spinal cord, and intrathecal or epidural administration provides long-lasting analgesia with fewer systemic side effects. Morphine (0.1 mg/kg), fentanyl (4 μ/kg), pethidine, and methadone have been used successfully by way of the epidural route in cats.[31,55,95–98] Morphine is probably the most appropriate with regard to duration of action and quality of analgesia combined with the fewest systemic effects. Epidural injection is technically more challenging in cats because of their small size, and because the spinal cord ends more caudally, entering the subarachnoid space is more likely. If this occurs, half of the epidural dose may still be administered.[66]

NONSTEROIDAL ANTI-INFLAMMATORY DRUGS

The use of this group of analgesics in cats has recently been extensively reviewed.[99] They can provide up to 24 hours of analgesia and are not subject to the legal regulations of opioids. These drugs act to inhibit cyclo-oxygenase (COX) enzymes, and because there is considerable species variation in COX expression, the efficacy and safety of a drug in one species cannot be assumed in another. It was believed that COX-1 was responsible for normal homeostatic functions, such as maintenance of gastric mucosal integrity, platelet function, and renal autoregulation, whereas COX-2 was associated with inflammation. The development of COX-2–selective, or –preferential, NSAIDs was hailed as a breakthrough in preventing toxicity from these drugs, but continued reports of problems associated with their use suggest that the simple COX-1/COX-2 concept is flawed and much more complex than previously believed. It is now known that constitutive COX-2 is produced in the kidney and central nervous system in some species and is required for normal function.

As a group, NSAIDs have a lower safety margin than opioids or α_2-agonists and are not reversible. There is potential for toxicity with NSAID use in cats because their limited ability to glucuronidate exogenous drugs results in prolonged duration of effect with the potential for drug accumulation. The mean half-life of carprofen in cats is approximately 20 hours, twice that of the dog, but it can vary from as short as 9 hours up to 49 hours.[100,101] Meloxicam seems to be metabolized by oxidative enzymes, however, with less variable results.[99] Carprofen, meloxicam, and ketoprofen are now widely used in cats.[64,77,78,102,103]

As in other species, the contraindications to NSAID use are gastrointestinal ulceration or bleeding, platelet dysfunction, renal dysfunction, and concurrent corticosteroid use. Renal autoregulation is prostaglandin dependent in the face of hypotension, and NSAIDs must not be given in the face of volume depletion (vomiting, diarrhea, hemorrhage, or other fluid losses) or in situations, such as sepsis, in which low blood pressure is likely or has been confirmed. Cats seem to be particularly susceptible to the adverse renal effects of NSAIDs.

In some situations, however, for example, the stable normovolemic trauma or surgical patient, these drugs can be valuable for alleviating acute pain. Carprofen has a long history in the United Kingdom, where the injectable formulation (4 mg/kg administered subcutaneously) is licensed for a single treatment; however, lower doses are also effective.[78] There have been reports of gastrointestinal toxicity, generally associated with concurrent disease and prolonged administration of the oral formulation.[104]

Problems with repeated dosing are likely a result of individual variation in pharmacokinetics.

Meloxicam is a COX-2–preferential NSAID with market authorization for use in cats in many countries, including the United States. In the United States, the injectable formulation is approved for a single preoperative dose at 0.3 mg/kg administered subcutaneously. Many veterinarians use lower doses (0.1–0.2 mg/kg) with good effect, and if there are concerns that the cat may become hypotensive or lose blood during surgery, its use can be reserved until the early recovery period without much loss of efficacy; however, if this approach is used, the cat should receive other preoperative analgesics, such as an opioid.

Ketoprofen is available as an injectable formulation, but oral preparations are commonly compounded. The pharmacokinetics and clinical efficacy of ketoprofen are well documented,[64,102,105] and it has been used for up to 5 days to treat cats with musculoskeletal pain.[106] Because it is a potent COX-1 inhibitor, it may interfere with platelet function; therefore, its preoperative use is not recommended.

There seems to be little difference in the efficacy of the NSAIDs described previously for the treatment of acute surgical pain.[102] Comparison of four injectable NSAIDs given subcutaneously at extubation after ovariohysterectomy (carprofen, ketoprofen, meloxicam, and tolfenamic acid) resulted in 9 of 10 cats in each group having desirable overall clinical assessment scores for 18 hours. Despite the cats' apparent comfort, none of the NSAIDs prevented postoperative wound tenderness.[102]

COMPARISON OF OPIOIDS AND NONSTEROIDAL ANTI-INFLAMMATORY DRUGS FOR SURGICAL PAIN

Carprofen and meperidine have been compared when given subcutaneously at the end of surgery. Two hours after ovariohysterectomy, meperidine (10 mg/kg administered intramuscularly) provided better analgesia than carprofen, but from 2 to 20 hours, carprofen was superior and the cats that received carprofen required less "rescue analgesia".[78] Injection of carprofen before castration or ovariohysterectomy was found to be more effective than meperidine given at the end of surgery[77] and seemed to offer good analgesia for 24 hours. A single dose of ketoprofen (2 mg/kg administered subcutaneously) given at the end of anesthesia outperformed a single dose of buprenorphine or meperidine.[64]

LONG-TERM USE OF NONSTEROIDAL ANTI-INFLAMMATORY DRUGS IN CATS

NSAIDs form the basis for managing many types of chronic pain, particularly OA, in most species. Recent data confirm that NSAIDs are also effective for this disease in cats. Clarke and Bennett[9] reported a marked improvement in 61% of cats, a moderate improvement in 14%, and a slight improvement in 25%, as reflected by an increased willingness to jump, the ability to jump higher, a decrease in stiffness, and increased activity within 4 weeks after initiating treatment with oral meloxicam. An increase in activity was recorded in cats diagnosed with OA when they were given meloxicam for 1 week compared with placebo.[23] The approved dosing regimen for chronic use is 0.05 mg/kg/d (Metacam, Ingelheim/Rhein, Germany [0.5 mg/mL] package insert, European Union approval); however, many cats improve on lower doses ($\leq$0.025 mg/kg) or on a dosing regimen of every other day. It is recommended by the author (and others) that after an initial dose of 0.05 mg/kg, the daily dose should be lowered to 0.025 mg/kg or less to identify those cats that are managed with lower dosages—the lowest effective dose should be used. This cautious approach protects cats from potential adverse effects in those that may be susceptible. Compliance is an important issue to address, especially in cats that require long-term treatment and are notoriously difficult for owners to medicate; therefore, it is encouraging that 96% of cats readily accepted meloxicam orally or in their food.[9] In another study, there was no difference in response to treatment between meloxicam and ketoprofen in cats with chronic musculoskeletal disease, but meloxicam was significantly more palatable.[106]

As in dogs, cats receiving NSAIDs for chronic pain should be monitored for side effects related to renal and hepatic function and gastrointestinal erosions. There are no universally accepted monitoring guidelines, but a biochemistry panel, complete blood cell count, and urine analysis before initiating treatment and repeated at 1 and 4 weeks and then at every 4 to 6 months are recommended. Continual reassessment of the patient by the veterinarian and owner is important so that the dose can be tapered to the lowest effective amount, and owners should be educated on the potential side effects and how to recognize these in their cat. The most common side effect of long-term meloxicam administration is intermittent gastrointestinal upset. Vomiting, diarrhea, or both were seen in 18% of cats in one study,[9] whereas only 2% of cats vomited in another report[106]; however, none of these problems persisted, and none were severe enough to warrant withdrawal of the drug.[9]

LOCAL ANESTHETIC DRUGS

Local anesthetics can be used for regional blockade (epidural analgesia), to block specific nerves (intercostal, limbs, and digits [107]), and for infiltration into wounds or fractures (surgical or traumatic).[66,108] The value of these techniques is underestimated, and they are underused in trauma and surgical patients, in which they can provide complete analgesia with minimal side effects.Whenever possible, the clinician should use local anesthetics. Lamont [66] offers a good review of techniques, including brachial plexus block. A particularly useful technique is to implant a "soaker" catheter in a wound (eg, postamputation wound or after large tumor removal) to provide a method for maintaining continuous analgesia. After fibrosarcoma removal in cats, the use of a wound infusion catheter significantly reduced the time the cat was hospitalized, suggesting that this technique improves mobility and time to resume eating (the criteria used for discharge).[109] Lidocaine (2–4 mg/kg) can be repeated every 2 to 3 hours or as needed based on wound palpation. Bupivacaine is longer acting, and 2 mg/kg would be expected to last 4 to 5 hours. Both of these drugs can be diluted with sterile saline to provide a suitable volume. Some researchers recommend a combination of lidocaine plus bupivacaine to achieve a fast onset and longer duration of action; in this case, the total dose of local anesthetic should not exceed 2 mg/kg.

Topical anesthetic creams can be applied to shaved skin to provide analgesia for venipuncture, large-bore catheter placement, bone marrow aspiration, or a variety of other critical care procedures. The two commercially available agents are an over-the-counter liposome-encapsulated formulation of lidocaine (L-M-X; Ferndale Laboratories, Ferndale, Minnesota) and a prescription-only mixture of lidocaine and prilocaine (EMLA cream; AstraZeneca LP, Wilmington, Delaware). Transdermal absorption did occur after application of L-M-X at a dose of 15 mg/kg, but plasma concentrations remained significantly lower than toxic values.[110] There was no systemic uptake of the components of EMLA cream, and its use subjectively eliminated the usual signs of discomfort seen with jugular catheter placement.[111] In another study, 60% of jugular catheters were successfully placed when EMLA cream was used compared with 38% when it was not.[112] Another topical technique is the use of lidocaine patches (Lidoderm 5%, Endo Pharmaceuticals, Chadds Ford, Pennsylvania), which are marketed for alleviating postherpetic neuralgia pain in human patients. Systemic uptake is low in cats, and this technique can provide good wound analgesia and can be used as part of a multimodal approach to pain management.[113]

In dogs, systemic lidocaine infusion has shown beneficial effects as an analgesic in surgical patients[114] and as an anesthetic-sparing technique with no adverse cardiovascular effects.[115,116] In cats, increasing plasma concentrations of lidocaine caused a dose-dependent decrease in isoflurane requirements.[117] Despite a significant reduction in the dose of inhalant agent, lidocaine produced more cardiovascular depression than an equipotent dose of isoflurane alone and was associated with an increase in blood lactate concentration;[118] for these reasons, it cannot be recommended in cats. This study emphasizes once again the importance of species-specific studies.

α_2-ADRENOCEPTOR AGONISTS

This group of drugs, which includes xylazine, medetomidine, and, more recently, dexmedetomidine, provides sedation, muscle relaxation, and analgesia in cats. These drugs are not commonly used for their analgesic effect alone because of the profound sedation and cardiovascular depression that accompanies their use. The use of xylazine should now be discouraged because it has been identified as a risk factor for perioperative mortality in cats, whereas medetomidine has not.[119]

Medetomidine (racemic mixture) and dexmedetomidine (the D-isomer) are excellent when used as part of the anesthetic protocol for healthy surgical patients because they make cats easier to handle, decrease anesthetic requirements,[120] and provide analgesia. Currently, medetomidine is not licensed for use in cats in the United States but dexmedetomidine is. On a mg/kg basis, the dose of dexmedetomidine is half that of medetomidine to achieve the same effect, and similar to medetomidine, atipamezole fully reverses its effects.[121] Dexmedetomidine has been combined with butorphanol and with ketamine, which resulted in better sedation than when it was used alone.[122]

Medetomidine and dexmedetomidine can also be given by CRI; analgesia is dose related, but muscle relaxation is not, and high infusion rates decrease the level of sedation.[123]

After ovariohysterectomy, medetomidine at a dose of 15 μg/kg provided similar pain relief as butorphanol at a dose of 0.1 mg/kg and was better than placebo treatment.[124] In painful and fractious cats, oral administration of medetomidine, which likely results in transmucosal uptake, is a useful technique,[125] and, more recently, dexmedetomidine (40 μg/kg) was effective by the buccal route and analgesia lasted longer compared with the same dose given intramuscularly.[126]

Epidural administration of medetomidine (10 μg/kg) was found to be superior to fentanyl (4 μg/kg),[31] and systemic effects were mild and short-lived.[97] This technique may be an option for cats undergoing caudal abdominal, pelvic, or hind limb surgery.

KETAMINE

Ketamine has traditionally been viewed as a dissociative anesthetic used for chemical restraint in cats. More recently ketamine, an NMDA antagonist, has been studied for its analgesic properties, because spinal NMDA receptors are involved in the process of central sensitization and "wind-up".[127] In a feline research model, a weak visceral analgesic effect of ketamine was reported.[128] Anesthetic protocols incorporating ketamine provide better postoperative analgesia in cats after ovariohysterectomy.[129] Ketamine (2 mg/kg administered intravenously) resulted in a brief increase in thermal antinociception followed by a later period of significant hyperalgesia.[130] It should be noted that in the latter study, cats did not undergo any painful procedures, and the effect of ketamine may be different when used for sedation alone compared with its use in surgical patients. Although popular and effective for reducing postoperative opioid requirements in dogs undergoing major surgery, low-dose ketamine infusions have not been critically evaluated in cats in a clinical setting. Ketamine infusion sufficient to cause unconsciousness abolished arousal as measured by electroencephalography (EEG) and autonomic responses during nociceptive stimulation in cats, but reflex responses to paw pinch remained.[131] These findings suggest that clinical assessment of ketamine's analgesic properties may prove to be difficult.

Other NMDA antagonists, such as amantadine at a dose of 3 to 5 mg/kg administered orally, have been suggested by Gaynor[132] for treating chronic pain in cats, and there are anecdotal reports of its success.

MULTIMODAL APPROACH TO PAIN RELIEF

The use of several different analgesic agents is logical; a multimodal approach may produce better results than a single agent because each drug works at a different part of the pain pathway. In addition, combining drugs may permit lower doses of each to be used. A successful outcome was not correlated to the number of analgesics used in cats after fibrosarcoma removal,[109] but combining a wound infusion catheter with other analgesic agents was beneficial, as reflected in a shorter hospital stay. Recently, the combination of buprenorphine and carprofen performed better than either drug alone for cats undergoing ovariohysterectomy (P.V. Steagall, personal communication, 2007). Other combinations of analgesics remain to be critically evaluated. Widespread clinical experience supports using analgesics from different groups, however.

OTHER ANALGESIC AGENTS AND TREATMENT MODALITIES

Tricyclic antidepressants, including amitriptyline, clomipramine, and imipramine, can provide relief in human beings with chronic neuropathic pain.[133] Amitriptyline (2.5–12.5 mg/kg administered orally once daily) has been used to treat feline interstitial cystitis with few side effects[134] and may be effective for other chronic pain syndromes, including OA and inflammatory bowl disease. The anticonvulsant gabapentin is an effective treatment for neuropathic pain in people;[135] based on individual case reports, this drug shows promise in cats[136] and suggested doses have been published.[132] Interestingly, gabapentin is now also thought to be an effective treatment for postsurgical pain, and when used around the time of surgery, it may reduce the incidence of chronic pain.

Nutraceuticals and chondroprotective agents are widely used in the treatment of OA in cats despite the lack of good evidence-based data in their favor,[137] and "joint diets" are now available for cats.

Many cats tolerate acupuncture, massage, and physical therapy surprisingly well, and these treatment modalities can provide significant pain relief. It is difficult to document the efficacy of acupuncture, because each patient is unique and is treated differently, even if the underlying cause (eg, OA) is the same. Large-scale prospective trials of complimentary therapies should be undertaken in veterinary medicine as they have been in human medicine.

ROUTE AND EASE OF ADMINISTRATION OF ANALGESIC AGENTS

Cats are notoriously difficult to medicate, especially for owners; therefore, route of administration and palatability of analgesic drugs must always be considered to achieve optimal compliance. The efficacy of transmucosal delivery of buprenorphine has been validated,[51] and it is well tolerated; oral meloxicam was easily administered to 96% of cats with OA.[9] Sedation and analgesia can be achieved with buccal dexmedetomidine, which is especially useful for fractious cats.[126] Despite their popularity, there is little evidence to support the use of transdermal creams,[49,138] but further research on this mode of delivery is warranted.

SUMMARY

Great strides continue to be made in the field of feline analgesia. A better understanding of the cat's unique metabolism has led researchers to realize that extrapolation across species boundaries is unwise, and this has resulted in many feline-specific studies. Opioids are now used more commonly in cats with good analgesic effect and few side effects. Excellent acute pain management is achievable in cats by using opioids, NSAIDs, α_2-agonists, and local anesthetics; the latter are the most underused technique. A multimodal approach using agents that work at different places in the pain pathway is encouraged because this can have added benefits, and more studies in this area that look at the best combinations of drug classes are eagerly awaited. Compared with dogs, few pain scoring systems have been developed for cats, and this remains an important goal. Management of chronic pain in cats can be challenging, but there is now an approved NSAID for long-term use, at least in some countries. As we gain experience with less traditional analgesics, such as gabapentin, and critically evaluate complimentary therapies, our ability to provide comfort to this population of cats should improve.

REFERENCES

1. Bernstein P. The human-cat relationship. In: Rochlitz I, editor. The welfare of cats. Dordrecht (The Netherlands): Springer; 2005. p. 47–89.
2. Joubert KE. Anaesthesia and analgesia for dogs and cats in South Africa undergoing sterilisation and with osteoarthritis—an update from 2000. J S Afr Vet Assoc 2006;77(4):224–8.
3. Hewson CJ, Dohoo IR, Lemke KA. Perioperative use of analgesics in dogs and cats by Canadian veterinarians in 2001. Can Vet J 2006;47(4):352–9.
4. Williams VM, Lascelles BD, Robson MC. Current attitudes to, and use of, perioperative analgesia in dogs and cats by veterinarians in New Zealand. N Z Vet J 2005;53(3):193–202.
5. Coleman DL, Slingsby LS. Attitudes of veterinary nurses to the assessment of pain and the use of pain scales. Vet Rec 2007;160(16):541–4.
6. Hellyer P, Rodan I, Brunt J, et al. AAHA/AAFP pain management guidelines for dogs and cats. J Feline Med Surg 2007;9(6):466–80.
7. Godfrey DR. Osteoarthritis in cats: a retrospective radiological study. J Small Anim Pract 2005;46(9):425–9.
8. Clarke SP, Mellor D, Clements DN, et al. Prevalence of radiographic signs of degenerative joint disease in a hospital population of cats. Vet Rec 2005;157(25): 793–9.
9. Clarke SP, Bennett D. Feline osteoarthritis: a prospective study of 28 cases. J Small Anim Pract 2006;47(8):439–45.
10. Hewson CJ, Dohoo IR, Lemke KA. Factors affecting the use of postincisional analgesics in dogs and cats by Canadian veterinarians in 2001. Can Vet J 2006; 47(5):453–9.

11. Paul-Murphy J, Ludders JW, Robertson SA, et al. The need for a cross-species approach to the study of pain in animals. J Am Vet Med Assoc 2004;224(5):692–7.
12. Montagna P. Recent advances in the pharmacogenomics of pain and headache. Neurol Sci 2007;28(Suppl 2):S208–12.
13. Lascelles BD, Robertson SA. Use of thermal threshold response to evaluate the antinociceptive effects of butorphanol in cats. Am J Vet Res 2004;65(8):1085–9.
14. Johnson JA, Robertson SA, Pypendop BH. Antinociceptive effects of butorphanol, buprenorphine, or both, administered intramuscularly in cats. Am J Vet Res 2007;68(7):699–703.
15. Cambridge A, Tobias K, Newberry R, et al. Subjective and objective measurements of postoperative pain in cats. J Am Vet Med Assoc 2000;217(5):685–90.
16. Smith J, Allen S, Quandt J, et al. Indicators of postoperative pain in cats and correlation with clinical criteria. Am J Vet Res 1996;57(11):1674–8.
17. Smith J, Allen S, Quandt J. Changes in cortisol concentration in response to stress and postoperative pain in client-owned cats and correlation with objective clinical variables. Am J Vet Res 1999;60(4):432–6.
18. Romans CW, Conzemius MG, Horstman CL, et al. Use of pressure platform gait analysis in cats with and without bilateral onychectomy. Am J Vet Res 2004;65(9):1276–8.
19. Romans CW, Gordon WJ, Robinson DA, et al. Effect of postoperative analgesic protocol on limb function following onychectomy in cats. J Am Vet Med Assoc 2005;227(1):89–93.
20. Robinson DA, Romans CW, Gordon-Evans WJ, et al. Evaluation of short-term limb function following unilateral carbon dioxide laser or scalpel onychectomy in cats. J Am Vet Med Assoc 2007;230(3):353–8.
21. Slingsby L, Jones A, Waterman-Pearson AE. Use of a new finger-mounted device to compare mechanical nociceptive thresholds in cats given pethidine or no medication after castration. Res Vet Sci 2001;70(3):243–6.
22. Waran N, Best L, Williams V, et al. A preliminary study of behaviour-based indicators of pain in cats. Anim Welf 2007;16(S):105–8.
23. Lascelles BD, Hansen BD, Roe S, et al. Evaluation of client-specific outcome measures and activity monitoring to measure pain relief in cats with osteoarthritis. J Vet Intern Med 2007;21(3):410–6.
24. Lascelles BD, Hansen BD, Thomson A, et al. Evaluation of a digitally integrated accelerometer-based activity monitor for the measurement of activity in cats. [Epub date]. Vet Anaesth Analg Oct 10 2007.
25. Court M, Greenblatt D. Molecular basis for deficient acetaminophen glucuronidation in cats. An interspecies comparison of enzyme kinetics in liver microsomes. Biochem Pharmacol 1997;53(7):1041–7.
26. Court M, Greenblatt D. Biochemical basis for deficient paracetamol glucuronidation in cats: an interspecies comparison of enzyme constraint in liver microsomes. J Pharm Pharmacol 1997;49(4):446–9.
27. Court M, Greenblatt D. Molecular genetic basis for deficient acetaminophen glucuronidation by cats: UGT1A6 is a pseudogene, and evidence for reduced diversity of expressed hepatic UGT1A isoforms. Pharmacogenetics 2000;10(4):355–69.
28. Borron SW, Monier C, Risede P, et al. Flunitrazepam variably alters morphine, buprenorphine, and methadone lethality in the rat. Hum Exp Toxicol 2002;21(11):599–605.

29. Dixon MJ, Robertson SA, Taylor PM. A thermal threshold testing device for evaluation of analgesics in cats. Res Vet Sci 2002;72(3):205–10.
30. Dixon MJ, Taylor PM, Steagall PV, et al. Development of a pressure nociceptive threshold testing device for evaluation of analgesics in cats. Res Vet Sci 2007; 82(1):85–92.
31. Duke T, Cox AM, Remedios AM, et al. The analgesic effects of administering fentanyl or medetomidine in the lumbosacral epidural space of cats. Vet Surg 1994; 23(2):143–8.
32. Briggs SL, Sneed K, Sawyer DC. Antinociceptive effects of oxymorphone-butorphanol-acepromazine combination in cats. Vet Surg 1998;27(5):466–72.
33. Brosnan RJ, Pypendop BH, Siao KT, et al. Effects of remifentanil on measurements of analgesia and anesthetic immobility in cats. Proceedings of the 13th Annual IVECCS Conference. New Orleans: 2007. Available at: http://www.acva.org/professional/abstract/. Accessed December 10, 2007.
34. Fertziger AP, Stein EA, Lynch JJ. Letter: suppression of morphine-induced mania in cats. Psychopharmacologia 1974;36(2):185–7.
35. Clark WG, Cumby HR. Hyperthermic responses to central and peripheral injections of morphine sulphate in the cat. Br J Pharmacol 1978;63(1):65–71.
36. Booth N, Rankin AL. Evaluation of meperidine hydrochloride in the cat. Vet Med 1954;49:249–52.
37. Ilkiw JE, Pascoe PJ, Fisher LD. Effect of alfentanil on the minimum alveolar concentration of isoflurane in cats. Am J Vet Res 1997;58(11):1274–9.
38. Gellasch KL, Kruse-Elliott KT, Osmond CS, et al. Comparison of transdermal administration of fentanyl versus intramuscular administration of butorphanol for analgesia after onychectomy in cats. J Am Vet Med Assoc 2002;220(7):1020–4.
39. Niedfeldt RL, Robertson SA. Postanesthetic hyperthermia in cats: a retrospective comparison between hydromorphone and buprenorphine. Vet Anaesth Analg 2006;33(6):381–9.
40. Wegner K, Robertson SA. Dose-related thermal antinociceptive effects of intravenous hydromorphone in cats. Vet Anaesth Analg 2007;34(2):132–8.
41. Posner LP, Gleed RD, Erb HN, et al. Post-anesthetic hyperthermia in cats. Vet Anaesth Analg 2007;34(1):40–7.
42. Robertson S, Wegner K, Lascelles BDX. Antinociceptive and side-effects of hydromorphone after subcutaneous administration in cats. 2008, JFMS; in press.
43. Sparkes AH, Papasouliotis K, Viner J, et al. Assessment of orocaecal transit time in cats by the breath hydrogen method: the effects of sedation and a comparison of definitions. Res Vet Sci 1996;60(3):243–6.
44. Mogil JS. The genetic mediation of individual differences in sensitivity to pain and its inhibition. Proc Natl Acad Sci U S A 1999;96(14):7744–51.
45. Klepstad P, Dale O, Skorpen F, et al. Genetic variability and clinical efficacy of morphine. Acta Anaesthesiol Scand 2005;49(7):902–8.
46. Billet O, Billaud JN, Phillips TR. Partial characterization and tissue distribution of the feline mu opiate receptor. Drug Alcohol Depend 2001;62(2):125–9.
47. Sawyer DC, Rech RH. Analgesia and behavioral effects of butorphanol, nalbuphine, and pentazocine in the cat. J Am Anim Hosp Assoc 1987;23:438–46.
48. Taylor PM, Robertson SA, Dixon MJ, et al. Morphine, pethidine and buprenorphine disposition in the cat. J Vet Pharmacol Ther 2001;24(6):391–8.
49. Robertson SA, Taylor PM, Sear JW, et al. Relationship between plasma concentrations and analgesia after intravenous fentanyl and disposition after other routes of administration in cats. J Vet Pharmacol Ther 2005;28:1–7.

50. Robertson SA, Taylor PM, Sear JW. Systemic uptake of buprenorphine by cats after oral mucosal administration. Vet Rec 2003;152(22):675–8.
51. Robertson SA, Lascelles BD, Taylor PM, et al. PK-PD modeling of buprenorphine in cats: intravenous and oral transmucosal administration. J Vet Pharmacol Ther 2005;28(5):453–60.
52. Pypendop BH, Pascoe PJ, Ilkiw JE. Effects of epidural administration of morphine and buprenorphine on the minimum alveolar concentration of isoflurane in cats. Am J Vet Res 2006;67(9):1471–5.
53. Valverde A, Dyson DH, McDonell WN. Epidural morphine reduces halothane MAC in the dog. Can J Anaesth 1989;36(6):629–32.
54. Pypendop BH, Siao KT, Pascoe PJ, et al. Effects of epidurally administered morphine or buprenorphine on the thermal threshold in cats. Am J Vet Res 2008; 69(8):983–7.
55. Troncy E, Junot S, Keroack S, et al. Results of preemptive epidural administration of morphine with or without bupivacaine in dogs and cats undergoing surgery: 265 cases (1997–1999). J Am Vet Med Assoc 2002;221(5):666–72.
56. Dohoo SE, Dohoo IR. Postoperative use of analgesics in dogs and cats by Canadian veterinarians. Can Vet J 1996;37(9):546–51.
57. Wagner AE. Is butorphanol analgesic in dogs and cats? Vet Med 1999;94: 346–51.
58. Robertson SA, Taylor PM, Lascelles BD, et al. Changes in thermal threshold response in eight cats after administration of buprenorphine, butorphanol and morphine. Vet Rec 2003;153(15):462–5.
59. Lascelles BD, Capner C, Waterman-Pearson AE. A survey of current British veterinary attitudes to peri-operative analgesia for cats and small mammals. Vet Rec 1999;145(21):601–4.
60. Watson AD, Nicholson A, Church DB, et al. Use of anti-inflammatory and analgesic drugs in dogs and cats. Aust Vet J 1996;74(3):203–10.
61. Joubert KE. The use of analgesic drugs by South African veterinarians. J S Afr Vet Assoc 2001;72(1):57–60.
62. Stanway G, Taylor P, Brodbelt D. A preliminary investigation comparing preoperative morphine and buprenorphine for postoperative analgesia and sedation in cats. Vet Anaesth Analg 2002;29:29–35.
63. Dobbins S, Brown NO, Shofer FS. Comparison of the effects of buprenorphine, oxymorphone hydrochloride, and ketoprofen for postoperative analgesia after onychectomy or onychectomy and sterilization in cats. J Am Anim Hosp Assoc 2002;38(6):507–14.
64. Slingsby LS, Waterman-Pearson AE. Comparison of pethidine, buprenorphine and ketoprofen for postoperative analgesia after ovariohysterectomy in the cat. Vet Rec 1998;143(7):185–9.
65. Murrell JC, Robertson SA, Taylor PM, et al. Use of a transdermal matrix patch of buprenorphine in cats: preliminary pharmacokinetic and pharmacodynamic data. Vet Rec 2007;160(17):578–83.
66. Lamont LA. Feline perioperative pain management. Vet Clin North Am Small Anim Pract 2002;32(4):747–63, v.
67. Robinson TM, Kruse-Elliott KT, Markel MD, et al. A comparison of transdermal fentanyl versus epidural morphine for analgesia in dogs undergoing major orthopedic surgery. J Am Anim Hosp Assoc 1999;35(2):95–100.
68. Franks JN, Boothe HW, Taylor L, et al. Evaluation of transdermal fentanyl patches for analgesia in cats undergoing onychectomy. J Am Vet Med Assoc 2000; 217(7):1013–20.

69. Glerum LE, Egger CM, Allen SW, et al. Analgesic effect of the transdermal fentanyl patch during and after feline ovariohysterectomy. Vet Surg 2001;30(4):351–8.
70. Lee DD, Papich MG, Hardie EM. Comparison of pharmacokinetics of fentanyl after intravenous and transdermal administration in cats. Am J Vet Res 2000;61(6):672–7.
71. Pettifer GR, Hosgood G. The effect of rectal temperature on perianesthetic serum concentrations of transdermally administered fentanyl in cats anesthetized with isoflurane. Am J Vet Res 2003;64(12):1557–61.
72. Davidson CD, Pettifer GR, Henry JD Jr. Plasma fentanyl concentrations and analgesic effects during full or partial exposure to transdermal fentanyl patches in cats. J Am Vet Med Assoc 2004;224(5):700–5.
73. Riviere JE, Papich MG. Potential and problems of developing transdermal patches for veterinary applications. Adv Drug Deliv Rev 2001;50(3):175–203.
74. Egger CM, Glerum L, Michelle Haag K, et al. Efficacy and cost-effectiveness of transdermal fentanyl patches for the relief of post-operative pain in dogs after anterior cruciate ligament and pelvic limb repair. Vet Anaesth Analg 2007;34(3):200–8.
75. Pettifer G, Dyson D. Hydromorphone: a cost-effective alternative to the use of oxymorphone. Can Vet J 2000;41(2):135–7.
76. Wegner K, Robertson SA, Kollias-Baker C, et al. Pharmacokinetic and pharmacodynamic evaluation of intravenous hydromorphone in cats. J Vet Pharmacol Ther 2004;27(5):329–36.
77. Balmer TV, Irvine D, Jones RS, et al. Comparison of carprofen and pethidine as postoperative analgesics in the cat. J Small Anim Pract 1998;39(4):158–64.
78. Lascelles BD, Cripps P, Mirchandani S, et al. Carprofen as an analgesic for postoperative pain in cats: dose titration and assessment of efficacy in comparison to pethidine hydrochloride. J Small Anim Pract 1995;36(12):535–41.
79. Kukanich B, Lascelles BD, Aman AM, et al. The effects of inhibiting cytochrome P450 3A, p-glycoprotein, and gastric acid secretion on the oral bioavailability of methadone in dogs. J Vet Pharmacol Ther 2005;28(5):461–6.
80. Steagall PV, Carnicelli P, Taylor PM, et al. Effects of subcutaneous methadone, morphine, buprenorphine or saline on thermal and pressure thresholds in cats. J Vet Pharmacol Ther 2006;29(6):531–7.
81. Rohrer Bley C, Neiger-Aeschbacher G, Busato A, et al. Comparison of perioperative racemic methadone, levo-methadone and dextromoramide in cats using indicators of post-operative pain. Vet Anaesth Analg 2004;31(3):175–82.
82. Mollenhoff A, Nolte I, Kramer S. Anti-nociceptive efficacy of carprofen, levomethadone and buprenorphine for pain relief in cats following major orthopaedic surgery. J Vet Med A Physiol Pathol Clin Med 2005;52(4):186–98.
83. Lascelles D, Waterman A. Analgesia in cats. In Pract 1997;19(4):203–13.
84. Palminteri A. Oxymorphone, an effective analgesic in dogs and cats. J Am Vet Med Assoc 1963;143:160–3.
85. Lascelles BD, Robertson SA. Antinociceptive effects of hydromorphone, butorphanol, or the combination in cats. J Vet Intern Med 2004;18(2):190–5.
86. Liehmann L, Mosing M, Auer U. A comparison of cardiorespiratory variables during isoflurane-fentanyl and propofol-fentanyl anaesthesia for surgery in injured cats. Vet Anaesth Analg 2006;33(3):158–68.
87. Mendes GM, Selmi AL. Use of a combination of propofol and fentanyl, alfentanil, or sufentanil for total intravenous anesthesia in cats. J Am Vet Med Assoc 2003;223(11):1608–13.

88. Pypendop BH, Brosnan RJ, Siao KT, et al. Pharmacokinetics of remifentanil in conscious and isoflurane anesthetized cats. Proceedings of the 13th Annual IVECCS Conference: New Orleans, 2007. Available at: http://www.acva.org/professional/abstract/. Accessed December 10, 2007.
89. Correa Mdo A, Aguiar AJ, Neto FJ, et al. Effects of remifentanil infusion regimens on cardiovascular function and responses to noxious stimulation in propofol-anesthetized cats. Am J Vet Res 2007;68(9):932–40.
90. Holzer P. Opioids and opioid receptors in the enteric nervous system: from a problem in opioid analgesia to a possible new prokinetic therapy in humans. Neurosci Lett 2004;361(1–3):192–5.
91. Pypendop BH, Ilkiw JE. Pharmacokinetics of tramadol, and its metabolite O-desmethyl-tramadol, in cats. J Vet Pharmacol Ther 2008;31(1):52–9.
92. Steagall PV. Evaluation of subcutaneous tramadol in cats. Presented at the Proceedings of the Association of Veterinary Anaesthetists Autumn Meeting; September 21–23rd. Newmarket: 2005. p. 78.
93. Chen HC, Radzi R, Rahman NA, et al. Analgesic effect of tramadol combined with tolfenamic acid in cats after ovariohysterectomy. Presented at the proceedings of the 13th Annual IVECCS Conference. New Orleans, September 27, 2007.
94. KuKanich B, Papich MG. Pharmacokinetics of tramadol and the metabolite O-desmethyltramadol in dogs. J Vet Pharmacol Ther 2004;27(4):239–46.
95. Tung A, Yaksh T. The antinociceptive effects of epidural opiates in the cat: studies of the pharmacology and the effects of lipophilicity in spinal analgesia. Pain 1982;12(4):343–56.
96. Golder F, Pascoe P, Bailey C, et al. The effect of epidural morphine on the minimum alveolar concentration of isoflurane in cats. Journal of Veterinary Anaesthesia 1998;25(1):52–6.
97. Duke T, Cox AM, Remedios AM, et al. The cardiopulmonary effects of placing fentanyl or medetomidine in the lumbosacral epidural space of isoflurane-anesthetized cats. Vet Surg 1994;23(2):149–55.
98. Jones RS. Epidural analgesia in the dog and cat. Vet J 2001;161(2):123–31.
99. Lascelles BD, Court MH, Hardie EM, et al. Nonsteroidal anti-inflammatory drugs in cats: a review. Vet Anaesth Analg 2007;34(4):228–50.
100. Taylor PM, Delatour P, Landoni FM, et al. Pharmacodynamics and enantioselective pharmacokinetics of carprofen in the cat. Res Vet Sci 1996;60(2):144–51.
101. Parton K, Balmer TV, Boyle J, et al. The pharmacokinetics and effects of intravenously administered carprofen and salicylate on gastrointestinal mucosa and selected biochemical measurements in healthy cats. J Vet Pharmacol Ther 2000;23(2):73–9.
102. Slingsby L, Waterman-Pearson AE. Postoperative analgesia in the cat after ovariohysterectomy by use of carprofen, ketoprofen, meloxicam or tolfenamic acid. J Small Anim Pract 2000;41:447–50.
103. Slingsby L, Waterman-Pearson AE. Comparison between meloxicam and carprofen for postoperative analgesia after feline ovariohysterectomy. J Small Anim Pract 2002;43(7):286–9.
104. Runk A, Kyles A, Downs M. Duodenal perforation in a cat following the administration of nonsteroidal anti-inflammatory medication. J Am Anim Hosp Assoc 1999;35(1):52–5.
105. Lees P, Taylor PM, Landoni FM, et al. Ketoprofen in the cat: pharmacodynamics and chiral pharmacokinetics. Vet J 2003;165(1):21–35.

106. Lascelles B, Henderson A, Hackett I. Evaluation of the clinical efficacy of meloxicam in cats with painful locomotor disorders. J Small Anim Pract 2001;42(12): 587–93.
107. Curcio K, Bidwell LA, Bohart GV, et al. Evaluation of signs of postoperative pain and complications after forelimb onychectomy in cats receiving buprenorphine alone or with bupivacaine administered as a four-point regional nerve block. J Am Vet Med Assoc 2006;228(1):65–8.
108. Duke T. Local and regional anesthetic and analgesic techniques in the dog and cat: part II, infiltration and nerve blocks. Can Vet J 2000;41(12):949–52.
109. Davis KM, Hardie EM, Martin FR, et al. Correlation between perioperative factors and successful outcome in fibrosarcoma resection in cats. Vet Rec 2007;161(6): 199–200.
110. Fransson BA, Peck KE, Smith JK, et al. Transdermal absorption of a liposome-encapsulated formulation of lidocaine following topical administration in cats. Am J Vet Res 2002;63(9):1309–12.
111. Gibbon KJ, Cyborski JM, Guzinski MV, et al. Evaluation of adverse effects of EMLA (lidocaine/prilocaine) cream for the placement of jugular catheters in healthy cats. J Vet Pharmacol Ther 2003;26(6):439–41.
112. Wagner KA, Gibbon KJ, Strom TL, et al. Adverse effects of EMLA (lidocaine/prilocaine) cream and efficacy for the placement of jugular catheters in hospitalized cats. J Feline Med Surg 2006;8(2):141–4.
113. Weil AB, Ko J, Inoue T. The use of lidocaine patches. Compendium 2007;29(4): 208–16.
114. Smith LJ, Bentley E, Shih A, et al. Systemic lidocaine infusion as an analgesic for intraocular surgery in dogs: a pilot study. Vet Anaesth Analg 2004;31(1): 53–63.
115. Muir WW 3rd, Wiese AJ, March PA. Effects of morphine, lidocaine, ketamine, and morphine-lidocaine-ketamine drug combination on minimum alveolar concentration in dogs anesthetized with isoflurane. Am J Vet Res 2003;64(9): 1155–60.
116. Valverde A, Doherty TJ, Hernandez J, et al. Effect of intravenous lidocaine on isoflurane MAC in dogs. Vet Anaesth Analg 2004;31(4):264–71.
117. Pypendop BH, Ilkiw JE. The effects of intravenous lidocaine administration on the minimum alveolar concentration of isoflurane in cats. Anesth Analg 2005; 100(1):97–101.
118. Pypendop BH, Ilkiw JE. Assessment of the hemodynamic effects of lidocaine administered IV in isoflurane-anesthetized cats. Am J Vet Res 2005;66(4):661–8.
119. Brodbelt DC, Pfeiffer DU, Young LE, et al. Risk factors for anaesthetic-related death in cats: results from the confidential enquiry into perioperative small animal fatalities (CEPSAF). Br J Anaesth 2007;99(5):617–23.
120. Mendes GM, Selmi AL, Barbudo-Selmi GR, et al. Clinical use of dexmedetomidine as premedicant in cats undergoing propofol-sevoflurane anaesthesia. J Feline Med Surg 2003;5(5):265–70.
121. Granholm M, McKusick BC, Westerholm FC, et al. Evaluation of the clinical efficacy and safety of dexmedetomidine or medetomidine in cats and their reversal with atipamezole. Vet Anaesth Analg 2006;33(4):214–23.
122. Selmi AL, Mendes GM, Lins BT, et al. Evaluation of the sedative and cardiorespiratory effects of dexmedetomidine, dexmedetomidine-butorphanol, and dexmedetomidine-ketamine in cats. J Am Vet Med Assoc 2003;222(1):37–41.
123. Ansah OB, Raekallio M, Vainio O. Correlation between serum concentrations following continuous intravenous infusion of dexmedetomidine or medetomidine in

cats and their sedative and analgesic effects. J Vet Pharmacol Ther 2000;23(1): 1–8.
124. Ansah OB, Vainio O, Hellsten C, et al. Postoperative pain control in cats: clinical trials with medetomidine and butorphanol. Vet Surg 2002;31(2):99–103.
125. Ansah O, Raekallio M, Vainio O. Comparing oral and intramuscular administration of medetomidine in cats. J vet Anaesth 1998;25(1):41–6.
126. Slingsby LS, Taylor PM, Waterman-Pearson AE. Efficacy of buccal compared to intramuscular dexmedetomidine for antinociception to a thermal nociceptive stimulus in the cat. Presented at the 9th World Congress of Veterinary Anaesthesia: Santos, Brazil. September 12–16, 2006. p. 163.
127. Petrenko AB, Yamakura T, Baba H, et al. The role of N-methyl-D-aspartate (NMDA) receptors in pain: a review. Anesth Analg 2003;97(4):1108–16.
128. Sawyer D, Rech R, Durham RA. Does ketamine provide adequate visceral analgesia when used alone or in combination with acepromazine, diazepam, or butorphanol in cats. J Am Anim Hosp Assoc 1993;29:257–63.
129. Slingsby LS, Lane EC, Mears ER, et al. Postoperative pain after ovariohysterectomy in the cat: a comparison of two anaesthetic regimens. Vet Rec 1998; 143(21):589–90.
130. Robertson S, Lascelles BD, Taylor P. Effect of low dose ketamine on thermal thresholds in cats. Vet Anaesth Analg 2003;30(2):110.
131. Taylor JS, Vierck CJ. Effects of ketamine on electroencephalographic and autonomic arousal and segmental reflex responses in the cat. Vet Anaesth Analg 2003;30(4):237–49.
132. Gaynor JS. Other drugs used to treat pain. In: Gaynor JS, Muir SS, editors. Handbook of veterinary pain management. St. Louis: Mosby; 2008. p. 260–76.
133. Finnerup NB, Otto M, Jensen TS, et al. An evidence-based algorithm for the treatment of neuropathic pain. MedGenMed 2007;9(2):36.
134. Chew DJ, Buffington CA, Kendall MS, et al. Amitriptyline treatment for severe recurrent idiopathic cystitis in cats. J Am Vet Med Assoc 1998;213(9):1282–6.
135. Gilron I. Gabapentin and pregabalin for chronic neuropathic and early postsurgical pain: current evidence and future directions. Curr Opin Anaesthesiol 2007; 20(5):456–72.
136. Lamont LA, Tranquilli WJ, Mathews KA. Adjunctive analgesic therapy. Vet Clin North Am Small Anim Pract 2000;30(4):805–13.
137. Beale BS. Use of nutraceuticals and chondroprotectants in osteoarthritic dogs and cats. Vet Clin North Am Small Anim Pract 2004;34(1):271–89.
138. Marks SL, Taboada J. Transdermal therapeutics. J Am Anim Hosp Assoc 2003; 39(1):19–21.

Pain Management for the Pregnant, Lactating, and Neonatal to Pediatric Cat and Dog

Karol A. Mathews, DVM, DVSc

KEYWORDS

• Pregnant • Lactating • Neonates • Pediatric • Pain • Analgesia

The science and management of pain is extremely broad, and investigation into all aspects takes time. Because most cats and dogs requiring analgesia to manage pain are mature and not pregnant or lactating, it stands to reason that this majority would be studied and emphasized in most textbooks and journal articles. Unfortunately, neonatal, pediatric, and pregnant or lactating animals have received little attention in veterinary investigations. As a consequence, analgesics are often avoided in these animals, because the effects of these drugs on the developing fetus, the nursing animals, and developing young are not known to many. The purpose of this review is to focus on commonly used analgesics and their safety in these animals and to touch on the associated pharmacologic aspects of these drugs.

ANALGESIA FOR PREGNANT DOGS AND CATS

Pregnant animals may incur injury, undergo a surgical procedure, or experience chronic pain, requiring management with analgesics. Unfortunately, there are no clinical studies investigating the safety of any analgesics in the pregnant dog or cat. Although many peri-cesarean section analgesic and anesthetic regimens have been recommended and used with no apparent ill effects, the more subacute to chronic use of analgesics in pregnant dogs and cats has not been studied. A comprehensive source of information cited in relation to analgesia in pregnant women classifies all drugs to risk factor category A, B, C, D, or X based on evidence of risk to the fetus and nursing infant.[1] The A category declares no risk to the fetus, whereas B, C, and D represent progressive risk to the fetus and recommendations for extenuating use. Category X indicates contraindication in women who are or may become pregnant.

Emergency and Critical Care Medicine, Department of Clinical Studies, Ontario Veterinary College, University of Guelph, Guelph, Ontario, Canada N1G 2W1
E-mail address: kmathews@ovc.uoguelph.ca

Vet Clin Small Anim 38 (2008) 1291–1308
doi:10.1016/j.cvsm.2008.07.001 vetsmall.theclinics.com

Because of a lack of appropriate studies in animals and human beings, no drugs are listed in category A. Many studies in pregnant women have shown minimal to no fetal or neonatal compromise, however, with some opioids administered for variable periods.

The pharmacologic features of pregnant animals differ from those of the nonpregnant animal; various physiologic changes associated with the maternal-placental-fetal unit can alter pharmacodynamics, pharmacokinetics, and distribution to the fetus.[2] The maternal factors that may alter drug absorption in women are decreased gastrointestinal motility and esophageal reflux and vomiting in addition to increased cutaneous blood flow, which may enhance absorption of transdermally administered drugs.[2] Whether these factors occur with some frequency, or are applicable to dogs and cats, is not known. Cutaneous blood flow potentially may increase in the late stage of cat and dog pregnancy, and enhanced absorption of transdermal medication may occur in this setting. As total body water is increased with distribution throughout the maternal tissues, amniotic fluid, placenta, and fetus, the volume for distribution of drugs is also increased.[3] Total body fat may also be increased, resulting in a larger volume of distribution for lipid-soluble drugs with less available in the plasma. Reduced serum albumin, which may occur in pregnancy in women, could result in more free normally protein-bound drug, which would then be available for action on maternal receptor sites and transport across the placenta to the fetus. In dogs and cats, however, albumin levels may drop to low normal values, but it is thought that this is secondary to the increased plasma volume and dilution in normal pregnancy and is not attributable to reduced albumin load (Catherine Gartley, personal communication, 2005). Hepatic enzymatic activity may be altered, and renal function is gradually increased with increased elimination of water-soluble drugs and metabolites.[2]

The placental barrier is considered to be a lipoprotein; therefore, drugs with high lipid solubility are permeable.[4] Lipophilic compounds diffuse passively along a concentration gradient to the fetus. Equilibrium is reached as the concentration increases within the fetus, limiting further transport. Drugs that are polar, ionized, protein bound, or water soluble are less likely to cross the placenta into the fetus. Should free drug bind immediately to fetal proteins, a favorable concentration gradient persists until protein binding is saturated and increased free drug equilibrates with the maternal plasma concentration. Molecules smaller than 600 d, which applies to many pharmacologic compounds, readily cross the placenta. The placenta is an enzymatically active organ. Cytochrome P-450 enzymes, *N*-acetyltransferase, glutathione transferase, and sulfating enzymes can alter the activity of drugs into their active or inactive forms with variable activity in the fetus. Blood flow also determines the rate of drug entering the placenta, and increased or decreased placental flow influences delivery of drugs to the fetus.[4] As the placenta ages, its thickness decreases, facilitating further diffusion into the fetus. In vitro studies examining transfer of morphine across the term human placenta have shown that the cotyledon acts as a storage depot for morphine and that morphine is released for approximately 60 minutes after the maternal administration of the drug ceases, effectively prolonging fetal exposure to morphine.[5] Because of species differences in anatomy, the site of potential placental storage of analgesics will differ in dogs and cats, because these species do not have placental cotyledons.

The stage of gestation of the fetus influences the effects of the various analgesics. The same drug administered in the early stage has a different effect when administered at the later stages of gestation.[1,2] The human fetal liver can perform many enzymatic and metabolic activities as it matures; however, it cannot perform glucuronidation, which is important for the metabolism of many lipophilic drugs, such as some opioids.[1] These effects would be similar to those in our veterinary patients. Unlike the human fetus, the liver of the dog fetus (not known for cats) has no drug-metabolizing capabilities; therefore, elimination of drugs from the canine fetal circulation is by means of fetal immature renal mechanisms or diffusion back through the placenta to the mother.[6] Fetal body water and albumin increase, and body fat decreases, during development, all of which influence plasma concentrations of various drugs.[2]

Opioids

Currently, opioids are the analgesic of choice in pregnant women and animals. With prolonged use (several weeks) during pregnancy, however, the fetus may be adversely affected. An increased incidence of babies born with low birth weight and behavioral deficits has been reported in human mothers taking opioids during pregnancy. Similar findings have been reported in laboratory animals.[7] The behavioral problems incurred with chronic use may be a result of reduced nervous system plasticity secondary to the opioid action on the development of normal synaptic connections, neurotransmitter production, and metabolism.[8] Chronic use during pregnancy would be extremely rare in veterinary patients. Based on the human literature, short-term opioid analgesic administration should not, and does not, seem to be a problem in veterinary patients. Again, long-term use may result in adverse effects on the fetus; however, the benefit to the mother must be considered. Of interest, a review of the addiction medicine literature, with experience gained from pregnant women seeking recovery from opioid addiction, concluded that methadone seemed to be safe for the treatment of pain during pregnancy.[2] Methadone is a good analgesic with efficacy comparable to that of morphine. Only parenteral methadone can be administered to dogs, because this opioid is not absorbed by way of the oral route in this species. Oral absorption has not been reported in the cat.

Studies investigating the transplacental transfer and metabolism of buprenorphine in the isolated placenta observed low transplacental transfer of buprenorphine to the fetal circulation with a single “dose”.[9] Because buprenorphine is deposited into the intervillous space, it acts as a depot and transplacental transfer to the fetal circuit is low. The direct effects of buprenorphine on the fetus depend on its concentration in the fetal circulation. Because less than 10% of placental buprenorphine, which is slowly released from the placenta, reaches the fetal circulation, little would be available to the fetal circulation.[9] With repeated administration, however, an increased depot of the drug would result in continuous release into the fetal circulation, which may contribute to neonatal withdrawal in a small number of neonates.[10]

Another study examining the rate of transfer from the maternal circulation of fentanyl reported that fentanyl rapidly crossed the placenta and entered the fetal brain during the first and early second trimesters in aborted human fetuses.[11] The concentration of fentanyl was still present in the fetal brain after clearance from the maternal blood. A study investigating human fetal and maternal plasma opioid concentrations after epidural sufentanil-bupivicaine or fentanyl-bupivicaine mixtures administered for analgesia during labor and delivery noted that sufentanil placental transfer was greater than that of fentanyl.[12] There was significant reuptake of sufentanil to the maternal circulation, however, which may considerably reduce neonatal opioid exposure. In this study, fentanyl administration was associated with lower neurobehavioral test scores at 24 hours of life, although none of the neonates had clinically significant depression. The investigators concluded that both drugs are acceptable for use with epidural bupivicaine during labor but that reduced neonatal opioid exposure with sufentanil suggests that it may have some advantages over fentanyl.[12]

No reports linking therapeutic use of morphine with major congenital defects have been published.[1] Maternal addiction to morphine with subsequent neonatal withdrawal syndrome is well documented, however. Morphine was widely used during labor in women until the 1940s, when it was replaced by meperidine. The clinical impression was that less respiratory depression was noted with meperidine when compared with that when morphine was used.[1] For continuing analgesia, however, morphine is recommended and not meperidine.

Opioids are frequently used in veterinary medicine to control pain associated with cesarean section. For the most part, puppies and kittens are successfully delivered and vigorous. If the puppies or kittens are depressed after delivery, a small drop of naloxone placed sublingually should reverse the depressant effects of the opiate. Repeat dosing in 30 minutes may be required if the neonates become depressed again. If continual renarcotization in the newborn is a concern, the owner should be given instructions on sublingual administration of a drop of naloxone dispensed in a tuberculin syringe. Other potential causes for perioperative depression must be considered if the cesarean section was not routine.

Opioid Antagonist

When "overdose" or adverse effects of an opioid are noted in the mother after any surgical procedure required during pregnancy, reversal by titration with naloxone is effective. One approach is to combine naloxone (0.4 mg/mL) 0.1 mL or 0.25 mL (for larger animals) with 10 mL saline and titrate at 1 mL/min only until unwanted affects are eliminated; with this technique, the analgesia still persists. Because naloxone may only last for 30 minutes, however, redosing in the same manner may be required.

It is not known whether the placenta retains naloxone. If this is the case, naloxone may have the effect of counteracting prolonged fetal exposure to morphine, because placental leaching of the drug would negate the need for repeated maternal naloxone dosing strictly as a fetal protectant.[5] It is known that naloxone does not alter the transfer or clearance of morphine across the placenta and that naloxone's effects are likely antagonism of morphine by direct actions on fetal μ-receptors.[5]

When opioid analgesia is required, as in any other painful situation, one should dose to effect (**Table 1**) and treat the underlying problem. It is also important to ensure that there are no other stresses and the patient has an environment that is comfortable, clean, and at normal ambient temperature.

Nonsteroidal Anti-Inflammatory Analgesics

The nonsteroidal anti-inflammatory analgesics (NSAIAs) are used extensively in human and veterinary medicine. In addition to administration for pain management, NSAIAs are prescribed to reduce significant abnormal right-to-left shunting of blood across the ductus arteriosus or foramen ovale when this is identified before birth of human babies.[13] The NSAIAs inhibit cyclooxygenase (COX) production, with a subsequent reduction in prostaglandin synthesis, which normally maintains ductal patency and regulates the pulmonary vasculature.[14] Adverse effects associated with this maneuver include pulmonary hypertension[13] in the fetus. A comorbid condition associated with NSAIA administration in this setting is nephrotoxicity of the fetus,[15] although a single injection does not seem to cause adverse effects. Earlier reports on adverse effects of NSAIAs in human medicine are inconsistent; however, there does seem to be some association of these drugs with teratogenesis,[16] especially during the first trimester, during which much fetal organogenesis takes place.[17] Orofacial clefts in the fetus may also be associated with NSAIA administration.[18] From earlier reports, a renal embryopathy syndrome in babies when mothers were administered

Table 1
Analgesic dosages for pregnant cats and dogs

Opioid Agonists	Dose (mg/kg)	Route of Administration	Dosing Interval (Hours)
Morphine	Dog:		
	0.1–0.5	Extremely slow IV bolus	1–4
	0.1–0.5	IV per hour	CRI
	0.5–1	IM, SC	1–4 (6)
	0.1–0.3	Epidural	4–8 (12)
	0.5–2	PO titrate to effect	4–6
	Cat:	IV, extremely slowly	
	0.05–0.2	IM, SC	2–6
Oxymorphone	Dog:		
	0.02–0.2	IV	2–4
	0.05–0.2	IM, SC	2–4 (6)
	0.05–0.3	Epidural	4–6
	Cat:		
	0.02–0.1	IV	2–4
	0.05–0.1	IM, SC	2–4
Hydromorphone	Dog:		
	0.04–0.2	IV	4–6
	0.05–0.2 (extreme cases)	IM, SC	4–6
	Cat:		
	0.02–0.1 (extreme cases)	IV	4–6
	0.05–0.1	IM, SC	4–6
Oxycodone	Dog:		
	0.1–0.3	PO	6–8
Methadone	Dog and cat:		
	0.1–0.5	IV, IM, SC	2–4
Codeine	Dog:		
	1–2	PO titrate to effect	6–8
	Cat:		
	0.5–1	PO titrate to effect	12

Naloxone is an opioid antagonist, and it should always be available when opioids are used. The dose depends on the administered opioid, dose, and duration of action. Because the dose required for reversal is never known, the author starts by slowly titrating naloxone intravenously in 0.004- to 0.04-mg/kg (0.01–0.1 mL of 0.4-mg/mL solution) increments until the desired clinical response is achieved. For easy titration, one can combine naloxone, 0.1 to 0.25 mL, with 0.9% saline (10 mL). It may be necessary to redose at varying intervals, because the duration of opioid action is longer than that of naloxone.

The dosages given in **Table 1** are those recommended for the nonpregnant cat or dog and are given here as a guide. The dose used in the pregnant animal should be dosed according to lean (nonpregnant) weight; however, the goal is to relieve pain, so titration to effect would be the most prudent method of dosing.

Abbreviations: IM, intramuscular; IV, intravenous; PO, per os; SC, subcutaneous.

Adapted from Mathews KA, editor. PAIN HURTS: how to understand, recognize, treat, and stop [CD-ROM]. Guelph, Ontario, Canada: Jonkar Computer Systems; 2003; with permission.

indomethacin for more than 48 hours has been recognized.[19] The NSAIAs may also have adverse effects on the reproductive tract and fetus because they block prostaglandin activity, resulting in cessation of labor and disruption of fetal circulation.[20] Other complications include transient renal insufficiency that can measurably decrease fetal urinary output and lead to oligohydramnios; fetal abnormalities in hemostasis that extend into the neonatal period, predisposing to intraventricular hemorrhage; and reduction in mesenteric blood flow predisposing to necrotizing enterocolitis.[21] More recent studies have identified the importance of COX-2 for maturation of the embryologic kidney; potential placental transfer of the NSAIAs may cause arrest of nephrogenesis in the fetus.[22] NSAIDs should not be administered to pregnant animals. A single injection after cesarean section is acceptable, however, and is frequently administered at the author's institution.

Because COX-2 induction is necessary for ovulation and subsequent implantation of the embryo,[20] NSAIAs should be avoided in breeding female animals during this stage of the reproductive cycle. A recent study in women taking aspirin, other NSAIAs, or acetaminophen showed an 80% miscarriage rate in those exposed to aspirin or other NSAIAs for 7 days or longer but not in those exposed to acetaminophen during the first 20 weeks of gestation. Because acetaminophen has a different mechanism of action than other NSAIAs, this may be why miscarriage did not occur.[23] The 20 weeks of gestation in human beings may equate to approximately 4 to 5 weeks in dogs and cats.

Because there are no studies specifically examining the safety or potential adverse effects of the more recently approved NSAIAs in veterinary medicine (eg, meloxicam, carprofen, deracoxib, firocoxib, tolfenamic acid, ketoprofen) to pregnant cats or dogs, it is suggested that administration be restricted to a single dose after cesarean section. Based on the Ontario Veterinary College (OVC) experience over several years, where meloxicam, 0.1 mg/kg, administered intravenously is administered after cesarean section, follow-up by the theriogenology department has not noted abnormalities potentially associated with NSAIAs in the offspring at any time, suggesting that other similar veterinary-approved NSAIAs would also be appropriate. The COX-2–specific NSAIAs have not been used in this setting at the OVC, however.

Ketamine

Ketamine, an *N*-methyl-D-aspartate (NMDA) receptor antagonist, rapidly crosses the placenta to the fetus in animals and human beings.[1] Ketamine has become a useful adjunctive analgesic for severe pain in hospitalized patients. In this setting, it is necessary to administer ketamine as a constant rate infusion (CRI) because of its short duration of action. There are no reports in the veterinary or human literature examining the effects on the mother or fetus at doses used in this setting (0.2–1.0 mg/kg/h). Based on ketamine's effect on uterine contractions and tone, maternal discomfort and potential for miscarriage may be a concern. When administered at anesthetic dosages, no teratogenic or other adverse fetal effects have been observed in reproduction studies during organogenesis and near delivery with rats, mice, rabbits, and dogs.[1] Doses of 2 mg/kg administered to mothers before delivery resulted in profound respiratory depression and increased muscle tone of the infant at birth, however; lower doses (0.25–1.0 mg/kg) were not associated with these complications. In human beings, low doses (0.275–1.1 mg/kg administered intravenously) of ketamine increased uterine contractions, whereas higher doses (2.2 mg/kg administered intravenously) resulted in a marked increase in uterine tone.[1] The effect of ketamine on intrauterine pressure varies depending on the stage of pregnancy. In full-term human patients, a 2-mg/kg intravenous dose of ketamine did not increase intrauterine pressure;

however, the same dose given to women before termination of an 8-to 19-week pregnancy increased intrauterine pressure, intensity, and frequency of contractions. The higher doses resulted in increased maternal systolic and diastolic pressure, and the low doses had no effect on fetal blood pressure.[1] Neurobehavioral tests demonstrate that human infants are depressed for up to 2 days after ketamine administration. If the anesthesia induction-to-delivery interval is less than 10 minutes, fetal abnormalities are greatly reduced.[1]

ANALGESIA FOR NURSING MOTHERS

Occasionally, nursing mothers require a surgical procedure or sustain injuries that are painful and require analgesic therapy. In addition to the humane aspect of treating the mother, analgesia is also important because a litter of pups or kittens may aggravate the painful state and may trigger aggression in the mother toward the pups or kittens. Clearly, analgesics must be administered; however, there is a lack of information on analgesic administration to lactating dogs or cats in the clinical setting. In addition to the pharmacokinetics of transfer and concentration of the various analgesics in breast milk, consideration must be given to the effects that the various analgesics may have on different stages of maturity of the puppies and kittens (ie, the neonate would potentially be more susceptible as a result of the immaturity of metabolizing functions). Characteristics of a drug that would facilitate secretion into milk are high lipid solubility, low molecular weight, and the non-ionized (charged) state. It is estimated that the neonate receives approximately 1% to 2% of the maternal dose of a drug.[24] The two classes of analgesics commonly used in veterinary patients are opioids and NSAIAs. These drugs are excreted in the milk; however, in most instances in people, the quantity is small. Nevertheless, there are differences that are important to note. Unfortunately, this information is not available for the commonly prescribed veterinary analgesics. Citations herein are therefore restricted to human and laboratory animal studies.

Nonsteroidal Anti-Inflammatory Analgesics

A potential concern regarding the administration of NSAIAs immediately after cesarean section, or even natural birth, is hemorrhage when the COX-1–preferential or COX-1–selective NSAIAs are used (ie, aspirin, ketoprofen, ketorolac, naproxen, ibuprofen). The continual presence of COX-2–preferential or COX-2–selective NSAIAs in milk may inhibit maturation of the kidney in puppies or kittens, because COX-2 is important in nephron maturation.[22] Complete maturation of the embryologic kidney does not occur until approximately 3 weeks after birth,[25] and normal function does not occur until approximately 6 to 8 weeks of age.[26–28] Because most NSAIAs may not be lipid soluble, are highly protein bound to plasma proteins, and may be present, to a great degree, in an ionized form in the plasma, theoretically, only a small amount may appear in breast milk, and thus would be safe to use. The NSAIAs have different characteristics that determine their secretion into milk and the metabolism and excretion in the suckling animal, however. For example, the low lipid solubility of the NSAIAs examined (ie, aspirin, ibuprofen, naproxen) results in a small amount being secreted in the milk; however, celecoxib has a high lipid solubility, which predicts potential ease of passage across biologic membranes.[29] It is suggested that celecoxib would readily pass through the mammary epithelium.[30] The molecular weight indicates that it is too large to pass through the pores of the mammary epithelium but could pass through the membranes.[30] Two breast milk peaks for the presence of celecoxib occurred at 5 and 35 hours after the last oral dose given to a human patient. The reason for the second peak is not clear and requires further investigation. Other NSAIAs, such as those with a long half-life (ie, naproxen, sulindac, piroxicam), can accumulate in the infant with prolonged use.[31] Meloxicam was excreted in the milk of rats at concentrations higher than those in plasma.[32] Acetaminophen is safe for use in human mothers, but aspirin should only be used occasionally, and for brief periods, because human infants eliminate salicylates slowly.[24] This would likely apply to kittens also. It is well established that acetaminophen cannot be administered to cats. It has been suggested that the single use of an NSAIA is safe in nursing human mothers.[33] Based on these individual characteristics of the NSAIAs prescribed for human mothers, studies investigating passage into breast milk of veterinary-approved drugs in cats and dogs are necessary to recommend guidelines for therapy. Until such studies are performed revealing no adverse affect on renal maturation and function at maturity, it is recommended that NSAIAs be reserved for single-dose use only after cesarean section. This recommendation is based on the experience of the theriogenologist at the OVC, where a single injection of meloxicam (COX-2–preferential NSAIA) is administered after cesarean section.

Opioids

As with the NSAIAs, there are no studies investigating the administration of various opioids in lactating cats and dogs. In the laboratory setting, morphine administration to mice with newborn pups may result in altered maternal behavior;[34] however, these changes have not been reported in the cat or dog despite the frequent administration of opioids around the time of surgery.[7] The author has not noted abnormalities with the mother or puppies after opioid administration for perioperative orthopedic or soft tissue pain; the mothers are attentive and the puppies are playful. The lipid solubility of the opioid influences its appearance in the milk; therefore, a more hydrophilic opioid, such as morphine, may appear in smaller amounts than a more lipid-soluble opioid, such as meperidine. A single dose of pethidine (meperidine) or morphine administered to nursing mothers did not seem to cause any risk to the suckling infant; however, repeated administration of pethidine, in contrast to morphine, had a negative impact on the infant.[33] Similarly, in another study, after receiving meperidine or morphine for 3 days after cesarean section, the babies of mothers receiving meperidine were less responsive than the babies of mothers receiving morphine.[35] This may be related to delayed metabolism or metabolites of the opioid rather than to a high concentration through the milk, however. Short-term use of codeine in nursing mothers was also noted to be safe; however, infant plasma samples 1 to 4 hours after feeding (20–24 minutes after administration to the mother) showed codeine levels to be higher than those of morphine.[36] Intrathecal administration of morphine to a woman, before and for 7 weeks after the birth of her baby, proved to be safe with no alterations in sleep, arousal behavior, or general development in the infant.[37] Prolactin[38] and oxytocin[39] levels may be altered after morphine administration; however, there was no apparent clinical effect in milk production or infant feeding in a human trial. A 15-day study of human mothers on a methadone maintenance program, receiving 40 to 105 mg/d, concluded that methadone is "safe" to use in breastfeeding mothers.[40] This was based on detection of a total relative dose of less than 5% for both the *S*-methadone and *R*-methadone enantiomers in the neonates. An arbitrary cutoff level of predicted infant exposure of less than 10% of the maternal dosage is recommended. Methadone should be administered only parentally in dogs and cats. Butorphanol in human beings passes into breast milk in concentrations paralleling levels in maternal serum.[41] At doses of 2 mg per person (estimated at 60–70 kg) every 6 hours, the American Academy of Pediatrics considers butorphanol compatible with breastfeeding;[42]

however, as with any analgesic, allowing suckling to occur after peak levels of drug have waned is advised. Hydromorphone hydrogen chloride (HCl) at a dose of 2 mg administered intranasally to breastfeeding human mothers revealed a rapid distribution from plasma into breast milk; however, the drug did not partition into the milk fat. It was estimated that the infant would receive approximately 0.67% of the maternal dose, which is considered a limited exposure.[43]

Rather than withhold opioid analgesic therapy because of potential concern for the puppies and kittens, when there is no published evidence to support this, administration of analgesics (**Table 2**) with observation of behavior is suggested. To prevent potential for drug side effects, avoid nursing during peak drug levels; when possible, time nursing immediately before the next dose, and avoid sedatives with long half-lives.[44] Should lack of vigor or respiratory depression attributable to opioid administration occur in puppies or kittens, one drop of naloxone (0.4 mg/mL) under the tongue, with titration to effect, should reverse these adverse effects.

Ketamine

No reports on the passage of ketamine into breast milk were found.

ANALGESIA FOR PEDIATRIC PATIENTS

An important fact to consider is that an unmanaged painful experience, especially when the nervous system is developing, may have a permanent negative impact on the animal. Studies in neonates and infants have revealed that when anesthesia or analgesia was withheld during circumcision, altered pain sensitivity and increased anxiety occurred with subsequent painful experiences, such as vaccination, when compared with children who had undergone circumcision but received local anesthesia.[45] Such studies suggest that infants retain a "memory" of a previous painful experience and their response to a subsequent painful stimulus is altered. This has also been shown in laboratory animals,[46] and there is no reason to believe this to be any different in cats and dogs.

In this discussion, the term *pediatric* generally refers to the first 6 months of life. Because of important physiologic changes that occur during this time frame, a further demarcation is defined for this review: neonatal (0–2 weeks), infant (2–6 weeks), weanling, (6–12 weeks), and juvenile (3–6 months). This distinction is made to make the reader aware of the metabolic changes that are occurring during these periods of maturation.[47] Animals between 3 and 6 months of age seem to require adult dosing regimens to effect analgesia.

There tends to be apprehension in administering analgesic drugs, especially opioids, to young animals because of the often cited "decreased drug metabolism and high risk for overdose." Although this may be a potential concern in the neonate, it is not necessarily so through all stages of maturation. Based on the human literature, the analgesic requirement may be higher at a certain stage of development, especially in the pediatric human patient, than in the adult.[48] Children 2 to 6 years of age have greater weight-normalized clearance than adults for many drugs. Higher rates of drug metabolism by cytochrome P-450 in children compared with adults have been attributed to a larger liver mass per kilogram of body weight rather than to age-related changes in intrinsic enzyme catalytic rates.[49] More rapid clearance in children may require more frequent dosing.[50] Although there are no reports in the veterinary literature suggesting that increased dosing should be considered in the young cat or dog, personal experience with intensive monitoring of the rare young (4–6-month-old) animal that inadvertently received 10 times the recommended opioid dose revealed no

Table 2
Analgesic dosages for nursing mothers

Opioid Agonists	Dose (mg/kg)	Route of Administration	Interval (Hours)
Morphine	Dog:		
	0.1–0.5	Extremely slow IV	1–4
	0.1–0.5	IV per hour	CRI
	0.5–1	IM, SC	1–4 (6)
	0.1–0.3	Epidural	4–8 (12)
	0.5–2	PO titrate to effect	4–6
	Cat:		
	0.05–0.2	IV, extremely slowly	2–6
	0.5–1	IM, SC	8–12
Hydromorphone Increased temperature frequently noted with administration in cats	Dog:		
	0.04–0.2	IV	4–6
	0.05–0.2	IM, SC	4–6
	Cat:		
	0.04–0.1	IV	4–6
	0.05–0.1	IM, SC	4–6
Oxycodone	Dog:		
	0.1–0.3	PO	6–8
Methadone	Dog and cat:		
	0.1–0.5	IV, IM, SC	2–4
Fentanyl	Cat and dog:		
	0.001–0.005+	IV loading	0.5–1
	0.001–0.005	IV for 20–60 minutes	CRI
	0.05 anesthesia	IV for 60 minutes	CRI
Fentanyl transdermal patch	Should be avoided due to potential ingestion by puppies or kittens		
Codeine	Dog:		
	1–2	PO titrate to effect	6–8
	Cat:		
	0.5–1	PO titrate to effect	12

The dosages given here are those recommended for the nonlactating cat or dog and are given here as a guide. The dose used in these animals should be that required to relieve pain; thus, titration to effect would be the most prudent method of dosing.

For opioid reversal, see naloxone in **Table 1**.

Abbreviations: IM, intramuscular; IV, intravenous; PO, per os; SC, subcutaneous.

Adapted from Mathews KA, editor. PAIN HURTS: how to understand, recognize, treat, and stop [CD-ROM]. Guelph, Ontario, Canada: Jonkar Computer Systems; 2003; with permission.

adverse effects; on the contrary, these animals seemed to be quite comfortable. This is not to suggest that the opioid dose should be increased but to emphasize that administering the analgesic to effect, rather than at a predetermined dose, is the most important method by which to manage pain (**Table 3**). Opioids can be reversed with naloxone (see **Table 3**) should there be clinical evidence of central nervous system (CNS) depression with associated respiratory depression, hypotension, and bradycardia. If bradycardia (heart rate <60 beats per minute) is noted and is associated with poor perfusion only, glycopyrrolate may be administered rather than reversing the opioid. Increasing the heart rate in this setting increases cardiac output. Maintaining a normal heart rate to ensure appropriate cardiac output is important in pediatric patients. Most animals that are comfortable and sleeping have low heart rates, especially the larger breeds. This does not warrant concern. Because the effects of the opioid occur quite rapidly after administration, it is wise to monitor for potential adverse effects rather than to reverse a "potential" problem that may not happen.

Neonates, and potentially infants, need to be considered separately from the weanling or juvenile patient when considering analgesics.[7] Neonates do feel pain, and the nociceptive threshold may be lower than in the adult. This has been attributed to a potential delay in development of the descending inhibitory mechanism. Because of the slower development of some neurotransmitters or receptors, certain drugs may not be effective at this stage of development. Because the NMDA system seems to be underdeveloped in the neonate, ketamine may not be effective. In a review of sedatives and analgesics used in children between the ages of 1–18 years of age, ketamine combined with a benzoiazepine was noted to be a safe and effective analgesic/sedative combination for emergency procedures.[51] Neonates have reduced clearance of many drugs as compared with infants, children, and adults largely because of the (1) greater water composition of their body weight, (2) larger fraction of body mass that consists of highly perfused tissues, (3) lower plasma concentration of proteins that bind drugs, and (4) incomplete maturation of their hepatic enzyme systems.[52] The hepatorenal system continues to develop until 3 to 6 weeks of age; this may result in reduced metabolism and excretion, which may require alterations in dosing and dosing intervals.[47] For all young animals, the presence of milk in the stomach may inhibit the absorption of some drugs, potentially resulting in lower blood levels.

Opioids

Lower doses of fentanyl or morphine are required for analgesia in the neonate when compared with the 5-week-old puppy.[52] Extremely young puppies are also more sensitive to the sedative and respiratory depressant affects of morphine, and it is recommended that fentanyl may be a more suitable opioid in the extremely young, especially the neonate.[53,54] This would likely apply to kittens. Sedative and opioid combinations should be avoided in this young age group, because the sedation is extremely profound. If further sedation is required, a low dose of the sedative may be administered after the opioid has had time for full effect. Fentanyl was found to be an effective analgesic in children between 1-18 years of age undergoing emergency room procedures. The addition of midazolam to fentanyl increased sedation and reduced respiratory rate.[51]

Morphine is the standard opioid for relief of severe pain in children; however, meperidine, fentanyl, and sufentanil are also administered when appropriate.[52,55,56] In veterinary patients, others have recommended administering half of the usual adult dose of these agents to puppies and kittens when used as a premedication before anesthesia.[57] For use as an analgesic, however, this may not be appropriate. Based on human pediatric studies, dosing depends on the degree of pain and the phase of maturation.[48] Neonates require less; however, animals a few weeks old may require an adult dose regimen. Starting at lower dosages and increasing to effect is recommended. Reversal of any adverse effects may be titrated using naloxone (see **Table 3**). The following dosing recommendations are ranges published for dogs and cats. Fentanyl transdermal patches and fentanyl "lollipops" (transmucosal) are administered to

Table 3
Analgesic dosages for pediatric patients

Drug	Species	Dose (mg/kg) (Lower Dosages in Patients less than 4 Weeks of Age)	Route of Administration (SC Suggested for Patients less than 4 Weeks of Age)	Interval (Hours)
Mild to moderate pain				
Opioid agonists				
Morphine	Dog			
		0.1–0.5	IM, SC, extremely slowly IV	1–4
		0.05+	IV, SC per hour	CRI
		0.25+	PO titrate to effect	4–6 (8)
	Cat			
		0.05–0.1	IM, SC	1–4
		0.025+	IV, SC per hour	CRI
		0.25+	PO titrate to effect	4–6 (8)
Methadone	Dog and cat	0.1–0.5	IV, IM, SC	1–4
Fentanyl	Dog and cat	0.002–0.010	IV loading	0.5–1
		0.001–0.005	IV/20–60 min	CRI
Meperidine	Dog and cat	2–5	IM	0.5–1
Opioid agonist-antagonists				
Butorphanol	Dog	0.1–0.2	IV, IM, SC	1–4
	Cat	0.1–0.2 (or to effect)	IV, IM, SC	1–4
	Dog and cat	0.05–0.01+	IV, SC per hour	CRI
Opioid partial agonists				
Buprenorphine		0.005–0.010	SC	~6

Moderate to severe pain				
Opioid agonists				
Morphine	Dog	0.5–1+	IM, SC, extremely Slowly IV	1–4
		0.05+	IV, SC per hour	CRI
		0.5+	PO titrate to effect	4–6 (8)
	Cat	0.1–1	IM, SC	1–4
		0.05+	IV, SC per hour	CRI
		0.5+	PO titrate to effect	4–6 (8)
Methadone	Dog	0.5-1+	IM, SC, IV	1–4
Hydromorphone	Dog and cat	0.05–0.1	IV, IM, SC	2–4 (6)
Fentanyl	Dog and cat	0.005–0.010+	IV loading	0.5–1
		0.001–0.005	IV for 20–60 minutes	CRI
Meperidine	Dog and cat	2–5	IM	0.5–1
Sedatives				
Midazolam	Cat and dog	0.05–0.1	IV, IM	Dog up to 6 hours
				Cat can be >6 hours
Diazapam	Cat and dog	0.05–0.1	IV	Dog up to 6 hours
				Cat can be >6 hours
Acepromazine	Cat and dog	0.01–0.025	IM, SC	2–6

Naloxone is an opioid antagonist. Naloxone should always be available when opioids are used. The dose required depends on the administered opioid, dose, and duration of action. Because a definitive dose for reversal is never known, the author starts by slowly titrating naloxone intravenously in 0.004- to 0.04-mg/kg (0.01–0.1 mL of 0.4-mg/mL solution) increments until the desired clinical response is achieved. For easy titration, combine naloxone, 0.05 to 0.1 mL, with 0.9% saline (10 mL). You may have to redose at varying intervals, because the duration of opioid action is longer than that of naloxone.

Abbreviations: IM, intramuscular; IV, intravenous; PO, per os; SC, subcutaneous.

Adapted from Mathews KA, editor. PAIN how to understand, recognize, treat, and stop [CD-ROM]. Guelph, Ontario, Canada: Jonkar Computer Systems; 2003; with permission.

children.[56] No veterinary studies are available in this young group of patients assessing these routes of administration.

Nonsteroidal Anti-Inflammatory Analgesics

The NSAIAs are not recommended for animals less than 6 weeks of age based on developing hepatorenal systems. The COX-2 is required for renal maturation and sodium and water balance at the level of the kidney. It is important to ensure that this system is fully developed before administration of NSAIAs. Therefore, until studies confirm the safety of these agents in animals less than 6 yo 8 weeks of age, their use should be avoided.

Sedatives

Sedatives should be used with caution in young animals, especially when they are less than 12 weeks of age.[58] The phenothiazine tranquilizers (ie, acetylpromazine) undergo little hepatic biotransformation and may cause prolonged CNS depression. These agents are not analgesic; in fact, they may mask an increase in the level of pain if analgesics are not coadministered. These drugs induce peripheral vasodilation, and hypotension and hypothermia may result; however, this is dose dependent. If these drugs are required and there may be occasion for their use, the dosage for acetylpromazine should be reduced to 0.005 to 0.025 mg/kg administered intramuscularly or subcutaneously. It is advised that the concentration of 10-mg/mL commercial product be diluted to 1 mg/mL before withdrawing for administration to facilitate accurate dosing. Opioids have sedating effects, especially in young animals; therefore, if these drugs are required, the addition of a sedative may not be necessary in animals younger than 4 months.

LOCAL ANESTHETICS FOR ALL AGE GROUPS: GENERAL CONSIDERATIONS

The most frequently used local anesthetic in human medicine is lidocaine, and this also seems to be the case in veterinary medicine. Infiltration of lidocaine is extremely painful even with 27- to 30-gauge needles, especially in the neonate or pediatric patient.[55] To reduce pain, buffering, warming (37°–42° C), and slow administration are recommended. Buffering can be accomplished by mixing 1% lidocaine with sodium bicarbonate at a 10:1 ratio (1% lidocaine at a rate of 1 mL combined with sodium bicarbonate at a rate of 0.1 mEq [0.1 mL of 1 mEq/mL]). Because most veterinary practices have a 2% solution, this can be diluted to a 1:1 ratio with 0.9% sodium chloride (1% = 10 mg/mL) and mixed with sodium bicarbonate to a further 10:1 ratio (lidocaine/sodium bicarbonate) before administration. It might be advisable to use a maximum dose of lidocaine in kittens of 3 mg/kg in the neonate to 6 mg/kg in the older pediatric patient and a dose of 6 mg/kg in the neonatal pup to 10 mg/kg in the older pediatric patient. The lower dose is required because of the immaturity of peripheral nerves and not because the younger animals are at any greater risk for toxic side effects. This dose should be diluted in 0.9% saline for accurate dosing, ease of administration, and distribution over the site. Bupivacaine may also be used with a 2-mg/kg maximum dose in the older kitten and puppy, with half of this dose advised for the neonate and weanling. Buffering of a 0.5% bupivicaine solution (5 mg/mL) requires a 20:1 mixture with sodium bicarbonate, 1 mEq/mL (~0.5 mL bupivacaine and 0.025 mL sodium bicarbonate), and warming as described for lidocaine.

Previously, the most frequently used topical cream local anesthetic in our institution was EMLA (eutectic mixture of local anesthetic) cream. This is a prescription-only mixture of lidocaine, 2.5%, and prilocaine, 2.5%, combined with thickening agents to form an emulsion (EMLA cream; AstraZeneca LP, Wilmington, Delaware). Dosing is calculated in a similar manner to the injectable formulation. Local anesthetic concentrations are described as weight by volume (grams per 100 mL) or weight by weight (grams per 100 g); therefore, the 2.5% cream is 2500 mg per 100 g (25 mg/g). This product is not sterile and should be used only in intact skin to provide anesthesia for intravenous catheter placement, blood collection, lumbar puncture, and other minor superficial procedures. EMLA cream should be covered with an occlusive dressing for at least 30 minutes and preferably longer. In children, the peak effect is at 2 hours; however, the author's experience in animals is that 30 minutes facilitates such procedures as jugular catheter placement using the Seldinger technique; however a longer dwell time might be necessary in the more active animal. In one veterinary study, there was no systemic uptake of the components of EMLA cream and its use seemed to be effective in preventing signs of discomfort during jugular catheter placement.[59] Another product is an over-the-counter liposome-encapsulated formulation of 4% lidocaine (ELA-Max or L.M.X; Ferndale Laboratories, Ferndale, Michigan).Transdermal absorption did occur after application of 15 mg/kg of this product, but plasma concentrations remained significantly lower than toxic values.[60] The area was covered to prevent licking, with subsequent absorption through the oral mucous membrane and concerns for lidocaine toxicity. A similar product containing 4% lidocaine (MAXILINE 4; Ferndale Laboratories, Ferndale, Michigan) is currently used at the author's institution and is preferred to EMLA cream, because the local anesthetic effect occurs faster. This product is only used in intact skin. Another solution, in gel form, is a mixture of 4% lidocaine, 0.1% epinephrine, and 0.5% tetracaine, which can be applied to broken or intact skin.[55] Because of the epinephrine content, this should be avoided in end-arterial regions and mucous membranes. The author has no experience with the use of this product, and there are no published pediatric veterinary studies. The advantage with these products is that no injection is required, but they should be covered after application for approximately 30 minutes.

Two percent lidocaine is also available in a sterile gel in a cartridge and is useful for sterile local desensitization. This is frequently used at the author's institution for desensitization of the vaginal vault before urinary catheter placement in female cats and dogs, and it may also be applied to the penis before urinary catheter placement.

CONCLUSIONS

The opioids seem to be the safest class of analgesic in this population of veterinary patients. Specific drug selection, dosage, and timing of administration all have to be considered. Although the NSAIAs may seem safe in certain settings in the human patient, their use in veterinary patients should be withheld until studies specifically investigating the veterinary-approved drugs prove their safety.

SUMMARY

Little information on the approach to analgesia in pregnant, nursing, or extremely young animals is available in the veterinary literature. The unique physiologic characteristics in this group of patients must be considered when selecting analgesics. As with mature cats and dogs, the origin and severity of pain in this group of animals may be similar; however differences do exist. The diagnosis and assessment of pain in pregnant and nursing animals is based on the problem at hand and is similar that of mature animals. The diagnosis in the extremely young, however, may be more challenging but should be suspected based on history and clinical signs. Response to analgesic therapy is advised in all animals to confirm the presence and degree of pain. Various analgesics and analgesic modalities are discussed, with emphasis placed on preference and caution for each group. Management of pain is extremely important in all animals but especially in the extremely young, in which a permanent hyperalgesic response to pain may exist with inadequate therapy. Inappropriate analgesic selection in pregnant and nursing mothers may result in congenital abnormalities of the fetus or neonate. Inadequate analgesia in nursing mothers may cause aggressive behavior toward the young. Review of the human and veterinary literature on the various analgesics available for use in this group of patients is discussed.

REFERENCES

1. Briggs GG. Instructions for use of the reference guide. In: Briggs GG, Freeman RK, Yaffe SJ, editors. Drugs in pregnancy and lactation. 5th edition. Baltimore (MD): William & Wilkins; 1998. p. xxi–xxii, p. 746–47, p. 578–81.
2. Wunsch MJ, Stanard V, Schnoll SH. Treatment of pain in pregnancy. Clin J Pain 2003;19(3):148–55.
3. Loebstein R, Lalkin A, Koren G. Pharmacokinetic changes during pregnancy and their clinical relevance. Clin Pharmacokinet 1997;33:328–43.
4. Ward R. Maternal-placental-fetal unit: unique problems of pharmacologic study. Pediatr Clin North Am 1989;36:1075–88.
5. Kopecky EA, Simone C, Knie B, et al. Transfer of morphine across the human placenta and its interaction with naloxone. Life Sci 1999;65(22):2359–71.
6. Papich M. Effects of drugs on pregnancy. In: Bonagura JD, editor. Kirk's current veterinary therapy X small animal practice. Philadelphia: WB Saunders Co.; 1989. p. 1291–9.
7. Pascoe PJ. Perioperative pain management. Vet Clin North Am Small Anim Pract 2000;30(4):917–32.
8. Di Giulio AM, Tenconi B, Malosio ML, et al. Perinatal morphine: I. Effects on synapsin and neurotransmitter systems in the brain. J Neurosci Res 1995;42: 479–85.
9. Nanovskaya T, Deshmukh S, Brooks M, et al. Transplacental transfer and metabolism of buprenorphine. J Pharmacol Exp Ther 2002;300(1):26–33.
10. Fischer G, Rolley JE, Eder H, et al. Treatment of opioid-dependent pregnant women with buprenorphine. Addiction 2000;95:239–44.
11. Cooper J, Jauniaux E, Gulbis B, et al. Placental transfer of fentanyl in early human pregnancy and its detection in fetal brain. Br J Anaesth 1999;82:929–31.
12. Loftus JR, Hill H, Cohen S. Placental transfer and neonatal effects of epidural sufentanil and fentanyl administered with bupivicaine during labor. Anesthesiology 1995;83:300–8.
13. Alano MA, Ngougmna E, Ostrea EM, et al. Analysis of non-steroidal anti-inflammatory drugs in meconium and its relation to persistent pulmonary hypertension of the newborn. Pediatrics 2001;107:519–23.
14. Philips JB, Lyrene RK. Prostaglandins, related compounds and the perinatal pulmonary circulation. Clin Perinatol 1984;11:565–79.
15. Cuzzolin L, Cere MD, Fanos V. NSAID-induced nephrotoxicity from the fetus to the child. Drug Safety 2001;24(1):9–18.
16. Schoenfield A, Bar Y, Merlob P, et al. NSAIDS: maternal and fetal considerations. Am J Reprod Immunol 1992;28:141–7.
17. Lee VC, Rowlingson JC. Pre-emptive analgesia: update on nonsteroidal anti-inflammatory drugs in anesthesia. Advances in Anesthesia 1995;12:69–110.

18. Ericson A, Kallen BAJ. Nonsteroidal anti-inflammatory drugs in early pregnancy. Reproductive Toxicology 2001;15:371–5.
19. Kaplan BS, Restaino I, Raval DS, et al. Renal failure associated with in utero exposure to non-steroidal anti-inflammatory agents. Pediatr Nephrol 1994;8: 700–4.
20. Dubois RN, Abramson SB, Crofford L, et al. Cyclooxygenase in biology and disease. FASEB J 1998;12:1063–73.
21. van der Veyver IB, Moise KJ. Prostaglandin synthetase inhibitors in pregnancy. Obset Gynecol Surv 1993;48:493–502.
22. Harris RC. Cyclooxygenase-2 in the kidney. J Am Soc Nephrol 2000;11:2387–94.
23. De-Kun L, Liyan L, Odouli R. Exposure to non-steroidal anti-inflammatory drugs during pregnancy and risk of miscarriage: population based cohort study. BMJ 2003;327:368–73.
24. Britt R, Pasero C. Pain control: using analgesics during breastfeeding. Am J Nurs 1999;99(9):20.
25. Horster M, Kember B, Valtin H. Intracortical distribution of number and volume of glomeruli during postnatal maturation in the dog. J Clin Invest 1971;50:796–800.
26. Aschinberg LC, Goldsmith DI, Olbing H, et al. Neonatal changes in renal blood flow distribution in puppies. Am J Physiol 1975;228:1453–61.
27. Horster M, Valtin H. Postnatal development of renal function: micropuncture and clearance studies in the dog. J Clin Invest 1971;50:779–95.
28. Kleinman LI, Lubbe RJ. Factors affecting the maturation of glomerular filtration rate and renal plasma flow in the newborn dog. J Physiol 1972;223:395–409.
29. Pharmacia Canada Inc. and Pfizer Canada Inc. Celebrex (celecoxib) product monograph. Mississauga, Ontario and Kirland, Quebec, Canada, May 8, 2002.
30. Knoppert DC, Stempak D, Baruchel S, et al. Celecoxib in human milk: a case report. Pharmacotherapy 2003;23(1):97–100.
31. Spencer JP, Gonzalez Luis S III, Barnhart DJ. Medications in the breast-feeding mother. Am Fam Physician 2001;64(1):119–26.
32. Boehringer Ingelheim product monograph. Compendium of pharmaceuticals and specialties. Canadian Pharmacists Association 2002.
33. Spigset O, Hagg S. Analgesics and breast-feeding: safety considerations. Paediatr Drugs 2000;2(3):223–38.
34. Haney M, Miczek KA. Morphine effects on maternal aggression, pup care and analgesia in mice. Psychopharmacology (Berl) 1989;98:68.
35. Wittels B, Scott DT, Sinatra RS. Exogenous opioids in human breast milk and acute neonatal neurobehavior: a preliminary study. Anesthesiology 1990;73(5): 864–9.
36. Meny RG, Naumburg EG, Alger LS, et al. Codeine and the breastfed neonate. J Hum Lact 1993;4:237–40.
37. Oberlander TF, Robeson P, Ward V, et al. Prenatal and breast milk morphine exposure following maternal intrathecal morphine treatment. J Hum Lact 2000; 16:137–42.
38. De Rensis F, Cosgrove JR, Willis HJ, et al. Ontogeny of the opioidergic regulation of LH and prolactin secretion in lactating sows. II: interaction between suckling and morphine administration. J Reprod Fertil 1999;116:243–51.
39. Lindow SW, Hendricks MS, Nugent FA, et al. Morphine suppresses the oxytocin response in breast-feeding women. Gynecol Obstet Invest 1999;48:33–7.
40. Begg EJ, Malpas TJ, Hackett LP, et al. Distribution of *R*- and *S*-methadone into human milk during multiple, medium to high oral dosing. Br J Clin Pharmacol 2001;52(6):681–8.

41. Pittman KA, Smyth RD, Losada M, et al. Human perinatal distribution of butorphanol. Am J Obstet Gynaecol 1980;138:797–800.
42. Committee on Drugs, American Academy of Pediatrics. The transfer of drugs and other chemicals into human milk. Pediatrics 1994;93:137–50.
43. Edwards JE, Rudy AC, Wermeling DP, et al. Hydromorphone transfer into breast milk after intranasal administration. Pharmacotherapy 2003;23(2):153–8.
44. Bond GM, Holloway AM. Anesthesia and breast-feeding—the effect on mother and infant. Anaesth Intensive Care 1992;20(4):426–30.
45. Taddio A, Katz J, Ilersich AL, et al. Effect of neonatal circumcision on pain response during subsequent routine vaccination. Lancet 1997;349:599–603.
46. Lee BH. Managing pain in human neonates—application for animals. J Am Vet Med Assoc 2002;221(2):233–7.
47. Boothe DM, Bucheler Jorg. Drug and blood component therapy and neonatal isoerythrolysis. In: Hospkins J, editor. Veterinary pediatrics: dogs and cats from birth to six months. Philadelphia: WB Saunders Co; 2001. p. 35–56.
48. Collins JJ. Palliative care and the child with cancer. Hematol Oncol Clin North Am 2002;16:657–70.
49. Blanco JG, Harrison PL, Evans WE, et al. Human cytochrome P450 maximal activities in pediatric versus adult liver. Drug Metab Dispos 2000;28:379–82.
50. Hunt A, Joel S, Dick G, et al. Population pharmacokinetics of oral morphine and its glucuronides in children receiving morphine as immediate-release liquid or sustained-release tablets for cancer pain. J Pediatr 1999;135:47–55.
51. Mace SE, Barata IA, Cravero JP, et al. Clinical policy: evidence-based approach to pharmacologic agents used in pediatric sedation and analgesia in the emergency department. J Pediatr Surg 2004;39(10):1472–84.
52. Berde CB, Sethna NF. Analgesics for the treatment of pain in children. N Engl J Med 2002;347(14):1094–103.
53. Luks AM, Zwass MS, Brown RC. Opioid-induced analgesia in neonatal dogs: pharmacodynamic differences between morphine and fentanyl. J Pharmacol Exp Ther 1998;284:136–41.
54. Bragg P, Zwass MS, Lau M. Opioid pharmacodynamics in neonatal dogs: differences between morphine and fentanyl. J Appl Physiol 1995;79:1519–24.
55. Rodriguez E, Jordan R. Contemporary trends in pediatric sedation and analgesia. Pediatric emergency medicine: current concepts and controversies. Emerg Med Clin North Am 2002;1:199–222.
56. Ball AJ, Ferguson S. Analgesia and analgesic drugs in paediatrics. Br J Hosp Med 1996;55(9):586–90.
57. Grandy JL, Dunlop CI. Anesthesia of pups and kittens. J Am Vet Med Assoc 1987;1991:1244–9.
58. Hosgood G. Surgical and anesthetic management of puppies and kittens. Compendium on Continuing Education for the Small Animal Practitioner 1992;14(5):345–57.
59. Gibbon KJ, Cyborski JM, Guzinski MV, et al. Evaluation of adverse effects of EMLA (lidocaine/prilocaine) cream for the placement of jugular catheters in healthy cats. J Vet Pharmacol Ther 2003;26(6):439–41.
60. Fransson BA, Peck KE, Smith JK, et al. Transdermal absorption of a liposome-encapsulated formulation of lidocaine following topical administration in cats. Am J Vet Res 2002;63(9):1309–12.

Perioperative Pain Management in Veterinary Patients

Doris H. Dyson, DVM, DVSc

KEYWORDS

• Analgesia • Surgical pain • Dog • Cat

As veterinarians in the twenty-first century, we have an ethical responsibility to our patients and clients to avoid, or at least to reduce significantly, pain in animals under our care. The American Animal Hospital Association and the American Association of Feline Practitioners have joined to promote an emphasis in veterinary medicine on pain management.[1] Although this mandate can be stretched to cover a range from "less than appropriate" management to "unnecessary extremes" in analgesia administration, this article attempts to define a safe, practical, and yet suitable approach to management of pain in the perioperative period. Treatment for pain that approaches either extreme should be addressed by observation and refinement, because exact recipes do not suit all individuals, even animals that have undergone a similar procedure. Veterinarians must use their best judgment related to a starting point (often beginning with guidelines), monitor the patient's response to such treatment, and adjust accordingly. Clearly, the veterinarian's role in pain management is not complete after establishment of an analgesic plan.

ADJUNCTS TO PAIN MANAGEMENT

Usually, we think of analgesic drugs when the topic of pain management is mentioned, but it is important to keep in mind the other aspects that contribute to successful pain control. Anxiety, stress, and uncomfortable surroundings have an impact on the individual 's ability to handle pain. We recognize the comfort of our own bed in a quiet home with loving people, familiar objects nearby, and appetizing food as significant determinants in our overall feeling of well-being. Research has also shown that psychologic and physical aspects have an impact on the achievement of pain control.[2] Veterinarians may be able to reduce anxiety and uncomfortable surroundings with simple actions. Noise, temperature, and light can be maintained at a more optimal level for our patients. Quiet rooms can be defined to isolate the patient to keep it from disturbing others or to provide a calmer environment for the more sensitive

Department of Clinical Studies, Ontario Veterinary College, University of Guelph, Guelph, Ontario, Canada N1G 2W1
E-mail address: ddyson@ovc.uoguelph.ca

Vet Clin Small Anim 38 (2008) 1309–1327
doi:10.1016/j.cvsm.2008.06.006 vetsmall.theclinics.com

animal. Nursing care that includes provision of clean bedding, comforting words, petting, cuddling, and playing with the pet should contribute significantly to the management of mild pain and supplement the pharmacologic treatment of more severe pain, as has been reported in human infants.[3] Many practices encourage family visits during hospital stays to help reduce patient stress and gain insight on other interventions toward analgesia for the individual involved. Further information on good nursing care for surgical patients can be found in the article by Shaffron, Fagella, and Taylor elsewhere in this issue.

Nonanalgesic pharmacologic approaches can also provide calming effects that intensify the pain relief from specific analgesic drugs. This is the principle behind neuroleptanalgesia, which is able to provide better results than analgesia alone when minor surgical procedures are required. Therefore, the use of sedatives and tranquilizers is considered along with the administration of analgesic drugs, when appropriate.

ADVANCE APPLICATION OF ANALGESIA

Fentanyl patches require advance application to be effective for perioperative pain management. Animals that are admitted the night before can have a patch placed if this is an option for postoperative management. The advantage of this method is achievement of a steady-state level of analgesia in 12 hours (cats) to 24 hours (dogs) and lasting 72 hours. Fentanyl plasma concentrations vary significantly among individuals, however, and it may not be possible to guarantee achievement of good analgesic levels at the time of surgery. The impact of a fentanyl patch on inhalant requirements during surgery has been estimated by minimum alveolar concentration (MAC) measurement. A MAC reduction of 18% in cats[4] and 37% in normothermic dogs is expected, with no significant MAC reduction in hypothermic (34.5°C) dogs.[5] The reduction in MAC in cats is not much different than after administration of butorphanol,[6] and because hypothermia, which is commonly expected during longer and more painful surgical procedures, reduces the impact on MAC as well, further intramuscular opioid administration in premedication should not cause concerns. If clinical signs of opioid administration are apparent in advance of premedication (eg, panting, mild sedation), one may elect to give only half of the opioid dose planned. Further opioid can be administered if needed during the operation. Many anesthetists believe that these results and the safety associated with opioid use during surgery provide little reason to reduce opioid doses significantly in the premedication period, however (**Table 1**). Thus, the entire dose is usually used for premedication when fentanyl patches are used.

Some nonsteroidal anti-inflammatory analgesics (NSAIAs) may also be administered in advance of premedication if there are no present or expected contraindications for use (see the article by Papich and the article by Mathews elsewhere in this issue). This preoperative use may be a reasonable option to ensure analgesia at the time of recovery if the operation is unlikely to be associated with excessive blood loss or hypotension. A complete history from the owner and careful assessment of the patient are critical to ensure that NSAIA use is actually safe, however, irrespective of time of administration. For example, owners may administer aspirin to their pet and yet not consider this when asked indirectly if the animal is on any medication. Related to considering use before surgery, not all NSAIAs can be recommended. Carprofen, meloxicam, and tepoxalin have been assessed and found to be safe in healthy dogs when given in advance of anesthesia.[7–10] Recommendations on timing of NSAIA administration varies according to the route selected. If oral drugs are selected, they are usually not given with premedication but at the last meal, although oral administration can result in a rapid effect similar to that achieved with intravenous dosing

(30–60 minutes). Research indicates that the achievement of maximum plasma concentrations is longer, and that onset of analgesia for acute synovitis is slower, after meloxicam administration when compared with other NSAIAs,[11] although clinical experience associated with treatment of surgical pain shows an onset that is typical of other NSAIAs. Subcutaneous administration of any NSAIA may result in a longer onset, however.

The analgesic efficacy of NSAIAs has been documented for several surgical procedures in dogs[12–15] and cats,[16–19] but this should not eliminate consideration of additional analgesic drugs. Because no significant MAC reduction results from the preoperative administration of NSAIAs,[20,21] the addition of opioid analgesics can provide this and other benefits, such as prevention of wind-up.

PREMEDICATION

Most surgical procedures performed in general practice are elective; thus, the patient is presented without pain. The ideal approach to managing pain in these patients is to prevent it, and this usually starts with the premedication analgesics. Other patients presented for surgery may have accompanying pain and have analgesia on board as discussed previously or may be receiving continuous rate infusions (CRIs; as discussed elsewhere in this article) according to the level of pain on admission to the hospital. The anesthetist or practitioner must consider any present opioid effects at time of presentation for surgery in addition to the impact of other drugs on board when deciding on premedication requirements. If the analgesic administered during the preoperative period is effective, it should never be assumed that the intraoperative and postoperative pain is going to be managed equally as well. For some surgical procedures, the pain may be less after surgery (eg, cervical disk surgery), whereas for others, the pain may be greater during and after surgery (eg, most fracture repairs, peritonitis).

Opioid analgesics are the most commonly selected drugs for perioperative pain prevention or treatment. The specific drug selection and dose should be based on the level of expected pain. Butorphanol or buprenorphine is appropriate for mild (to moderate) pain (likely that involved in an ovariohysterectomy or castration performed by an experienced veterinarian). Buprenorphine has the advantage of a 6-hour duration of effect compared with as little as 2 hours with butorphanol. Morphine or hydromorphone could be selected for a longer effect as well, but low doses (eg, 0.2–0.3 mg/kg, 0.02–0.03 mg/kg, respectively) may be more appropriate for milder pain. Occasionally the "harder to handle" patient requires use of these more profound opioids at higher doses for the additional sedating effect that they achieve; however, dysphoria and panting may be a disadvantage. It is important to keep in mind that elective surgery is not always associated with mild pain. Surgical skill (ie, inexperienced) and patient condition (eg, severe obesity) can change the expected pain level of a procedure. Onychectomy in a cat is an elective procedure associated with a greater level of pain. Good analgesia has been shown after administration of buprenorphine (0.01 mg/kg),[22] although hydromorphone (0.05 mg/kg) could also be chosen for premedication for such procedures. When other surgical procedures are required that involve more extensive tissue trauma or take longer to perform (thus increasing inflammation from tissue handling), the μ-agonists are usually selected, and typical doses in dogs are 0.3 to 0.5 mg/kg and 0.03 to 0.05 mg/kg for morphine and hydromorphone, respectively, or fentanyl at a dose of 3 to 5 μg/kg. Extremely painful operations or those in which significant wind-up may be present may require up to 1.0 mg/kg and 0.1 mg/kg, respectively, especially when performed in smaller patients (surface area impact on drug dosing). Cats are safely

Table 1
Common analgesic drugs are listed with suggested doses and expected duration of effect based on various indications

Drug	Indication	Dose	Duration
Buprenorphine	Minor procedures (eg, castration, joint tap, laceration)	0.003–0.005 mg/kg	4–8 hours
	Mild to moderate pain (eg, ovariohysterectomy)	0.005–0.1 mg/kg	4–8 hours
Butorphanol	Minor procedures (eg, castration, joint tap, laceration)	0.1–0.2 mg/kg	3–6 hours
	Mild to moderate pain (eg, ovariohysterectomy)	0.2–0.4 mg/kg	2–4 hours
Fentanyl	Premedication or loading dose	2–10 μg/kg	15–20 minutes
	Moderate pain associated with most orthopedic procedures (eg, fracture repair, back surgery)	2–5 μg/kg/h	Infusion duration + 20 minutes
	Moderate to severe pain associated with major surgery (eg, thoracotomy, amputation)	3–10 μg/kg/h	Infusion duration + 20 minutes
Fentanyl patch	Painful procedures that may benefit from extended duration of effect (eg, declawing) or from steady level of underlying analgesia (eg, trauma surgery, orthopedic surgery) in association with other analgesic techniques	Cats, dogs <10 kg: 25 μg/h	3–5 days
		10–20 kg: 50 μg/h	3 days
		20–30 kg: 75 μg/h	3 days
		>30 kg: 100 μg/h	3 days
Hydromorphone	Mild to moderate pain associated with straightforward abdominal surgery (eg, ovariohysterectomy) or elective orthopedic surgeries (eg, dew claw removal)	0.02–0.03 mg/kg	3–6 hours
	Moderate pain associated with most orthopedic procedures (eg, cruciate surgery, declawing)	0.03–0.05 mg/kg	3–4 hours
	Moderate to severe pain associated with major surgery (eg, thoracotomy, amputation)	0.05–0.1 mg/kg. (monitor for hyperthermia in cats if high doses are given)	3–4 hours
Ketamine	Used as premedication (usually in combination) for good restraint and somatic analgesia	Cat: 5–7 mg/kg Dog: 3–5 mg/kg	20–30 minutes
	Short-term analgesia	0.2–4 mg/kg	10–30 minutes
	Analgesic infusion (usually with other drugs)	0.1–2 mg/kg/h	Infusion duration
Ketamine with diazepam (1:1 or 2:1)	Used to supplement premedication effect	0.03–0.04 mL/kg	4–6 minutes

Lidocaine	Used in association with any induction for analgesia and MAC reduction; often given before induction and then infusion used	2 mg/kg => 50–200 μg/kg/min (reduce dose in 1 hour or stop 20 minutes before recovery)	Infusion duration
	Used in association with any induction for antiarrhythmic effect, analgesia and MAC reduction; bolus often given before and after induction and then infusion used	2 mg/kg (twice in 10 minutes) + 120 μg/kg/min (reduce dose in 1 hour)	Infusion duration
Medetomidine	Used as premedication in healthy animals for more profound restraint and associated analgesia	Dog: 10–20 μg/kg Cat: 20 μg/kg	1–2 hours
	Supplementation of analgesia (and sedation)	1–2 μg/kg/h	Infusion duration
	Used immediately after surgery (in close association with extubation)	1–2 μg/kg	0.2–0.5 hour
Meperidine	Short-term mild to moderate analgesia for intramuscular use only	5–10 mg/kg	0.5–2 hours
Morphine	Mild to moderate pain associated with straightforward abdominal surgery (eg, ovariohysterectomy) or elective orthopedic operations (eg, dew claw removal)	Dog: 0.2–0.3 mg/kg Cat: 0.2 mg/kg	3–4 hours
	Moderate pain associated with most orthopedic procedures (eg, cruciate surgery, declawing)	Dog: 0.3–0.5 mg/kg (not in cats)	3–4 hours
	Moderate to severe pain associated with major surgery (eg, thoracotomy, amputation)	Dog: 0.5–1 mg/kg (not in cats)	3–4 hours
Nonsteroidal anti-inflammatory analgesics	Possibly alone in mild to moderately painful procedures and as supplementation of other analgesia in moderate to severe pain Loading dose is rarely needed in elective procedures (without wind-up and less painful) Injectable formulations are noted as follows:		
	Carprofen	Cat: 4 mg/kg once Dog: 4 mg/kg/d => 2 mg/kg/d	>24 hours 12–24 hours
	Ketoprofen (postoperative use only)	2 mg/kg/d => 1 mg/kg/d	24 hours
	Meloxicam	0.2 mg/kg/d => 0.1 mg/kg/d	24 hours

Range noted relates to surface area adjustment or degree of effect required. A separate cat dose is noted when needed. An extended list of drugs and more detail are found in this article and in the other article by Dyson elsewhere in this issue.

premedicated with hydromorphone for procedures associated with moderate to severe pain, using a starting dose of 0.05 mg/kg and considering that the duration of effect may be longer in cats than in dogs. Caution related to use of high doses or early repeat dosing is warranted to avoid hyperthermia (see section on preparation for recovery for more detail). Fentanyl can also be used in the cat at similar doses as used in the dog. Morphine, however, is rarely used at a dose higher than 0.2 mg/kg in the cat.

Ketamine is a somatic analgesic that may be added to the premedication. Telazol contains tiletamine, another *N*-methyl-D-aspartate (NMDA) antagonist with similar analgesic properties. Hyperalgesia associated with surgery in people seems to be less with ketamine, and the requirement for postoperative analgesia is reduced.[23,24] Ketamine is a useful premedication in cats (5–7 mg/kg), although it is more often selected in those that are hard to handle. Although ketamine is rarely used in dogs for premedication, evidence for incorporation as an intraoperative infusion is presented elsewhere in this article.

At the time of premedication, this author often administers sedatives to reduce anxiety from the handling involved (**Table 2**). Acepromazine is quite effective in most cats and dogs. Even low doses can be helpful (0.01–0.02 mg/kg) when selected in the quiet or older dog. Cats typically require a minimum of 0.05 mg/kg if an effect is to be achieved by its addition to the premedication, whereas more may be required after surgery to produce an improvement in analgesia (discussed in the section on preparation for recovery). The older cat or dog may be managed without acepromazine as part of the premedication in most situations, however, with the option of adding this for recovery if necessary. Compromised patients are best managed without using acepromazine. Preliminary evidence indicates that treatment of hypotension may be more difficult when acepromazine is on board.[25] Benzodiazepines (diazepam or midazolam at a dose of 0.2 mg/kg) can produce an anxiolytic effect and are occasionally

Table 2
Drugs (dosages listed reflect combination use) that are useful in combination with some of the analgesics in Table 1

Acepromazine	Preoperative use in young healthy animals	Cat: 0.05–0.15 mg/kg Dog: 0.02–0.05 mg/kg	3–4 hours
	Preoperative use in geriatric patients	Cat: 0.02–0.05 mg/kg Dog: 0.01–0.02 mg/kg	3–4 hours
	Immediate postoperative use (in close association with extubation)	Cat: 0.02–0.05 Dog: 0.01–0.02	0.5–2 hours
Diazepam or midazolam	Used with premedication	0.2–0.5 mg/kg	10–20 minutes
	Used intravenously in association with induction, during surgery, or with recovery	0.2 mg/kg	5 minutes
Propofol	Used to supplement premedication effect	0.5–1 mg/kg	2–3 minutes

These are typically used with opioids and have no analgesic properties but enable the analgesic to be more effective because of the calming effect achieved.

selected in place of acepromazine in more critical patients when an additional sedative effect beyond that of the opioid alone is desired. In most critical cases, however, it is not necessary to include a benzodiazepine, because opioid use in these patients usually is associated with a good level of sedation.

α_2-Agonists can also be used for analgesia and sedation in healthy dogs and cats. Those animals showing any potential for cardiovascular compromise or organ dysfunction should not be given this class of drug because of its peripheral vasoconstriction effects and depression of cardiac output. Medetomidine is the most commonly used α_2-agonist in small animals (5–20 μg/kg for dogs, 10–20 μg/kg for cats). At these doses, one can expect significant MAC reduction and analgesia for approximately 1 hour, although some animals show a more prolonged sedative effect. Low doses reduce the duration of cardiovascular depression rather than the degree.[26] During the postoperative period, microdoses (as discussed elsewhere in this article) may be used, and such low doses (<2 μg/kg) have less effect on the cardiovascular system.

NSAIAs can be administered at this time (if not given earlier) if no contraindications exist, but it must be recognized that the full effect may not be present at the completion of short procedures. Patients need to be covered with other means of analgesia for 30 to 60 minutes before an NSAIA is effective.

INDUCTION

Such drugs as opioids, ketamine, α_2-agonists, or lidocaine may be components of the induction protocol; as such, they result in analgesia at this time.

Only in critical cases do opioids facilitate induction (usually combined with diazepam at a dose of 0.2 mg/kg). The opioid dose required is at the high end (hydromorphone at 0.05–0.1 mg/kg administered intravenously, fentanyl at a dose of 10–20 μg/kg administered intravenously) and provides good analgesia, although respiratory depression and bradycardia are to be expected. Fortunately, the associated negative effects from opioids are managed easily with positive-pressure ventilation or anticholinergic administration. The higher doses suggested previously are more likely required when minimal premedication or analgesia is on board in advance. Such patients are often continued on opioid infusions (as described elsewhere in this article) to maximize MAC reduction.

For the more common situations, ketamine is frequently used for induction, combined with opioids, acepromazine, α_2-agonists, or benzodiazepines. The dose used for intravenous administration may have a short duration of analgesia, whereas typical doses that are used intramuscularly, as often performed in cats, should provide some analgesia for the duration of surgery. Nevertheless, it must be recognized that the analgesia associated with ketamine is more somatic than visceral, so further analgesia may be required. Teletamine (in Telazol) would have similar effects.

α_2-Agonists may be administered intramuscularly with ketamine to achieve induction. Postoperative analgesia was apparent after ovariohysterectomy in cats that received ketamine and medetomidine intramuscularly for anesthesia.[27] Comments and concerns related to this combination are similar to those given for premedication. It is important to recognize that although good analgesia is associated with these drugs, the duration is limited to, and often less than, the sedative effect.[28]

Lidocaine is discussed in greater detail related to use in CRIs. A single dose (2 mg/kg) should result in a short period of analgesia and MAC reduction. For this reason, it may be used as part of the induction.

MAINTENANCE

Inhalants, propofol, and thiopental do not produce analgesia, although excessive depth of anesthesia may allow painful procedures to be performed. These depths are associated with significant respiratory and cardiovascular depression, however, and wind-up is unlikely to be avoided. Thus, a more balanced method of anesthesia is preferred.

Local anesthesia should be included in procedures in which a significant benefit is possible. Digital (onychectomy), dental (extractions), intercostal (thoracotomy), epidural (hind limb fractures), and brachial plexus (forelimb fractures) blockade has been used to improve intraoperative and postoperative analgesia in small animals. Readers are referred to the articles by Lemke and Valverde elsewhere in this issue for details on techniques.

Single-dose administration of any of the analgesics previously mentioned can be performed as needed during maintenance of anesthesia. If the premedication dose is waning or was poorly judged, another dose can be given to bring the level up to what may be effective. For example, one may see that the hydromorphone effect is not as good 2 hours into a procedure. At least half of the dose has been eliminated by this time, and another half-dose could be given. Repeat dosing of long-duration drugs (eg, hydromorphone) may be helpful during surgery but can create adverse effects in recovery if the dose on board is greater than required when the animal is recovering (ie, a full dose given at 2 hours may be beneficial for the surgery but results in too high a dose at recovery). For this reason and others, CRI administration has gained popularity. A CRI may be calculated as described under this topic elsewhere in this article.

Epidural administration of morphine or hydromorphone may reduce further analgesia requirements for 12 to 24 hours. The analgesia effect has been measured as far forward as the forelimbs and can be an excellent supplementation of analgesia for thoracotomy and peritonitis. More detail on this technique is found in the article by Valverde elsewhere in this issue.

Morphine has also been placed intra-articularly to affect receptors directly in joints. The evidence on its benefit is controversial,[29,30] but the addition of local anesthetic is effective and the technique is simple. Morphine (0.1 mg/kg) is added to bupivacaine (approximately 0.1 mL/kg [0.5% solution]) and placed intra-articularly at time of joint closure. With this technique and epidural administration, the dose of morphine is so low that systemic side effects are not significant.

Patient monitoring is invaluable in assessing patient analgesia during surgery. Increases in respiratory rate, heart rate, or blood pressure are typically noted when further analgesia is necessary. It is necessary to ensure that ventilation is adequate, however, because an increase in p_{CO_2} attributable to hypoventilation is a common confounder associated with similar physiologic changes.

CONTINUOUS RATE INFUSIONS

The following discussion covers the use of CRI analgesia administration in the preoperative, intraoperative, and postoperative situations. There are several advantages to this technique of administration in the management of pain. A steady level of analgesia is more likely to be achieved, because the mountains and peaks associated with intermittent analgesic use are avoided. A steady level is more likely to avoid significant adverse effects and is more easily titrated to achieve continuous comfort. When certain procedures or periods of time require a greater level of analgesia, it can be "dialed" to effect. Although the benefit of steady-state pain relief is difficult to measure, preemptive analgesia achieved in various ways has been shown to reduce postoperative analgesia demand in a multitude of studies (339 papers displayed in a recent search) ranging from local anesthetic[31] to nonsteroidal[32] and even inhaled opioid use.[33] Therefore, it is likely that our patients also reap such benefits with continuous analgesia control. Considering that infusions can be used during surgery, the anesthetist and the patient can gain from the impact on inhalant requirements (MAC reduction). Based on drug selection for these infusions, there may be other benefits that arise (discussed under the section on specific infusions).

Anyone can administer a CRI if he or she is capable of giving fluid therapy to a patient. A syringe pump is not required, although it is the simple way to manage infusions, especially when frequent adjustment of the dose is required. An ordinary fluid pump is usually capable of delivering drugs from a syringe, however. Test the consistency of fluid administration of the pump at hand with a saline infusion (watching the drips falling from an extension set) in advance of using this technique. If the consistency is limited to higher rates, the analgesic can be diluted in a part of, or the entire, hourly surgical or maintenance fluid to enable accurate administration. Only diazepam cannot be diluted because of concerns about precipitation. Midazolam can be used interchangeably with diazepam (same dosing recommendations would apply), and it can be diluted in fluids or mixed with other analgesics without such concerns. If neither a fluid pump nor a syringe pump is available, the use of a burrette inserted within the fluid line enables drug administration in a smaller volume of surgical or maintenance fluid (add analgesic to the volume to be given in 15–60 minutes). Another alternative is to reduce the volume in a bag of fluids to that appropriate for the duration of administration (eg, 250 or 500 mL rather than 1000 mL) and to spike this remaining volume with the expected drug requirement at the fluid rate to be administered. This last recommendation is more suitable for surgical patients than for awake patients, which would be less tolerant of fluid volume adjustment. The volume during surgery would be given at 10 mL/kg/h. A surgical fluid rate adjustment from 5 to 20 mL/kg/h could be safe in most animals, however, and would allow analgesia dose modification from half to double the starting point if deemed necessary. A second bag of fluids would have to be connected should fluid requirements dictate an increase in rate, as needed for blood loss correction.

Almost any analgesic can be adjusted to be given as an hourly rate by using the following calculation:[Effective Dose (mg)/Typical Duration of Effect (h)]

The calculation can be performed using pharmacologic data. For example, a dose of morphine at 0.5 mg/kg is likely to provide 4 hours of pain relief in a dog. This provides an estimate of the dose per hour (0.125 mg/kg/h), which can usually be adjusted as the effect is observed in the individual. In some situations, one might observe that a dose of 0.5 mg/kg given to a particular dog provides only 3 hours of analgesia. The calculation can use this clinical information to define the individual patient 's infusion guideline (0.17 mg/kg/h). Because there is a possibility of a reduced drug requirement with the CRI method of administration, either calculation may result in an overestimation of the dosage and require adjustment according to the patient 's response. Similar analgesic effects were observed in dogs administered half the dose as a CRI compared with intermittent intramuscular injection of morphine.[34] CRIs are usually limited to drugs with a duration of effect of 6 hours or less.

It must also be recognized that an hourly rate maintains analgesia that was achieved by an initial loading dose. As long as the expected duration of the loading dose is similar to that of the infusion drug, it does not have to be the same drug. Also, a short-duration drug like fentanyl can be easily used after a longer duration drug like morphine. Analgesia needs may increase over the first 4 hours (morphine 's expected duration) if the pain involved remains constant. Careful observation of the patient should indicate if this is the case. Because surgical pain may actually lessen over the first 4 to 24 hours after surgery, changes in fentanyl infusion may not be required, may be increased for only a few hours, or may actually decrease over time.

Veterinarians have several analgesic drug options for CRIs. Typically, an opioid is chosen first (eg, morphine, hydromorphone, fentanyl) in awake patients or during surgery. When a long-lasting opioid is on board during surgery (usually part of the premedication), however, lidocaine may be the first drug selected as a CRI to improve analgesia during surgery. The reasons for this are discussed elsewhere in this article. Other infusions (eg, ketamine, medetomidine) are usually added when these options alone are ineffective. These drugs are rarely selected alone for analgesia by CRI. One analgesic cocktail (morphine, lidocaine, and ketamine [MLK]) has gained popularity for surgery and is also discussed elsewhere in this article.

Opioid Continuous Rate Infusion

There are several reports on morphine CRI in dogs.[34–36] Although a rapid intravenous bolus of morphine is contraindicated because of histamine release,[37] a slow intravenous infusion can be used without concern. The doses that have been assessed range from 0.12 mg/kg/h[34] to 0.34 mg/kg/h.[36] The analgesia produced varied from mild to moderate. The higher dose resulted in plasma concentrations that were greater than the previously suggested analgesia range but were not associated with significant cardiovascular or respiratory side effects in healthy awake dogs. Because sedation is apparent at the higher CRI, it should be safe to assume that in the awake animal, undesirable central nervous system (CNS) depression would accompany any respiratory depression and provide a clue to overdosage. Sedation and mild hypothermia are expected consequences of using opioids for analgesia in the awake animal. In the anesthetized dog, bradycardia and respiratory depression are obvious, but both are easily treated in this setting, as mentioned previously. A conservative dose range for a morphine CRI may fall within the range of 0.12 to 0.25 mg/kg/h (corresponding roughly to the effect from 0.5–1.0 mg/kg as an intermittent dose) for dogs. Fentanyl is preferred in cats.

There are no published studies using hydromorphone as a CRI in dogs or cats. Considering the fact that the duration of effect tends to be similar to morphine and that hydromorphone is 10 times as potent as morphine, however, one should be able to extrapolate safely from the studies using a CRI with morphine. Thus, a dose range of 0.01 to 0.03 mg/kg/h should be effective. In either case, a loading dose of morphine from 0.3 to 1.0 mg/kg or a loading dose of hydromorphone from 0.03 to 0.1 mg/kg would be given to achieve appropriate analgesia in advance of starting the CRI. Hydromorphone, in contrast to morphine, is safe given rapidly intravenously at these doses.[38] The selected dose would vary with the procedure performed and the expected pain associated with it, in addition to the individual patient. Smaller patients would need a higher dose per kilogram than large dogs.

Fentanyl is presently the most popular opioid for CRI. The effectiveness and cardiovascular safety of this infusion in dogs have been reported.[39,40] Its short duration of effect makes it suitable for administration by this method. The dose-related MAC reduction and ceiling effect (42 μg/kg/h) from fentanyl CRI were first reported in 1982.[41] Doses of 3, 12, and 42 μg/kg/h showed a MAC reduction of 20%, 44%, and 65%, respectively. Practical intraoperative administration involves a loading dose of 3 to 5 μg/kg followed by a CRI of 10 μg/kg/h. This infusion can be halved or doubled based on the desired effect on the inhalant requirements. In rare critical cases in which isoflurane must be extremely low, fentanyl (50 μg/mL] and midazolam (5mg/mL)

(10:1 as vol/vol) have been administered at 1 mL/kg/h (45 μg/kg/h + 0.45 mg/kg/h, respectively). High intraoperative infusions of fentanyl (>5 μg/kg/h) need to be lowered in advance of recovery (approximately 20 minutes before the end of surgery). This should reduce the chance of postoperative dysphoria. Infusions used in the awake or recovering patient are usually 2 to 5 μg/kg/h, with doses as high as 10 μg/kg/h in extremely painful conditions.

Butorphanol has also been used as a CRI at 0.1 to 0.4 mg/kg/h. This infusion would be most appropriate for mild to moderate pain. A loading dose of 0.1 to 0.4 mg/kg would be appropriate.

Practical evidence for use of opioid CRIs in cats is nonexistent. Analgesia has been shown to be good after low-dose morphine administration (0.2 mg/kg),[42] and MAC reduction has been determined as significant at high (1.0 mg/kg) but not low (0.1 mg/kg) doses.[6] Morphine as a CRI is not likely to be suitable in cats, however, because of concerns for excitement with overdosing. If a μ-agonist is required, fentanyl would be the preferred drug because of its short duration of effect, thus reducing concerns for overdosing and excitement. Low doses of hydromorphone as a CRI can be used in the cat with assessment of effectiveness of the infusion, adjustment as needed, and monitoring for hyperthermia, however. An infusion based on a 6-hour duration of effect[43] rather than 4 hours, unless proved otherwise by individual response, may be a practical approach in cats (0.005–0.01 mg/kg/h). In general, butorphanol selection as a CRI would be a safe alternative for mild to moderate pain.

Lidocaine Continuous Rate Infusion

Lidocaine has been shown to reduce MAC in dogs, provide analgesia, and act as an antiarrhythmic. It is an excellent choice in cases in which these benefits are of value (eg, animals presented with gastric dilation/torsion, splenic tumors, chest trauma, cardiac disease). Such critical patients can be induced with the addition of 2 mg/kg as a bolus in advance of the induction agent, a second bolus of 2 mg/kg after intubation and stabilization onto an inhalant, and a CRI started at 120 μg/kg/min (7 mg/kg/h). This recommendation achieves immediate therapeutic levels for antiarrhythmic effects and an expectation for a MAC reduction of approximately 43%. This approach is extrapolated from studies performed in normal and cardiovascular-compromised patients.[44,45] Plasma levels from this method are similar to those achieved in longer than 30 minutes from a single 2-mg/kg dose followed by a 200-μg/kg/min (12 mg/kg/h) CRI. This second method would be suitable for dogs with no evidence of cardiovascular compromise, arrhythmia concern (requiring an immediate antiarrhythmic level), or possibly liver compromise (although lidocaine accumulation depends more on flow than on liver function). It is a simple method for intraoperative MAC reduction and analgesia in other cases (10 mg/kg/h simplifies calculations even more so with likely little difference), however. Before recovery or after 1 hour in long surgical procedures, the CRI should be reduced to 40 to 80 μg/kg/min (2–5 mg/kg/h) to reduce the chance of mildly toxic plasma levels. The infusion can simply be stopped if not needed for postoperative analgesia or arrhythmia management. At lower infusions, the MAC may be reduced by approximately 20%. Analgesia can be achieved with as little as 1 to 3 mg/kg/h, however. The effective loading dose for analgesia in the awake patient is similar to that during anesthesia (1–4 mg/kg).

Although MAC reduction has been measured in cats during lidocaine infusion, significant cardiovascular depression has been shown.[46] It has been suggested as an analgesic in the awake cat at a loading dose of 0.25 to 1 mg/kg followed by a CRI at 0.5 to 2 mg/kg/h.[47] At the Ontario Veterinary College, however, the author and her colleagues have no experience in this setting.

Ketamine Continuous Rate Infusion

Ketamine has been studied as a CRI in dogs and shown to provide an approximately 25% MAC reduction at 10 μg/kg/min (0.6 mg/kg/h).[35] Intraoperative CRI administration is suggested at 2 to 10 μg/kg/min (0.1–0.6 mg/kg/h) after a loading dose provided by ketamine in the induction or 2 mg/kg administered intravenously. At these doses, MAC reduction and somatic analgesia are expected without evidence of significant sympathetic drive. Doses between 0.1 and 2 mg/kg have been used for analgesia in the postoperative setting when other analgesics alone are not effective. CNS depression, muscle rigidity, and sympathetic drive may occur with higher doses, depending on coinciding drug use.

Morphine/Lidocaine/Ketamine Continuous Rate Infusion

A single report on the use of an MLK cocktail has been published.[35] Analgesia and MAC reduction are achieved with a mixture of morphine (12 mg), lidocaine (150 mg), and ketamine (30 mg) in surgical fluid (500 mL) dripped at the standard surgical fluid rate (10 mL/kg/h). This provides morphine at a rate of 4 μg/kg/min (0.24 mg/kg/h), lidocaine at 50 μg/kg/min (3 mg/kg/h), and ketamine at 10 μg/kg/min (0.6 mg/kg/h). The mixture produced the same MAC reduction (45%) and cardiovascular effects as morphine alone (same dose as in mixture). A multimodal approach to analgesia was suggested as the benefit of this cocktail. This view may not be taken by all anesthetists, however. If there is no measurable advantage, a simpler approach may be more appropriate.[48] The lack of benefit with the addition of ketamine along with opioids during orthopedic surgery was similar[35] to that shown in the study by Muir and colleagues. This MLK cocktail is not simpler to use and shows no clear advantage when compared with using higher lidocaine infusions or opioid infusions. Although no advantage has been shown at this point, it does not cause harm if mixed properly and inhalant adjustments are made appropriately. For severe postoperative pain, the concentrations of each drug in this mixture, and their combined potential effect, are unlikely to confer adequate analgesia.

PREPARATION FOR RECOVERY

Appropriate analgesia should be achieved in advance of recovery. This may require lowering or stopping infusions (as previously addressed), adding additional analgesics (eg, NSAIAs delayed for concerns about hypotension or those only used for postoperative administration), or bringing single-dose opioid injections up to therapeutic levels based on timing of last administration. There is no reason to avoid additional opioids until after recovery if the patient is expected to require more than the level on board. Delay in recovery associated with analgesia administration is more likely attributable to poor drug or dose selection. Calculate the dose required to produce the desired effect as described in the section on repeated intraoperative dosing during maintenance, and administer just before turning off the inhalant. If the drugs on board are likely to provide adequate analgesia, however, recovery can proceed with plans to provide more analgesia only if the patient seems to need such.

Sedatives should be preemptively administered if thought to be useful in recovery. The primary concern about acepromazine relates to intraoperative hypotension; however, a low dose in the premedication prevents this. Also, administration of low doses (0.01–0.02 mg/kg) at recovery does not seem to affect blood pressure adversely at this time. In hard-to-handle or stress-sensitive patients that were given acepromazine as part of their premedication, additional dosing before recovery may be appropriate to achieve significant sedation. The dose chosen depends on the residual premedication dose effect expected, but 0.01 to 0.02 mg/kg in dogs and 0.02 to 0.1 mg/kg in cats are suggested. In some cases, medetomidine may be preferred (1–2 μg/kg given as the patient is extubated). This is more likely to be chosen for the extremely aggressive animal.

POSTOPERATIVE ANALGESIA

Need for further analgesia is assessed after recovery. The patient must be carefully assessed to determine if excitement, whining, or agitation is pain, dysphoria, or disorientation. When in doubt, pain should be assumed, and the response to treatment defines if this judgment was correct. When pain is suspected or clearly displayed, rapid administration of hydromorphone, fentanyl, or butorphanol, as appropriate, should be performed. Morphine must be given intramuscularly or slowly intravenously. If necessary, propofol (0.5–1-mg/kg increments) can be used to return the animal to an anesthetized state until morphine is fully effective. Diazepam (0.2 mg/kg administered intravenously) is also effective in the short term to deepen the plane of sedation in a recovering animal that is showing signs of pain and provides time for the opioid to take effect. It is important to recognize that some dogs can become quite excited after benzodiazepine administration in the fully awake animal requiring analgesia. The opioid should always be given first in this circumstance.

Low doses of acepromazine (0.01–0.02 mg/kg for dogs, 0.02–0.05 mg/kg for cats) can be given if an animal is appearing only mildly uncomfortable or mildly dysphoric. Response to treatments (acepromazine or more opioid) may be the best method of diagnosis when uncertain. Occasionally, the treatment selected may be a reversal agent. If the patient is clearly dysphoric or returns to a whining state shortly after additional opioid administration, or if suspicion exists related to the use of high doses of opioid during surgery, a slow titration of naloxone can be given to effect (4 μg/kg diluted to 10 mL and given in 1-mL increments every minute).

For the animal that is thrashing and difficult to assess, medetomidine (1–2 μg/kg) can be helpful. Some analgesia is achieved, and when recovery occurs in 15 to 20 minutes, it is usually smooth if the initial recovery behavior was disorientation. This is an excellent approach in the "husky syndrome," wherein disorientation in this breed is associated with dramatic behavioral responses that are difficult to differentiate from pain.

After stabilization of the patient in an analgesic state at recovery, regular assessment is required to maintain this comfortable state. The patient may need no more analgesia, occasional single-dose injections of opioid, or CRI administration of one or more drugs to manage the pain.

ADVICE FOR SPECIFIC CASES

Not every case can be considered in this article, but a few special situations are discussed.

PEDIATRICS

Much evidence exists that human babies experience pain.[49,50] Responses to typical analgesics are not always as expected. A study in puppies revealed that newborn pups have a reduced requirement for analgesia and that, overall, puppies may be more sensitive to opioid-associated respiratory depression.[51] By 1 month of age, puppies have a significantly increased analgesic requirement. Based on this evidence, we must not ignore analgesia but must be cautious to monitor the effects of it.

Our primary analgesic choices for these cases include opioids and local anesthesia. Ketamine may be a consideration as well and seems to be a reasonable choice for short procedures in human infants,[52] although neonates may be less responsive to NMDA antagonists and ketamine is thus ineffective in providing analgesia.[53]

Opioids alone provide good restraint and sedation in addition to analgesia. In most situations, sedatives are not required in pediatric patients. The dose of opioid selected for premedication in healthy pediatric patients is often at the higher end of the range related to patient size, but redosing may be less frequent, and if profound sedation is associated with doses given, lower doses should be chosen. In sick patients or those younger than 1 month of age, low doses should be administered. The patient can be induced with propofol, diazepam/ketamine, or mask inhalant and then maintained on inhalant.

Local anesthesia is an excellent choice when possible. Eutectic mixture of local anesthetics (EMLA) cream is effective for local analgesia if given 30 minutes to penetrate the skin. The weight of the animal must be used to calculate a safe volume of injectable local anesthesia (2% lidocaine or 0.5% bupivicaine at approximately 0.4 mL/kg). Dilution to half strength with saline can be performed to allow more volume without risking toxicity. If laryngeal desensitization is performed, the use of 2% lidocaine drops rather than the 10% spray reduces the lidocaine dose by this route, allowing for a larger volume to be used in other specific local blockade.

NSAIAs are not recommended in patients younger than 8 weeks of age because of their effect on kidney development.

COMMON ELECTIVE SURGICAL PROCEDURES

Premade mixtures containing meperidine or butorphanol for premedication provide a low level of analgesia conferred by the opioid and are capable of producing a short-term mild to moderate analgesic effect. These mixtures are also dosed at the lowest end of the analgesic range, again making them most suitable for mild pain. With this in mind, further analgesia is required in many situations. NSAIAs are useful in these cases. In any elective procedure, the NSAIA loading dose (initial dose as double the maintenance dose) is usually not needed. The approved dosing of meloxicam at 0.3 mg/kg in cats (United States) is not recommended, because a dose of 0.1 or 0.2 mg/kg (orthopedic procedures) is adequate. Effective analgesia is common with use of the maintenance dose (0.1 mg/kg) for elective procedures, because wind-up is not established with any associated increased analgesic demands. If, however, the animal seems to be slightly uncomfortable later in the evening, a second dose can be given because this does not exceed label dosing.

Cat castrations are associated with mild pain and may not require more analgesia than that in the premedication period, provided that the procedure is performed within 15 to 30 minutes of administration. The administration of an NSAIA is a responsible approach to avoid any painful experience, however. Dog castrations should be managed adequately with an NSAIA, even if administered postoperatively, given the same conditions as for the cat. Ovariohysterectomies in dogs and cats may require an additional opioid dose for recovery if the NSAIA is withheld until the operation is over, however. The opioid dose should be calculated in the premedication period, and additional opioid should be added during or after surgery to achieve a total dose of butorphanol at 0.2 to 0.4 mg/kg or meperidine at 5 to 10 mg/kg. A more profound opioid dosed at the lower end of the range may be selected as part of the premedication (usually given with acepromazine), however. The use of NSAIAs for 1 to 3 days is a reasonable option for postoperative analgesia in these cases. If the

NSAIA is given 30 minutes or more before recovery, additional or more profound opioid administration is less likely to be required. Onychectomy in cats is best managed with buprenorphine or hydromorphone as part of the premedication and the addition of local blocks using bupivacaine or a lidocaine-bupivacaine mixture in advance of surgery (see the article by Lemke elsewhere in this issue). Postoperative NSAIA analgesia is indicated for 2 to 3 days. This technique seems to be effective, although fentanyl patches have also been applied for pain associated with the declawing procedure. In this case, because the fentanyl patch usually is removed on discharge and the effect quickly dissipates, analgesia can be continued with an NSAIA for 1 to 2 more days.

EMERGENCY CASES

The reader is referred to the article by Dyson elsewhere in this issue.

CESAREAN SECTION

There is little concern related to the use of opioids for premedication in patients requiring a cesarean section. If puppies or kittens are sedated or have respiratory depression from the expected placental transfer of the opioid, 1 drop of naloxone (0.4 mg/mL from a 1-mL syringe) can be administered under the tongue, and repeat doses can be sent home with the owner if longer acting opioids are involved. Doxapram may be helpful during resuscitation of the newborn if the response to naloxone is poor or if no opioids were used. Because of the analgesic effect of progesterone, which is at high levels at this time in the bitch or queen, butorphanol may be adequate as a premedication. Its short duration of effect can result in mild and short-duration respiratory depression on neonates but provides short-term analgesia in the bitch at recovery. A single dose of an NSAIA is often administered after surgery. Concerns for milk transfer and the impact on the neonate 's kidney development dictate the use of one dose only, however. If low-dose butorphanol is given for the premedication, the bitch could be provided a dose of hydromorphone for discharge, which can then provide several hours of analgesia. The antagonistic effect of the butorphanol is likely to be minimal when a μ-agonist is given approximately 1 hour after butorphanol. Although hydromorphone or morphine is suitable as a premedication in these cases, low-end doses should be given initially, with more given after removal of the puppies if deemed necessary (based on other analgesia present). There is a greater need to reverse the neonate when profound μ-agonists are selected, even when low doses are used. Local analgesia is also a reasonable choice, especially in cases in which inhalant use must be minimized because of cardiovascular instability. A local line block is quick and easy; epidural local analgesia can provide a longer duration of effect but involves more time and expertise.

GERIATRICS

In general, typical doses of analgesia are selected for the geriatric patient. Because of the slower elimination, however, redosing may be required less frequently. As in the pediatric patient, if excessive sedation is associated with the dose selected, lower doses would be administered thereafter. Partial reversal by careful titration with naloxone and saline, as previously described, can also be considered if an excessive effect of the opioid is noted.

SUMMARY

Pain exists; however, we can prevent it, and we can treat it. The fallacy that pain is protective and must be allowed to avoid risk for damage after surgery needs to be eradicated. Preoperative and postoperative analgesia is directed at aching pain, whereas sharp pain associated with inappropriate movements persists. Analgesia provides much more benefit than concern. Preoperative and intraoperative analgesia reduces wind-up and postoperative demands for analgesia, and during general anesthesia, it creates a more balanced plane associated with less cardiovascular depression. The advice given in this article provides guidelines for the veterinarian that can be adjusted according to the patient 's needs and responses. Suggestions are provided from the point of admission to discharge to give a starting point for individual tailoring of an analgesic plan.

REFERENCES

1. American Animal Hospital Association, American Association of Feline Practitioners, AAHA/AAFP Pain Management Guidelines Task Force Members, Hellyer P, Rodan I, Brunt J, et al. AAHA/AAFP pain management guidelines for dogs and cats. J Am Anim Hosp Assoc 2007;43:235–48.
2. de Jong AE, Middelkoop E, Faber AW, et al. Non-pharmacological nursing interventions for procedural pain relief in adults with burns: a systematic literature review. Burns 2007;33:811–27.
3. Golianu B, Krane E, Seybold J, et al. Non-pharmacological techniques for pain management in neonates. Semin Perinatol 2007;31:318–22.
4. Yackey M, Ilkiw JE, Pascoe PJ, et al. Effect of transdermally administered fentanyl on the minimum alveolar concentration of isoflurane in cats. Vet Anaesth Analg 2004;31:183–9.
5. Wilson D, Pettifer GR, Hosgood G. Effect of transdermally administered fentanyl on minimum alveolar concentration of isoflurane in normothermic and hypothermic dogs. J Am Vet Med Assoc 2006;228:1042–6.
6. Ilkiw JE, Pascoe PJ, Tripp LD. Effects of morphine, butorphanol, buprenorphine, and U50488H on the minimum alveolar concentration of isoflurane in cats. Am J Vet Res 2002;63:1198–202.
7. Kay-Mugford PA, Grimm KA, Weingarten AJ, et al. Effect of preoperative administration of tepoxalin on hemostasis and hepatic and renal function in dogs. Vet Ther 2004;5:120–7.
8. Crandell DE, Mathews KA, Dyson DH. Effect of meloxicam and carprofen on renal function when administered to healthy dogs prior to anesthesia and painful stimulation. Am J Vet Res 2004;65:1384–90.
9. Bergmann HM, Nolte IJ, Kramer S. Effects of preoperative administration of carprofen on renal function and hemostasis in dogs undergoing surgery for fracture repair. Am J Vet Res 2005;66:1356–63.
10. Fresno L, Moll J, Peñalba B, et al. Effects of preoperative administration of meloxicam on whole blood platelet aggregation, buccal mucosal bleeding time, and haematological indices in dogs undergoing elective ovariohysterectomy. Vet J 2005;170:138–40.
11. Borer LR, Peel JE, Seewald W, et al. Effect of carprofen, etodolac, meloxicam, or butorphanol in dogs with induced acute synovitis. Am J Vet Res 2003;64:1429–37.

12. Leece EA, Brearley JC, Harding EF. Comparison of carprofen and meloxicam for 72 hours following ovariohysterectomy in dogs. Vet Anaesth Analg 2005;32: 184–92.
13. Mathews KA, Pettifer G, Foster R, et al. Safety and efficacy of preoperative administration of meloxicam, compared with that of ketoprofen and butorphanol in dogs undergoing abdominal surgery. Am J Vet Res 2001;62:882–8.
14. Lascelles BD, Cripps PJ, Jones A, et al. Efficacy and kinetics of carprofen, administered preoperatively or postoperatively, for the prevention of pain in dogs undergoing ovariohysterectomy. Vet Surg 1998;27:568–82.
15. Welsh EM, Nolan AM, Reid J. Beneficial effects of administering carprofen before surgery in dogs. Vet Rec 1997;141:251–3.
16. Tobias KM, Harvey RC, Byarlay JM. A comparison of four methods of analgesia in cats following ovariohysterectomy. Vet Anaesth Analg 2006;33:390–8.
17. Gassel AD, Tobias KM, Egger CM, et al. Comparison of oral and subcutaneous administration of buprenorphine and meloxicam for preemptive analgesia in cats undergoing ovariohysterectomy. J Am Vet Med Assoc 2005;227: 1937–44.
18. Carroll GL, Howe LB, Peterson KD. Analgesic efficacy of preoperative administration of meloxicam or butorphanol in onychectomized cats. J Am Vet Med Assoc 2005;226:913–9.
19. Dobbins S, Brown NO, Shofer FS. Comparison of the effects of buprenorphine, oxymorphone hydrochloride, and ketoprofen for postoperative analgesia after onychectomy or onychectomy and sterilization in cats. J Am Anim Hosp Assoc 2002;38:507–14.
20. Turner PV, Kerr CL, Healy AJ, et al. Effect of meloxicam and butorphanol on minimum alveolar concentration of isoflurane in rabbits. Am J Vet Res 2006;67: 770–4.
21. Ko JC, Lange DN, Mandsager RE, et al. Effects of butorphanol and carprofen on the minimal alveolar concentration of isoflurane in dogs. J Am Vet Med Assoc 2000;217:1025–8.
22. Romans CW, Gordon WJ, Robinson DA, et al. Effect of postoperative analgesic protocol on limb function following onychectomy in cats. J Am Vet Med Assoc 2005;227:89–93.
23. Menigaux C, Guignard B, Fletcher D, et al. Intraoperative small-dose ketamine enhances analgesia after outpatient knee arthroscopy. Anesth Analg 2001;93: 606–12.
24. Stubhaug A. A new method to evaluate central sensitization to pain following surgery. Effect of ketamine. Acta Anaesthesiol Scand Suppl 1997;110:154–5.
25. Chen HC, Sinclair MD, Dyson DH. Use of ephedrine and dopamine in dogs for the management of hypotension in routine clinical cases under isoflurane anesthesia. Vet Anaesth Analg 2007;34:301–11.
26. Pypendop BH, Verstegen JP. Hemodynamic effects of medetomidine in the dog: a dose titration study. Vet Surg 1998;27:612–22.
27. Slingsby I, Lane E, Mears E, et al. Postoperative pain after ovariohysterectomy in the cat: a comparison of two anaesthetic regimens. Vet Rec 1998;143:589–90.
28. Kuo WC, Keegan RD. Comparative cardiovascular, analgesic, and sedative effects of medetomidine, medetomidine-hydromorphone, and medetomidine-butorphanol in dogs. Am J Vet Res 2004;65:931–7.
29. Sammarco JL, Conzemius MG, Perkowski SZ, et al. Postoperative analgesia for stifle surgery: a comparison of intra-articular bupivacaine, morphine, or saline. Vet Surg 1996;25:59–69.

30. Day TK, Pepper WT, Tobias TA, et al. Comparison of intra-articular and epidural morphine for analgesia following stifle arthrotomy in dogs. Vet Surg 1995;24:522–30.
31. Sekar C, Rajasekaran S, Kannan R, et al. Preemptive analgesia for postoperative pain relief in lumbosacral spine surgeries: a randomized controlled trial. Spine J 2004;4:261–4.
32. Martinez V, Belbachir A, Jaber A, et al. The influence of timing of administration on the analgesic efficacy of parecoxib in orthopedic surgery. Anesth Analg 2007;104:1521–7.
33. Onal SA, Keleş E, Toprak GC, et al. Preliminary findings for preemptive analgesia with inhaled morphine: efficacy in septoplasty and septorhinoplasty cases. Otolaryngol Head Neck Surg 2006;135:85–9.
34. Lucas AN, Firth AM, Anderson GA, et al. Comparison of the effects of morphine administered by constant-rate intravenous infusion or intermittent intramuscular injection in dogs. J Am Vet Med Assoc 2001;218:884–91.
35. Muir WW 3rd, Wiese AJ, March PA. Effects of morphine, lidocaine, ketamine, and morphine-lidocaine-ketamine drug combination on minimum alveolar concentration in dogs anesthetized with isoflurane. Am J Vet Res 2003;64:1155–60.
36. Guedes AG, Papich MG, Rude EP, et al. Pharmacokinetics and physiological effects of two intravenous infusion rates of morphine in conscious dogs. J Vet Pharmacol Ther 2007;30:224–33.
37. Robinson EP, Faggella AM, Henry DP, et al. Comparison of histamine release induced by morphine and oxymorphone administration in dogs. Am J Vet Res 1988;49:1699–701.
38. Guedes AG, Papich MG, Rude EP, et al. Comparison of plasma histamine levels after intravenous administration of hydromorphone and morphine in dogs. J Vet Pharmacol Ther 2007;30:516–22.
39. Steagall PV, Teixeira Neto FJ, Minto BW, et al. Evaluation of the isoflurane-sparing effects of lidocaine and fentanyl during surgery in dogs. J Am Vet Med Assoc 2006;229:522–7.
40. Schwieger IM, Hall RI, Hug CC Jr. Less than additive antinociceptive interaction between midazolam and fentanyl in enflurane-anesthetized dogs. Anesthesiology 1991;74:1060–6.
41. Murphy MR, Hug CC Jr. The anesthetic potency of fentanyl in terms of its reduction of enflurane MAC. Anesthesiology 1982;57:485–8.
42. Steagall PV, Carnicelli P, Taylor PM, et al. Effects of subcutaneous methadone, morphine, buprenorphine or saline on thermal and pressure thresholds in cats. J Vet Pharmacol Ther 2006;29:531–7.
43. Lascelles BD, Robertson SA. Antinociceptive effects of hydromorphone, butorphanol, or the combination in cats. J Vet Intern Med 2004;18:190–5.
44. Valverde A, Doherty TJ, Hernández J, et al. Effect of lidocaine on the minimum alveolar concentration of isoflurane in dogs. Vet Anaesth Analg 2004;31:264–71.
45. Nunes de Moraes A, Dyson DH, O 'Grady MR, et al. Plasma concentrations and cardiovascular influence of lidocaine infusions during isoflurane anesthesia in healthy dogs and dogs with subaortic stenosis. Vet Surg 1998;27:486–97.
46. Pypendop BH, Ilkiw JE. Assessment of the hemodynamic effects of lidocaine administered IV in isoflurane-anesthetized cats. Am J Vet Res 2005;66(4):661–8.
47. Gaynor JS, Muir WW. Handbook of veterinary pain management. St. Louis (MO): Mosby; 2002.

48. Reuben SS, Buvanendran A. Preventing the development of chronic pain after orthopaedic surgery with preventive multimodal analgesic techniques. J Bone Joint Surg Am 2007;89:1343–58.
49. Anand KJ, Johnston CC, Oberlander TF, et al. Analgesia and local anesthesia during invasive procedures in the neonate. Clin Ther 2005;27:844–76.
50. Taddio A, Katz J, Ilersich AL, et al. Effect of neonatal circumcision on pain response during subsequent routine vaccination. Lancet 1997;349:599–603.
51. Luks AM, Zwass MS, Brown RC, et al. Opioid-induced analgesia in neonatal dogs: pharmacodynamic differences between morphine and fentanyl. J Pharmacol Exp Ther 1998;284:136–41.
52. Herd D, Anderson BJ. Ketamine disposition in children presenting for procedural sedation and analgesia in a children 's emergency department. Paediatr Anaesth 2007;17:622–9.
53. Gibbs LM, Kendig JJ. Substance P and NMDA receptor-mediated slow potentials in neonatal rat spinal cord: age-related changes. Brain Res 1992;595:236–41.

Analgesia and Chemical Restraint for the Emergent Veterinary Patient

Doris H. Dyson, DVM, DVSc

KEYWORDS

- Emergency • Analgesia • Anesthesia • Sedation
- Dog • Cat

Pain level is considered the fifth vital sign in human patients,[1] and hospital accreditation may include the institution's approach to pain assessment and management.[2] This assertive approach emphasizes the importance of pain management and has also been included in the American Animal Hospital Association recommendations. Because animals feel and anticipate pain by similar mechanisms as people do,[3] this emphasis on pain management should also apply to animals. Continual painful experience in any animal is detrimental to the overall healing process and to the general well-being of any animal or person.[4–6] Pain often results in a prolonged hospital stay and increases the potential for secondary problems. Because there may be a link between acute pain and chronic pain in human beings with the hypothesis that if the acute pain were better controlled, the chronic pain would not develop,[7] this is also another factor to consider in animals. While considering all the negative physiologic effects associated with the experience of pain, above all, one's actions should be governed by the inhumane aspects of this unnecessary experience.

Frequently, analgesics are withheld in the emergent patient, because a common misconception is that analgesics "mask" physiologic indicators (eg, heart rate, respiratory rate) of patient deterioration. This is not the case. Evidence exists in the human literature,[8] and has also been an observation in veterinary patients,[9] that analgesics do not mask the signs of patient deterioration and should not be withheld for this reason. Even when large doses of opioids are used as a constant rate infusion (CRI) to treat pain, heart rate in response to hypotension, hypoxia, hypovolemia, or hypercarbia is still high. In fact, when the patient is treated adequately for pain, the potential for

Portions of this article were previously published in: Mathews KA, Dyson DH. Analgesia and chemical restraint for the emergent patient. Vet Clin North Am Small Anim Pract 2005;35: 481–515; with permission.
Department of Clinical Studies, Ontario Veterinary College, University of Guelph, Guelph, Ontario, Canada N1G 2W1
E-mail address: ddyson@ovc.uoguelph.ca

Vet Clin Small Anim 38 (2008) 1329–1352
doi:10.1016/j.cvsm.2008.06.007 vetsmall.theclinics.com
0195-5616/08/$ – see front matter

the tachycardia being pain related is eliminated and the clinician is alerted to patient deterioration. If analgesics are not used, the tachycardia may be presumed to be attributable to pain and other reasons are not considered.

Another major concern with analgesic use expressed by many veterinarians is the potential toxicity or adverse reactions associated with drug administration.[10–12] It is the impression of this author, and others, that these adverse effects, primarily those associated with opioid use, are overemphasized. With respect to ventilation, opioid administration after a traumatic incident may improve ventilation rather than impair it. A study performed in hypovolemic dogs (30% blood loss) confirmed that oxymorphone (no longer available) or hydromorphone does not result in deterioration in hemodynamics.[13] This concern for potential adverse effects of various analgesics is also a major reason for less frequent analgesic administration to cats.[10,11,14] Given our current level of understanding of the adverse effects of many analgesics in cats,[15] however, there is no longer an overriding reason for withholding them in this species (see the article by Robertson elsewhere in this issue). Throughout the veterinary literature, various analgesic regimens are suggested for many painful states in cats and dogs, and it is recommended that these "tried and true" guidelines be used rather than sticking to "traditional" or outdated single-study dogma.

The use of nonsteroidal anti-inflammatory analgesics (NSAIAs) in the emergent patient may be a concern, and they should be withheld until the volume, cardiovascular, and renal status of a patient is determined to be within normal limits and with no potential for deterioration.[16] For further detail on this topic, refer to the article by Papich elsewhere in this issue. As a guideline, until studies indicate safety in this group of patients, NSAIAs should not be administered to patients that have acute renal insufficiency, hepatic insufficiency, dehydration, hypotension, conditions associated with low "effective circulating volume," coagulopathies, evidence of gastric ulceration, or gastrointestinal disorders of any kind. Concurrent use of other NSAIAs (including aspirin) or corticosteroids is not recommended. NSAIAs are contraindicated in patients that have spinal injury (including herniated intervertebral disk) because of the potential for hemorrhage with associated neurologic deterioration. Cyclooxygenase (COX)-2 NSAIAs may not be a problem; however, even minor hemorrhage in the spinal cord may be deleterious. NSAIAs should never be administered to patients in shock, trauma cases on presentation, or patients with evidence of hemorrhage. Patients that have severe or poorly controlled asthma, or other moderate to severe pulmonary disease, may deteriorate with NSAIA administration. After further study in the future, COX-2 preferential or COX-1–sparing NSAIAs (eg, meloxicam, etodolac, carprofen, tolfenamic acid) may prove to be safe in some of these conditions. NSAIAs may have effects on the reproductive tract and fetus,[17] and therefore should not be administered during pregnancy and in breeding female animals during ovulation and subsequent implantation of the embryo (see the article by Mathews elsewhere in this issue).

In addition to analgesia for pain, many injured or ill animals require analgesia to facilitate restraint, diagnostic, and emergency procedures. Because each animal is presented with varying levels of injury or illness and is experiencing different degrees of pain (**Fig. 1**), individual drug selection and dosing to effect are essential rather than considering a standard regimen for all patients.

AGGRESSION

It is not uncommon for patients to be aggressive on presentation, preventing even the simplest of assessments or treatments. Cats are likely to be aggressive in a strange environment and after a fearful car trip. Animals may appear to be reasonably stable when

Severe to Excrutiating

Neuropathic pain – nerve entrapment, cervical intervertebral disc herniation, nerve inflammation

Central nervous system infarction/tumors

Meningitis

Inflammation – extensive (ie, peritonitis, fasciitis – especially *streptococcal,* cellulitis)

Multiple fractures repair where extensive soft tissue injury exists

Necrotizing pancreatitis

Necrotizing cholecystitis

Pathologic fractures

Bone cancer

Moderate to severe and severe (varies with degree of illness or injury)

Osteoarthritis, acute polyarthritis

Early or resolving stages of above soft tissue injuries/inflammation/disease

Peritonitis (ie,bacterial, urine, bile, pancreatic)

Capsular pain due to organomegally (ie, pyelonephritis, hepatitis, splenitis, splenic torsion)

Hollow organ distension

Mesenteric, gastric, testicular or other torsions

Ureteral/urethral/biliary obstruction

Pleuritis

Traumatic diaphragmatic hernia repair (associated with organ and extensive tissue injury)

Trauma (ie,orthopedic, extensive soft tissue, head)

Thoracolumbar disc disease

Re-warming after accidental hypothermia

Frostbite

Cancer pain

Mucositis after radiation therapy

Thrombosis/ischemia (arterial or venous), aortic saddle thrombosis

Hypertrophic osteodystrophy

Panosteitis

Corneal abrasion/ulceration

Glaucoma

Uveitis

Whelping/queening

Mastitits

Moderate

Diaphragmatic hernia repair (acute, simple with no organ injury)

Soft tissue injuries (ie,less severe than above)

Urethral obstruction

Early or resolving conditions mentioned above

Mild to moderate

Some dental problems

Some lacerations

Cystitis

Otitis

Chest drains

Early or resolving conditions mentioned above

Mild

Early, resolving or simple involvement of conditions mentioned above

Fig. 1. Expected level of pain associated with various emergent conditions.

acting aggressively, but this assumption should not be made hastily. Endorphin and epinephrine release can mask the seriousness of the patient's clinical condition. In the author's experience, for example, severely dehydrated cats can be so difficult to handle that a proper assessment is impossible without some chemical restraint (**Table 1**). These

Table 1
Commonly used drugs for most trauma patients

Drug	Dose	Route	Comments
Opioids			
Butorphanol	0.1–0.4 mg/kg	IM, IV	If concerns, titrate to effect in low doses initially Use if analgesia is necessary in neurologic cases regardless of potentiated respiratory depression; hand or mechanical positive-pressure ventilation can be instituted if this risk exists
Fentanyl	2–5 μg/kg/h	IM, IV	Titrated to effect as a CRI is recommended for moderate to severe pain Administration can be stopped periodically to allow for neurologic assessment in such cases
Hydromorphone	0.03–0.15 mg/kg	IM, IV	Preferred when upper gastrointestinal obstruction or significant CNS trauma is not present The younger and healthier an animal is, the higher is the dose that is required and the less sedative effect this opioid has if given alone If concerns, titrate to effect in low doses initially
Meperidine	3–10 mg/kg	IM	Suggested dose (low doses for giant breeds and high doses for cats and tiny dogs) If this is not effective, a more profound opioid or a mild sedative can be administered It may have less respiratory depression and rarely produces vomiting; thus, it is suitable in neurologic cases
Morphine	0.3–1 mg/kg	IM, SC	This is an alternative to hydromorphone but is limited by its route of administration Slow IV titration (diluted and given over 5 minutes at least) should reduce the chance of histamine release, while enabling administration to the desired effect

Other analgesics			
Ketamine	2–10 mg/kg	Preferably IV	Given by any route (including squirting a dose in the mouth) can easily and effectively restrain aggressive cats Avoid in animals with heart disease Recommended to be given with acepromazine, a benzodiazepine, or an opioid, if at all possible, to improve restraint and provide some relaxation
Medetomidine	0.01–0.02 mg/kg (for healthy animals)	—	Ability to reverse these drugs provides added safety and convenience for outpatients Can also be used in lower doses (0.005–0.01 mg/kg) with opioids to provide dependable and profound restraint in healthy animals
Sedatives			
Acepromazine	0.01–0.05 mg/kg 0.05–0.15 mg/kg (cats)	IM, IV, SC	Can be administered in combination with opioids or ketamine for more sedation and restraint when minor compromise is apparent and advanced age is not a concern Higher doses for smaller animals and when more restraint needed Lower doses in older or larger animals
Midazolam or diazepam	0.2–0.5 mg/kg	IV recommended	Safest supplements to opioid sedation IM absorption of midazolam is better than diazepam because of the solubility characteristics, and it is preferred, if available, when an IM route is chosen

This list is far from complete. These examples and their assessed levels of pain are only presumed. Please refer to **Tables 1–7** for suggested analgesic therapy with dose and interval adjustment based on the individual patient response.

Abbreviations: CNS, central nervous system; CRI, constant rate infusion; h, hours; IM, intramuscular; IV, intravenous; SC, subcutaneous.

Adapted from Mathews K, editor. PAIN how to understand, recognize, treat, and stop. CD-ROM ISBN0-9732655-0-7. Jonkar Computer Systems: Guelph, Ontario, Canada; 2003; with permission.

animals should be cautiously assessed from afar, and a thorough history should be taken before selecting a method of restraint. Chemical restraint rather than force is the humane and often safer way to deal with them. Once the reason for the aggression has been decided on, a more direct approach to the problem might be possible. Aggression may be secondary to significant pain and fear in traumatized animals. Respiratory distress may appear as a combination of panic and aggression.

If possible, place an oxygen mask on these animals or provide "flow-by" oxygen for supplementation when stress, poor perfusion, or respiratory compromise could exist. An oxygen mask provides a degree of protection to the handler as a type of muzzle for dogs. The aggressive cat could be allowed to settle down in an induction chamber with oxygen administration. If pain is a component of the aggression, opioid administration is a safe and effective approach to management. Opioids are considered extremely safe from the cardiovascular standpoint, with side effects that are usually easy to treat (anticholinergic administration in the case of bradycardia or titration of naloxone should other unwanted effects occur). Because the intravenous route is often not possible in these animals, drugs that can be administered intramuscularly, absorbed through mucous membranes, or inhaled are considered. The dose of opioid does not need to be reduced because of advanced or young age; rather, it is related to the clinical condition. When doubt exists as to the origin of the animal's illness, it may be wise to use meperidine initially (mild effect, short duration, minimal respiratory depression or panting, rarely producing nausea, and reversible). Meperidine at a dose of 3 to 10 mg/kg administered intramuscularly is suggested (lower doses for giant breeds and higher doses for cats and tiny dogs). If this is not effective, a more profound opioid or a mild sedative can be administered. When upper gastrointestinal obstruction or significant central nervous system (CNS) trauma is not present, a profound opioid, such as hydromorphone at a dose of 0.05 to 0.2 mg/kg administered intramuscularly or intravenously (maximum of 0.1 mg/kg in cats) or morphine at a dose of 0.5 to 1 mg/kg administered intramuscularly (dogs) or 0.2 mg/kg administered intramuscularly (cats, repeating the dose if needed) has a more calming effect. Mydriasis is noted in cats as the opioid effects occur. The young and healthier animal may require the higher dose, and a sedative is also usually required. When the physiologic status of the patient is not known, the safest supplement to opioid sedation is midazolam or diazepam (0.2–0.5 mg/kg). Absorption of midazolam is better than that of diazepam when given intramuscularly because of the solubility characteristics, and it is preferred when an intramuscular route is chosen. Occasionally, the benzodiazepines are unpredictable and excitement may occur, although this is more common in healthy young animals. When minor compromise is apparent and advanced age is not a concern, the aggressive animal can be most effectively and predictably sedated with a profound opioid and acepromazine at a dose of 0.02 to 0.05 mg/kg (dogs) and 0.05 to 0.15 mg/kg (cats). Aggressive cats can be restrained effectively and easily with ketamine (2–10 mg/kg) given by any route, including squirting a dose into the mouth. Midazolam, diazepam, or acepromazine should be combined with ketamine when an intramuscular route is possible to produce better restraint and relaxation with lower doses of ketamine. Avoid ketamine in cats if the possibility exists of significant renal compromise, because it requires renal excretion for recovery.[18] α_2-Agonists can be used in low doses with opioids to provide dependable and profound restraint in healthy animals. It is important to stress "healthy animals," because arrhythmias, cardiac output depression, and mortality have been associated with the use of xylazine in small animals when anesthesia follows.[19,20] Although the newer drugs in this class (eg, medetomidine) produce similar cardiac output effects and bradycardia, they may prove useful if used judiciously and combined with opioids to reduce the dose required. Healthy animals can be given xylazine at a dose of 0.05 to 0.2 mg/kg or medetomidine at a dose of 0.005 to 0.02 mg/kg with low to moderate doses of opioids. Cardiovascular effects are similar within these dose ranges of medetomidine, but the duration of the negative effects is shorter with lower doses. The sedation achieved is more predictable with higher doses of medetomidine, however. The ability to reverse these drugs provides some safety with their use and obvious convenience for outpatients or when daily procedures (eg, bandage changes) are required. Obtain intravenous access as soon as the animal allows it. Oxygen supplementation is also beneficial in patients with low cardiac output states.

An aggressive animal with unknown health status should not be given intramuscular doses of any drug at doses capable of producing anesthesia, even if anesthesia might be required. Attempt mild to moderate restraint with initial drug therapy, and if the animal then proves to be sensitive to the drugs, there is less chance of adverse effects or overdose. If you have achieved some restraint, you can then carry out the proper evaluation of the patient, allowing you to formulate a safe anesthetic plan if required.

Because of the potential for extremely sick cats to remain aggressive (sometimes in spite of opioid administration or restraint) for an intramuscular injection may be difficult and stressful, chamber inhalant induction is often required. This is a good choice in aggressive cats with suspected renal failure or in older cats with an unknown medical condition. Isoflurane and sevoflurane are suitable inhalants, but it is best to delay induction to general anesthesia until the cat's epinephrine release has minimized. Allow the animal to calm down in the tank before turning on the inhalant. Oxygen should be provided, and a towel over the chamber may initially help to reduce the animal's anxiety. Observe the animal frequently during induction, and move the tank to assess the level of restraint achieved. Remove the cat, and transfer it to a mask as soon as possible to allow better depth evaluation. Recognize that complete anesthetic induction is not always required for restraint and that sedation alone is possible with inhalants. If respiratory depression or obstruction occurs with this degree of restraint, complete induction and intubation are required; so be prepared. The patient requires cautious monitoring during this time (whether restraint or anesthesia is provided) while catheter placement, blood samples, and other diagnostic assessments may be occurring. An appropriate analgesic can be given after restraint if pain is a component of the problem or diagnostic procedure. The inhalant percent dialed should be reduced within 5 minutes of administration to avoid a deepened plane. If the cat is induced more rapidly (2–3 min) than expected, this may imply that significant cardiac output depression is present; thus, rapid crystalloid (10–30 mL/kg) or synthetic colloid (3–10 mL/kg) therapy given over 10 to 30 minutes, potentially with inotropic support (dopamine at a dose of 10 μg/kg/min or to effect), is advised. Suggested analgesics or sedatives for consideration after achieving restraint are listed in **Table 1**.

NEUROLOGIC COMPROMISE

Significant CNS depression can be present in cases admitted for emergency care. It is critical to provide oxygen and determine if positive-pressure ventilation is required. Increased respiratory depression with resultant increased $Paco_2$ from opioid drug therapy can result in an increase in intracranial pressure (ICP), as can nausea and vomiting, and could eventually result in brain herniation if not addressed. Although analgesia may seem to be adequate based on the level of CNS depression caused by head trauma, this must be well assessed, because pain also increases ICP. If analgesia is necessary, it should be administered by titrating low doses of an opiate slowly to effect. Fentanyl at a dosage of 2 to 5 μg/kg every 15 to 20 minutes is preferred, but butorphanol (0.1–0.4 mg/kg administered intravenously) or meperidine (3–5 mg/kg administered intramuscularly) is a reasonable alternative and is less likely to produce vomiting. Vomiting must be avoided, and is more common with a relative opioid overdose; titration of fentanyl may reduce the incidence of vomiting, because an overdose is avoided. Positive-pressure ventilation should be instituted if the risk for potentiated respiratory depression exists. Fentanyl CRI in cats and dogs is recommended for moderate to severe pain. Because fentanyl has a short duration of action (approximately 20 minutes), administration can be stopped periodically to allow for neurologic assessment. The response to these drugs must be monitored cautiously. When indicated, the use of a 2-mg/kg bolus of lidocaine, followed by 1 to 2 mg/kg/h for analgesia in these dogs, may be of value for up to 24 hours. A reduction in ICP may also occur with lidocaine administered intravenously[21–23] (K. Mathews, personal observation, 2007). Suggested analgesics are listed in **Table 1**.

RESPIRATORY COMPROMISE

Respiratory compromise is usually apparent directly on admission and is often associated with excitement, panic, or anxiety. If severe, it can progress rapidly to respiratory and cardiac arrest, and therefore must be dealt with immediately. Calming the animal facilitates therapy in mild situations, but anesthesia may be necessary for immediate treatment in severely distressed patients. In these situations, advanced preparation for intubation and ventilation should be performed; equipment and drugs should be available with doses calculated. Personnel who might be involved should be properly briefed on monitoring these patients and the need to respond quickly and efficiently if deterioration should occur. Recommendations for analgesia in the respiratory-compromised patient are listed in **Table 2**.

UPPER AIRWAY OBSTRUCTION

Although pain may not be experienced with most cases of airway obstruction, it is present with trauma to the upper airway. Typical causes of obstruction involve laryngeal paralysis, laryngeal or pharyngeal foreign bodies, tumors, inflammation or edema, brachycephalic syndrome, or collapsing trachea. Rapid intervention is usually necessary to guarantee oxygen delivery. Handling the animal may result in increased stress and anxiety that can worsen the situation. Calm the animal while attempting oxygen delivery by mask or flow-by. A mixture of oxygen and helium (Heliox, Linde Group [BOC], Guelph, Ontario, Canada) may be more effective because of ease of inspiration in the presence of increased airway resistance.[24] Use a low dose of acepromazine (0.01–0.05 mg/kg) adjusted for size and age combined with butorphanol (0.05–0.2 mg/kg) adjusted for size or hydromorphone (0.02–0.05 mg/kg) titrated slowly to effect. The intravenous route is preferred for the most rapid effect and ability to titrate, avoiding a relative overdose, which may result in panting or vomiting.

LOWER RESPIRATORY INJURY

Chemical restraint and analgesia are required to facilitate placement of a nasal oxygen cannula or chest tube, or for radiographic examination. The method of restraint selected should be the minimum required for the procedure with supplemental oxygen provided before, during, and after the procedure. Generous instillation of an ophthalmic local anesthetic into the nasal meatus is adequate for oxygen cannula placement in cats and dogs. Before chest tube placement in dogs, butorphanol or hydromorphone administered intravenously with low-dose acepromazine or diazepam, at doses suggested previously, is usually effective. Incremental doses of ketamine at 2 mg/kg administered intravenously to effect may be added, or slow titration (0.03–0.04-mL/kg increments) of diazepam and ketamine (a ratio of ketamine, 1 mL [100 mg/mL], to diazepam, 1 mL [5 mg/mL]) can provide good restraint. Cats should be anesthetized. Infiltration of a local anesthetic through skin to pleura should always be used before chest tube placement in cats and dogs even when anesthetized. A warmed 1% solution of lidocaine or 0.25% bupivicaine is recommended to avoid the "sting" of the more concentrated solution. Intrapleural and intraperitoneal placement of local anesthetics is a useful adjunct to opioid analgesics for thoracic incisional pain or pleuritis or pain associated with pancreatitis. Prepare a mixture of 0.5% bupivacaine (0.2 mL/kg) and sodium bicarbonate (0.01 mEq/kg), dilute with 0.9% saline (3 mL in cats and tiny dogs and 6–12 mL [relative to size of the dog] for larger dogs), and instill into the peritoneal or pleural space by means of a chest drain for intrapleural analgesia or a catheter for intraperitoneal analgesia. Be cautious to use aseptic technique. Flush with saline at a further dose of 3 to 12 mL (or a volume equal to the chest tube volume) to ensure placement into the pleural space. The addition of the sodium bicarbonate reduces the pain associated with local anesthetics at this site by increasing the pH of the solution. Do not add more sodium bicarbonate, because this makes the solution too alkaline; the ratio of drugs and saline must be adhered to. Without the sodium bicarbonate, local anesthetic instillation is painful. After intrapleural administration, the animal should be placed with the injured or incision side down for 5 minutes to enhance the effect at the desired site. The patient can also be rolled onto its back to allow the local anesthetic to flow into the paravertebral gutters to block nerves before entering the spinal cord. If the patient still appears uncomfortable, adjust its position to facilitate redistribution of the local anesthetic. Although the addition of sodium bicarbonate reduces the pain experienced, the positioning required and the local anesthetic itself can cause some pain; thus, be prepared for this.

DIAPHRAGMATIC HERNIA

Oxygen supplementation is critical to the safe management of cases of diaphragmatic hernia. Pleural fluid should be removed before any procedure to reduce ventilatory and oxygenation impairment. Significant cardiovascular compromise is also possible in these patients, and replacement of fluid deficits is important. Special concerns related to intestinal incarceration exist. Restraint may be required for radiography or thoracocentesis. Opioid or diazepam sedation is the safest approach when significant respiratory compromise is present.

MAJOR CHEST TRAUMA

Oxygen supplementation is a vital part of the treatment in these patients. These animals also need analgesia and may require some sedation to reduce movement and subsequent painful stimulation. Depending on the degree of pain associated with the injury, butorphanol (0.2–0.4 mg/kg), hydromorphone (03–0.1 mg/kg administered intravenously), or morphine (0.3–0.5 mg/kg administered intramuscularly [dogs] and 0.1–0.2 mg/kg administered intramuscularly [cats]) can be used. Although morphine can be given slowly intravenously, the possibility of histamine release with hypotension is a concern with the intravenous route of administration[25] and intramuscular administration is recommended (except if an infusion is used). Doses selected are primarily size related (smaller dose per kilogram for bigger dogs) and slowly titrated to effect when administered intravenously. An increased respiratory rate may be an early sign of a mild overdose, and the administration of the opioid can be stopped

Table 2
Respiratory compromise

Drug	Dose	Route	Comments
Upper airway obstruction or trauma			
Butorphanol with or without acepromazine	0.05–0.2 mg/kg 0.01–0.05 mg/kg	IM, IV	Doses should be adjusted for size and age Butorphanol may be selected for its antitussive effect Beneficial by IV route for rapid effect If unsuccessful, anesthetic induction and intubation are necessary
Diazepam and ketamine or propofol	2.5 mg/mL and 50 mg/mL of mixture at 0.02-mL/kg increments 1-mg/kg increments	IV IV	Chosen for the advantage of safe and slow induction to effect These animals may be sensitive to the dose used, especially if hypoxic Titrate to affect (0.25–0.20 of typical induction doses repeated in 15–20 seconds until intubation is possible
Diazepam	0.2 mg/kg	IV	Can be given to reduce the dose of propofol required and potential adverse cardiovascular effects (hypotension from vasodilation)
Dexamethazone	0.25 mg/kg	IV	Administration is advised to reduce edema
Butorphanol	0.05–0.2 mg/kg	IM, IV	As an antitussive and to assist recovery extubation if not already administered
Meperidine	2.5 mg/kg	IM	As an antitussive and to assist recovery extubation if not already administered
Placement of nasal cannula			
Generous instillation of an ophthalmic local anesthetic into the nasal meatus			
Chest tube placement (dogs)			
Butorphanol	0.05–0.2 mg/kg	IM, IV	Infiltration of a local anesthetic should be used in addition
or hydromorphone	0.05–0.1 mg/kg	IM, IV	Dose selected within the ranges provided should be based
or morphine	0.1–0.3 mg/kg	IM, IV	on required effect, size, and age
or methadone	0.1–0.3 mg/kg	IM, SC	
All with or without acepromazine	0.01–0.05 mg/kg	IV	
or diazepam	0.2 mg/kg	IV

Chest tube placement (cats)			
Butorphanol ±	0.1–0.4 mg/kg	IM, IV	Short-term anesthesia may be required for these procedures in cats
Diazepam	0.2 mg/kg	IV	—
With propofol	1-mg/kg increments	IV	Titrated for induction and isoflurane maintenance is preferred for such a short procedure because of the rapid recovery
Ketamine or diazepam and ketamine	2 mg/kg increments Slow titration of 2.5:50 mg/mL mixture at 0.02 mL/kg increments	IV to effect IV	This is a safe approach in cats with severe respiratory compromise and unknown cardiovascular status The sympathetic drive and lesser respiratory depression may offer a slight advantage of ketamine over propofol, although either may be used if cautious
Major chest trauma			
Butorphanol or hydropmorphone or morphine or methadone All with or without acepromazine or diazepam	0.2–0.4 mg/kg 0.05–0.2 mg/kg (titrate IV to effect) 0.3–0.5 mg/kg (dogs) 0.1–0.2 mg/kg (cats) 0.3-0.5 mg/kg 0.01-0.05 mg/kg 0.2 mg/kg	IM, IV IV IM IM IM, IV IV	Doses selected are primarily size related (smaller dose per kilogram for bigger dogs) Increased respiratory rate may be an early sign of a mild overdose, and drug should be stopped Although morphine can be given slowly IV, the possibility of histamine release can be a significant concern; IM administration is recommended (except if an infusion is used)
Ketamine	1–2 mg/kg	IV	This can provide short-term analgesia if morphine is selected for the long-term analgesic
Bupivacaine (for intercostal nerve blocks)	0.2 mL/kg of 0.5%	—	Divided between four to six nerves can provide analgesia for 3–6 hours and can be repeated as needed for rib fractures
Epidural analgesia with morphine (see **Table 4**)			

Abbreviations: IM, intramuscular; IV, intravenous; SC, subcutaneous.

Adapted from Mathews K, editor. PAIN how to understand, recognize, treat, and stop. CD-ROM ISBN0-9732655-0-7. Jonkar Computer Systems: Guelph, Ontario, Canada; 2003; with permission.

before panting occurs. Ketamine at a dose of 1 to 2 mg/kg administered intravenously can provide a short-term solution for analgesia if intramuscular morphine is selected for the long-term analgesic. Consider the use of local anesthesia to supplement systemic analgesia. Intercostal nerve blocks using 0.5% bupivacaine (0.2 mL/kg) divided between four to six nerves can provide excellent analgesia for 3 to 6 hours and can be repeated as needed for rib fractures. Epidural analgesia using morphine at a dosage of 0.1 to 0.3 mg/kg every 8 to 12 hours can impart reasonable analgesia in the thorax with limited adverse systemic effects.[26] For further information, see the article by Valverde elsewhere in this issue.

OTHER TRAUMA

Obviously, lacerations and fractures from trauma require analgesia. The drug and dose for initial management are determined by the severity and the instability of the injury (**Table 3**). The fractured limb should be immobilized until definitive repair is possible. Immobilization of fractures reduces pain significantly, and this should be performed as soon as possible. Few, if any, analgesics can stop incident pain produced by movement of fractured bones. Initially, opioids should be administered while determining cardiovascular and volume status. If there are no concerns for ongoing hemorrhage and hypovolemia or other contraindications for administration of an NSAIA, meloxicam, carprofen, or tolfenamic acid may be administered parenterally (**Table 4**). Analgesia recommendations for ongoing pain (after the initial acute management) are provided in **Table 4**.

Traumatic injury frequently results in muscle pain as well. We all have experienced this but tend to forget it in our veterinary patients. Even if lacerations and fractures are not identified, muscular pain can be present. This results from a direct blow to the muscle resulting in contusion. Hemorrhage or hematomas may compromise neural structures or result in muscle necrosis, which can be painful. Evidence of hemorrhage may be visualized as bruising, but if it is severe, blood seeps through the skin. Delayed-onset muscular pain is common in people and usually starts several hours after injury. Muscle contusions are painful, and activity should be reduced but not ceased unless there is a fracture present. To reduce swelling, and thus further discomfort, injuries to musculotendinous structures may benefit from local ice pack therapy (not directly placed onto the skin) for the first 24 hours; thereafter, heat application with gentle stretching of injured muscles is advocated.[27]

Injuries sustained to the abdomen, pelvis, hind limbs, and soft tissue of the posterior portion of the body may also benefit from epidural analgesia. Should parenteral opioids, combined with an NSAIA in the stable patient be inadequate to control pain until definitive repair, epidural analgesia is recommended. If this is not possible, consider the addition of the adjunct analgesics, lidocaine, or ketamine (**Table 5**). A urinary catheter should be placed in these animals.

CARDIOVASCULAR COMPROMISE

Avoid unnecessary sedation and anesthesia whenever possible, but recognize that excessive manual restraint with accompanying stress can be associated with epinephrine release and potential adverse effects. Drug doses selected should be low in most circumstances, and titration to effect is desirable (intravenous or inhalant administration) (**Table 6**). Any opioid alone is reasonable for sedation. Diazepam at a dose of 0.2 mg/kg administered intravenously can be added to improve the effect. The adverse effects are usually minimal. If bradycardia results, an anticholinergic, such as glycopyrrolate at a dose of 0.005 to 0.01 mg/kg administered intravenously,

Table 3
Suggested analgesics for the initial management of acute pain in cats and dogs

Severe to excruciating pain:
Requires high-dose opioids (titration to effect over 3–5 minutes is recommended)
Hydromorphone, 0.1 mg/kg (dogs and cats), or morphine, 1 mg/kg (dogs) and 0.2 mg/kg (cats), administered slowly IV or IM and give more if needed, to effect; use the effective dose divided by 2 to 4 to establish an hourly SC or IV CRI
or
Fentanyl, 10 to 50 μg/kg, administered IV titrated to effect (cats and dogs); use the effective dose as an hourly CRI
± NSAIAs when not contraindicated
Ketamine, 4 mg/kg, combined with the opioid previously recommended as a bolus (dogs and cats)
Lidocaine, 2–4 mg/kg bolus, followed by 2-4-mg/kg/h CRI (dogs); 0.25–1-mg/kg bolus and then 0.5–2 mg/kg/h (cats)
Caution with respect to overdose if local anesthetics have been administered by means of a different route
Tachycardia may persist and it may be impossible to control the pain. Consider combining these analgesics with epidurally placed analgesics or local blocks, or anesthetize the patient while attempting to find or treat the inciting cause. Remove the inciting cause immediately. This degree of pain can cause death.

Drug	Dose	Duration of Action or Dosing Interval
Moderate to severe pain		
Morphine or methadone Use low end of the dose for moderate pain	Cat: 0.1–0.2+ mg/kg IM, SC Dog: 0.5–1+ mg/kg IM, SC For IV dosing, use half the low-end dose, titrate over 3–5 minutes	2–6 h IM, SC 1–4 h IV
Hydromorphone Use low end of the dose for moderate pain	Cat and dog: 0.02– 0.1+ mg/kg IV, IM, SC	2–6 h
Fentanyl Use low end of the dose for moderate pain	Cat and dog: 0.001–0.01+ mg/kg	0.3 h
Ketamine Use low end of the dose for moderate pain	Cat and dog: 1–4 mg/kg IV Cat and dog: 2–10 mg/kg PO	prn (∼0.5 h)
Note: Opioids should be given to effect (previously cited dosing and frequency are the only guidelines).		
Mild to moderate pain: Use opioids listed previously for moderate pain at low end of dosage range for cats and dogs		
Butorphanol Use low end of dose for mild pain	Cat and dog: 0.1–0.4 IV Cat: 0.4–0.8 mg/kg IM, SC Dog: 0.1–0.4 mg/kg IM, SC	0.25–1 h 2–4 h 1–2 (3) h
Buprenorphine Use low end of dose for mild pain	Cat: 0.005–0.01 mg/kg IV, IM 0.02 mg/kg sublingual Dog: 0.005–0.02 mg/kg IV, IM	4–8 h 7 h 4–8 h
Meperidine (pethidine)	Cat and dog: 5–10 mg/kg IM, SC	20–30 min

Abbreviations: CRI, constant rate infusion; h, hours; IM, intramuscular; IV, intravenous; PO, per os; prn, as needed; SC, subcutaneous.

Adapted from Mathews K, editor. PAIN how to understand, recognize, treat, and stop. CD-ROM ISBN0-9732655-0-7. Jonkar Computer Systems: Guelph, Ontario, Canada; 2003; with permission.

Table 4
Suggested analgesia for various levels of ongoing pain

Severe to excruciating pain:
Requires high-dose opioids (titration to effect over 3–5 minutes is recommended) as described for initial treatment
This degree of pain can cause death.
Note: Opioids, ketamine, or lidocaine as a CRI can be combined in IV crystalloid fluids (fentanyl and ketamine have not been tested in lactated Ringer's solution or Ringer's solution, and therefore may not be compatible because of calcium content, using a burette in-line with the maintenance fluid rate). An additional individual drug can be placed in the burette, or additional fluids can be added to dilute if reduction is required.
Epidural analgesia/anesthesia: A 1:1 mixture of preservative-free morphine (1 mg/mL) and 0.25% bupivacaine is injected over 5 to 10 minutes (to avoid vomiting and development of a patchy block) at 0.1 mL/kg (sternal recumbency). Follow with a CRI at 0.4 to 0.8 mL/kg/d using a syringe pump. If lidocaine is given systemically, eliminate bupivacaine from this mixture to avoid overdose of local anesthetic. As an alternative to a CRI, intermittent injections (over 5–10 minutes) of 0.15 to 0.2 mL/kg every 6 hours may be administered. If hind limb weakness is encountered, the bupivacaine dose should be reduced by one half (0.125%) or one quarter (0.0625%) by diluting with sterile saline before mixing with the morphine.

Moderate to severe pain		
Morphine or methadone	Cat: 0.1–0.2+ mg/kg IV; titrate to effect over 3–5 minutes; 0.1–0.2 repeated as needed IM, SC	1–4 h 2–6 h
	Dog: 0.3–1 mg/kg IV, IM, SC Administer intermittently or follow with a CRI with effective dose over dosing interval	2–4 h
Hydromorphone	Cat and dog: 0.02–0.1+ mg/kg IV, IM, SC Administer intermittently or follow with a CRI with effective dose over dosing interval	2–6 h
Fentanyl	Cat and dog: 0.004–0.01+ mg/kg IV 0.001–0.010+ mg/kg/h	0.3 h CRI
Fentanyl patch	Cat: <10 kg; dog: 25 μg/h	3–5 days
	Dog: 10–20 kg to 50 μg/h 20–30 kg to 75 μg/h >30 kg to 100 μg/h	3 days
Ketamine (combined with an opioid or sedative)	Cat and dog: 1–4+ mg/kg/h IV, SC 0.2–4 mg/kg IV	5–30 minutes CRI
Note: The following NSAIAs should not be administered if any contraindications exist.		
Ketoprofen	Cat: <2 mg/kg SC, then <1 mg/kg	Once, then every 24 h up to 4 days
	Dog: <2 mg/kg IV, IM, SC, PO; then <1 mg/kg	Once, then every 24 h up to 4 days
Meloxicam	Cats: ≤0.2 mg/kg SC, PO; then ≤0.1 mg/kg	Once, then every 24 h up to 3 days
	Dogs: ≤0.2 mg/kg IV, SC, PO; then ≤0.1 mg/kg	Once, then every 24 h

(continued on next page)

Table 4 (*continued*)		
Carprofen	Cats: <4 (2 suggested) mg/kg SC Dogs: <4 mg/kg SC, IV, PO; then <2.2 mg/kg	Once Once, then every 12 h, preferably every 24 h
Bupivacaine 0.5%	Intrapleural and peritoneal use: 1 mg/kg (0.2 mL/kg lean weight) + 0.01 mEq/kg sodium bicarbonate diluted to 3, 6, or 12 mL (depending on size of the animal) with saline; for intrapleural use, flush this through tube with volume of 0.9% saline equal to volume of chest drain	6 h
Mild to moderate pain		
Opioids, as previously cited	Low dosages	Titrate down to lowest effective dose
Buprenorphine	Cat: 0.005–0.01 mg/kg IV, IM 0.01–0.002 mg/kg sublingual Dog: 0.005–0.02 mg/kg IV, IM	4–8 h 7 h 4–8 h
Butorphanol	Cat and dog: 0.1–0.4 mg/kg IV, IM, SC Administer intermittently or follow with a CRI with the effective dose over 2-h dosing interval	2 h
Codeine	0.5–2 mg/kg PO; titrate to effect	Every 6–12 h
Meperidine (pethidine)	5–10 mg/kg IM, SC for short-duration analgesia or administered at time of NSAIA injection	20–30 minutes
Morphine syrup	0.5 mg/kg PO; titrate to effect	Every 4–6 h
NSAIAs as previously cited	Low dosages	Titrate down to lowest effective dose
Bupivacaine 0.5%	Nerve blocks, infiltration or epidural use	3–6 h
Sedatives to combine with opioids		
Diazepam or midazolam	Cat and dog: 0.1–0.5 mg/kg IV, IM	Usually short-term effect
Acepromazine	Cat and dog: 0.01–0.05 mg/kg IV Cat and dog: 0.02–0.1 mg/kg IM, SC	1–2 h 2–6 h
Medetomidine	0.002–0.004 mg/kg IM, SC	15–60 minutes

Abbreviations: CRI, constant rate infusion; h, hours; IM, intramuscular; IV, intravenous; PO, per os; SC, subcutaneous.

Adapted from Mathews K, editor. PAIN how to understand, recognize, treat, and stop. CD-ROM ISBN0-9732655-0-7. Jonkar Computer Systems: Guelph, Ontario, Canada; 2003; with permission.

Table 5
Adjunctive analgesics suggested dosages

Drug	Species	Dosage	Route of Administration	Duration
Ketamine	Dogs and cats	0.2–4 mg/kg 0.2–4 mg/kg/h	IV IV	Bolus for control followed by CRI depending on severity of pain
Lidocaine	Dogs	1–4 mg/kg 1–5 mg/kg/h	IV IV	Bolus followed by CRI depending on severity of pain
	Cats	0.25–1 mg/kg 0.6–2 mg/kg/h	IV IV	Bolus followed by CRI
Gabapentin	Cats Dogs	2.5–5 (10) mg/kg 5–10 (25) mg/kg up to 12 mg/kg	PO PO PO	Every 12 h Every 8 h for pain Every 6 h for postseizure or post-CPR vocalization and thrashing; wean off slowly

Abbreviations: h, hours; IV, intravenous; PO, per os.

Adapted from Mathews K, editor. PAIN how to understand, recognize, treat, and stop. CD-ROM ISBN0-9732655-0-7. Jonkar Computer Systems: Guelph, Ontario, Canada; 2003; with permission.

Table 6
Cardiovascular compromise: shock and dehydration

Drug	Dose	Route	Comments
Butorphanol or	0.2–0.4 mg/kg	IM, IV	Doses selected are primarily size related (smaller dose per kilogram for bigger dogs); an increased respiratory rate may be an early sign of a mild overdose and should be stopped; although morphine can be given slowly IV, the possibility of histamine release can be a significant concern; IM administration is recommended (except if an infusion is used)
Hydromorphone or	0.05–0.2 mg/kg	Titrate IV to effect	
Methadone or	0.3–0.5 mg/kg (dogs)	IV, IM	
Morphine	0.1–0.2 mg/kg (cats)	IM, depending on the degree of pain	
Diazepam or midazolam	0.2 mg/kg	IV	Can be given to intensify effect of opioids

Abbreviations: IM, intramuscular; IV, intravenous.

Adapted from Mathews K, editor. PAIN how to understand, recognize, treat, and stop. CD-ROM ISBN0-9732655-0-7. Jonkar Computer Systems: Guelph, Ontario, Canada; 2003; with permission.

should be given to maintain cardiac output.[28] Low-dose ketamine (up to 5 mg per cat) with intravenously administered diazepam can be used to sedate cats while conferring some analgesia. Propofol should not be used in these animals because of the potential for significant hypotension.[29]

Opioids are generally considered the safest analgesic and are most effective in reducing the dose of other agents used for restraint and induction or maintenance of anesthesia should this be required. Fentanyl, alfentanil, and sufentanil are the drugs most widely accepted as safe in patients with cardiovascular compromise. Butorphanol has not been shown to have significant minimum alveolar concentration (MAC)–sparing effects in dogs.[30,31] Hydromorphone reduces the MAC and has minor cardiovascular depressive properties in hypovolemic dogs. Morphine, although it also reduces the MAC, is generally not advised because of its venodilation and potential for histamine release.[25] Recommended analgesic dosages for the various cardiovascular problems are listed in **Table 6**.

SHOCK

Provide oxygen by face mask, nasal cannula, tent, or flow-by while proceeding with assessments and treatment. These animals may be 10% to 15% dehydrated or have experienced a 30% to 45% intravascular fluid volume loss. Fluid resuscitation (with at least 50% of the loss corrected) should be achieved before profound chemical restraint or anesthesia is performed. The CNS depression associated with shock should allow catheter placement without any analgesia. Subcutaneous infiltration of a local anesthetic, such as 1% lidocaine (0.5–2 mL), should be used, if time permits, in any sedated, depressed, or stuporous animal before any emergency procedure (eg, chest drain placement, venous cutdown), because pain is still perceived but the animal cannot respond. This is also effective for jugular catheter placement in such patients. The crystalloid fluids should then be administered at a rate to restore perfusion as soon as possible. This varies with the individual patient and problem.

Once the animal is starting to respond, consider the need for analgesia (as noted previously). The persistent catecholamine release associated with pain further reduces oxygen delivery to the tissues and increases oxygen demand, and this detrimental effect is of greater concern than any adverse opioid effect. Partial reversal with naloxone (0.1–0.25 mL of a 0.4-mg/mL solution diluted in saline [10 mL] titrated in 1-mL increments to affect) is possible if any problem arises. Analgesia should not be reversed; only the unwanted adverse effects using this technique should be eliminated.

DEHYDRATION

If analgesia, restraint, or sedation is required in a dehydrated animal, do not use acepromazine. Start with a low-dose opioid, slowly increase, and add diazepam or midazolam as needed to effect.

ARRHYTHMIAS

Some trauma patients or other emergent patients may have premature ventricular contractions (PVCs). Traumatic myocarditis with associated arrhythmias is not uncommon and may be noted on presentation or within the following 48 hours. The rate of PVCs is not as much an issue as the effect of these arrhythmias (ie, poor cardiac output and perfusion). Initially, oxygen should be administered to improve oxygen delivery to the myocardium, especially to areas of poor perfusion (traumatized).

Analgesics should not be withheld. Careful titration of an opioid may be beneficial, because PVCs can be enhanced, or caused, by pain. Tachyarrhythmias are also frequently related to insufficient management of pain. Address pain with opioids in these cases, because enhanced vagal tone can also be advantageous.

Attempts to control these arrhythmias should be instituted before use of profound chemical restraint or anesthesia, which may cause further cardiovascular deterioriation. The advantage of treating PVCs in advance of anesthesia is to know that they are possible to treat so as to reduce the chance of a fatal arrhythmia during the stress of anesthetic induction and surgery and to maximize cardiac output. Mild sedation and a MAC-sparing effect occur with therapeutic levels of lidocaine (advantageous because the inhalant causes significant cardiovascular depression). Details on lidocaine administration around the time of surgery are found in the other article by Dyson elsewhere in this issue. Procainamide at a dose of 6 to 15 μg/kg administered intravenously over 20 minutes to avoid hypotension may be required if there is no response to lidocaine. Hypokalemia or metabolic acidosis may contribute to ventricular arrhythmias. If opioid use results in significant bradycardia in animals without cardiovascular compromise, atropine or glycopyrrolate could be used to treat the bradycardia. Glycopyrrolate is commonly chosen over atropine because of the increased duration of effect and slightly lower incidence of tachycardia and arrhythmias. It can take as long as 3 minutes to see the full effect of glycopyrrolate. Atropine has a more rapid onset of action than glycopyrrolate and is selected when significant bradycardia is immediately life threatening. If the patient is hypovolemic, treat the hypovolemia before treating opioid-induced bradycardia, because no benefit has been shown with pharmacologic treatment in the hypovolemic patient.[13]

GASTROINTESTINAL OR VISCERAL PAIN

α_2-Agonists, hydromorphone, and morphine have an increased incidence of vomiting when used for premedication or analgesia in the awake animal. These drugs should be avoided in cases in which a foreign body or other obstruction is suspected so as to avoid vomiting and subsequent worsening of the pain or when the potential for gastrointestinal rupture may occur. Butorphanol (0.2–0.4 mg/kg administered intramuscularly) or meperidine (3–5 mg/kg administered intramuscularly) can be used for premedication or mild sedation (for procedures like radiography) or for reducing stress and pain, in addition to reducing the dose of drugs used for induction. The more profound opioid that is available can be given after induction and stabilization when the vomiting center is less receptive to the opioids because of the depressant effects of general anesthesia at this site. Some antagonism may result from residual butorphanol effects, but this is rarely significant after approximately 1 hour. Analgesic recommendations for the various gastrointestinal problems are listed in **Table 7**.

Gastric or Dilation Volvulus

Cardiovascular compromise can present as a primary problem in these cases if shock, dehydration, or arrhythmias are present (refer to previous recommendations for cardiac compromise). Acid-base disorders (metabolic acidosis) and electrolyte disturbances (low potassium) may also be present. Occasionally, respiratory compromise may coexist because of abdominal enlargement and pressure on the diaphragm. Fentanyl or hydromorphone (with or without diazepam) is a popular choice for analgesia, although butorphanol or meperidine can be used as noted previously. Many of these dogs are large (eg, great danes); therefore, the effective dose is lower than typically used (eg, fentanyl at a dose of 2–3 μg/kg administered intravenously, hydromorphone

Table 7
Gastrointestinal compromise

Opioid Agonists	Dose	Route of Administration	Interval
Morphine	Dog: 0.1–0.5 mg/kg	Slow IV	1–4 h
	0.1–0.5 mg/kg	IV/h	CRI
	0.5–1 mg/kg	IM, SC	1–4 (6) h
	0.1–0.3 mg/kg	Epidural	4–8 (12) h
	0.5–2 mg/kg	PO, titrate to effect	4–6 h
	Cat: 0.05–0.2 mg/kg	IV slowly, IM, SC	2–6 h
	0.5–1 mg/kg	PO, titrate to effect	8–12 h
Hydromorphone	Dog: 0.04–0.2 mg/kg	IV (diluted and slowly titrated to effect in GDV)	2–4 h
	0.10–0.20 mg/kg	IM, SC	2–4 (6) h
	Cat: 0.04–0.10 mg/kg	IV, IM, SC	2–4 (6) h
Methadone	Dog and cat:	—	—
	0.1–0.5 mg/kg	IV, IM, SC	2–4 h
Fentanyl	Cat and dog:	—	—
	0.001–0.005+ mg/kg	IV loading	0.5–1 h
	0.001–0.005 mg/kg	IV 20–60 min	CRI

Abbreviations: CRI, constant rate infusion; GDV, gastric dilation volvulus; h, hours; IM, intramuscular; IV, intravenous; PO, per os; SC, subcutaneous.

Adapted from Mathews K, editor. PAIN how to understand, recognize, treat, and stop. CD-ROM ISBN0-9732655-0-7. Jonkar Computer Systems: Guelph, Ontario, Canada; 2003; with permission.

at a dose of 0.02–0.03 mg/kg administered intravenously), especially if cardiovascular compromise exists. The dose can be diluted in saline and slowly given over 5 minutes until the desired effect is reached. If panting or the appearance of nausea occurs, stop administration.

Pancreatitis and Peritonitis

Pancreatitis is a not an uncommon primary problem in dogs and cats, causing moderate to excruciating pain. Pancreatitis should be considered in patients presented with abdominal pain and in those recovering from a hypotensive event. Mild to moderate pain can be managed with butorphanol at a dose of 0.4 mg/kg given every 2 to 3 hours or an hourly CRI at a dose equal to the bolus dose that was effective in relieving pain, divided by 2 or 3. Monitoring the patient should dictate whether an increase or decrease is required. For patients that have pancreatitis, the question is often raised regarding the opioid effects on sphincter tone. Morphine and fentanyl, in decreasing order, increase intracommon biliary ductal pressure in human beings, which has been extrapolated to a similar potential affect on pancreatic ductal pressure in dogs. Hydromorphone likely has the same effect. Because moderate to severe pancreatitis is extremely painful, however, the opioids are required to control this pain. Experience in managing pain associated with pancreatitis indicates that the opioids work well with no apparent adverse effects (K. Mathews, personal communication, 2007). Buprenorphine (0.005–0.02 mg/kg in dogs and 0.005–0.01 mg/kg in cats administered every 8 hours) has less effect on intraductal pressure in people and may be the drug of choice in mild to moderate pain associated with pancreatitis. For more severe pancreatitis or pain associated with peritonitis attributable to abdominal wall–penetrating injuries, gastrointestinal perforation, biliary rupture, or urinary tract injury, hydromorphone or fentanyl can be administered in the same fashion as butorphanol, with the exception of the hydromorphone dose being divided by 4 for an hourly rate and fentanyl being administered at the effective bolus dose per hour. Again, monitoring the patient should indicate whether the dose should be changed. Lidocaine or ketamine may also be added as a CRI (see **Table 5**). Epidural analgesia by means of an epidural catheter is also an excellent method of controlling severe pain (see **Table 4**).[32] A 1:1 mixture of preservative-free morphine (1 mg/mL) and 0.25% bupivacaine is prepared and slowly injected over 5 to 10 minutes (to avoid vomiting and development of a patchy block) at 0.1 mL/kg while the animal is in sternal recumbency, followed by a continuous infusion at 0.4 to 0.8 mL/kg/d. A syringe pump is required to deliver these small volumes. If lidocaine is given systemically, strict adherence to calculations for bupivicaine is required to avoid overdose and it may be best to avoid bupivicaine when long-term lidocaine infusions have been used. The beneficial effect of continuous local anesthetic infusions is related to the proximity of the catheter tip to nerve roots involved. As an alternative to a constant infusion, intermittent injections (over 5–10 minutes) of 0.15 to 0.2 mL/kg every 6 hours may be administered. If hind limb weakness is encountered, the bupivacaine dose should be reduced by one half (0.125%) or one quarter (0.0625%) by diluting with sterile saline before mixing with the morphine. It is advised to prepare a single volume of the mixture for each 24 hours of treatment to avoid frequent disconnects of the syringe. Be reminded that the morphine is preservative-free; therefore, strict aseptic technique must be observed when withdrawing and mixing.

Intra-Arterial or Intravenous Catheter Placement

Most of the time, percutaneous catheter placement is a fast procedure with minimal discomfort; however, in difficult patients, when time permits, EMLA (eutectic mixture of local anesthetic [lidocaine 2.5% and prilocaine 2.5% combined with thickening agents to form an emulsion]) cream (Astra Zeneca Canada, Mississauga, Ontario, Canada) placed over the previously cleansed arterial or venipuncture site eliminates the pain of catheter placement. Dosing is calculated in a similar manner to the injectable formulation. Local anesthetic concentrations are described as weight by volume (grams per 100 mL); therefore, the 2% solution is 2g/100 mL (equals 20 mg/mL) which applies to the creams and gels. This product is not sterile and should be used only in intact skin to provide anesthesia for intravenous (peripheral and central) catheter placement, blood collection, lumbar puncture and other minor superficial procedures. EMLA cream should be covered with an occlusive dressing for at least 20 minutes and preferably longer, for optimum effect.

Urinary Catheter Placement

It is frequently necessary to place a urinary catheter in traumatized patients. This procedure rarely requires more than manual restraint in male patients; however, it is more difficult to carry out in female patients. Unless the male dog is struggling excessively or extremely small in size, chemical restraint is rarely needed. Female dogs and cats should receive an analgesic. Because the trauma patient is receiving analgesics attributable to pain from other injuries, no additional restraint is required, but topical local anesthetic should be used in female patients and all cats. A sterile 2% lidocaine gel in a tapered-end cartridge (Astra) can be introduced into the vaginal vault or the penile urethra 5 minutes before catheter placement.

ADJUVANT ANALGESIC DRUGS

Adjuvant analgesic drugs, such as lidocaine, ketamine, and tricyclic antidepressants, are not generally considered to be primary or first-choice analgesics. In fact, some of these drugs may have weak or nonexistent analgesic effects when used alone. Adjuvant analgesics are typically used in combination with other known analgesic drugs in acute pain states to manage severe pain, in which they seem to enhance their analgesic action, or to reduce the dose of the primary analgesic.[33] Suggested dosing regimens for these drugs are listed in **Table 5**.

Lidocaine

In addition to the local anesthetic effects, lidocaine has been shown to alleviate neuropathic pain and hyperalgesia and to reduce opioid requirements after surgery when administered as a CRI.[34]

Although not necessarily used as an adjunctive analgesic in this situation, lidocaine may be useful in managing patients that have head trauma during periods of increasing ICP, such as occurs during vomiting or "gagging." Lidocaine has been reported to lower ICP during a period of increasing ICP.[21–23] Patients that have head trauma experience pain, and the use of opioids may increase ICP in some instances if vomiting is induced or as a result of mild respiratory depression. The degree and significance of respiratory depression caused by opioids may be exaggerated in the patient that has head trauma. Lidocaine can be used in these cases, as a 1-mg/kg bolus, to treat impending tentorial herniation, followed by a CRI in some cases to reduce the opioid requirement in this acute setting for the ensuing 24 hours.

Ketamine

Ketamine is an *N*-methyl-D-aspartate (NMDA) antagonist, blocking the NMDA receptor wind-up and subsequent sensitization of dorsal horn neurons. Ketamine may also abolish established central sensitization. Ketamine should not be used alone for pain management, because there are no veterinary studies assessing efficacy and adverse effects of ketamine used as a sole analgesic agent in this setting. Ketamine, by means of CRI, is used as an adjunctive analgesic in severe pain states in combination with an opioid to enhance analgesia or reduce opioid requirements.[35] The infusion should be tapered down before being discontinued to prevent potential hyperalgesia. The hourly dosage varies considerably and depends on the pain experienced. The dosages in **Table 5** are those recommended; however, up to 4 mg/kg/h in dogs, in addition to high dosages of opioid (fentanyl or morphine), have been needed to achieve a level of comfort (similar to a light plane of anesthesia) facilitating sleep in patients with severe to excruciating pain. At the lower dosages required to relieve pain, the patient is alert and comfortable. Ketamine is excreted by way of the kidney in cats and is metabolized by the liver in dogs. It is essential that these organs are functioning normally before administration of ketamine. Only lower doses (up to 1 mg/kg) should be administered to animals with underlying cardiac disease.

Gabapentin

Gabapentin is used in human patients for management of neuropathic pain associated with diabetes, cancer, or primary nerve compression.[36] One of the classic features of this type of pain is the presence of abnormal pain induced by a nonnoxious stimulus (allodynia). Frequently, conventional analgesics, such as opioids and NSAIAs, show limited value in treating this type of pain. In dogs and cats that have neuropathic pain secondary to cervical or thoracolumbar intervertebral disk disease or pelvic trauma, gabapentin has reduced the pain in these severe pain states. In cases in which neuropathic pain was treated with gabapentin, it seemed that gabapentin contributed greatly to the analgesia that these animals were experiencing (K. Mathews, personal communication, 2007). Frequently, animals requiring this drug need several weeks to months for resolution, if ever, of their pain. Gabapentin is also useful in treating animals after cardiopulmonary arrest or seizures that are extremely restless, disoriented, vocalizing, or manic. Again, dosing to effect and resolution of these signs is the goal. Sedation in this instance is appropriate. There is an extremely wide dose range for gabapentin, and it should be given to effect. The dose-limiting affect generally observed is sedation. Careful lowering of the drug is recommended. Gabapentin is an antiepileptic agent, and recent studies suggest that the antiallodynic actions of gabapentin involve a central mechanism of action. It has been reported that gabapentin binds with the high-affinity $\alpha_2\delta$ subunits of voltage-dependent calcium channels, blocking calcium currents in isolated cortical neurons and blocking maintenance of spinal cord central sensitization.

Gabapentin is excreted by the kidneys; animals with renal insufficiency may require less frequent dosing because of slower elimination. Because dosing to effect is the method by which the appropriate dose is selected, once this effect is reached, treatment two times daily rather than three times daily may suffice. Nephrotoxicity is not an issue. Signs of overdose are reduced activity and excessive sleepiness, progressing to depression. Tapering the dose down is important, because stopping the drug abruptly may lead to rebound pain that may be severe.

NURSING CARE

Because a cold, damp, dirty, or noisy environment contributes to stress and anxiety, which, in turn, lowers the threshold to pain sensation, it is important that the patient be made comfortable, clean, warm, and dry. Stabilization of fractures and primary treatment of wounds and burns also reduce pain. Tender loving care is of utmost importance. Please refer to the article by SHaffron, Fagella, and Taylor elsewhere in this issue.

REFERENCES

1. McCaffrey M. Pain ratings: the fifth vital sign. Am J Nurs 1997;97:15–6.
2. Staats P. Pain: assessment and approach to practical pain management in the ICU. Society of Critical Care Medicine 29th Educational and Scientific Symposium; Orlando (FL), September 2000.
3. Vierck CJ. Extrapolation from the pain research literature to problems of adequate veterinary care. J Am Vet Med Assoc 1976;168:510–4.
4. Benson GJ, Wheaton LG, Thurmon JC, et al. Postoperative catecholamine response to onychectomy in isoflurane-anesthetized cats: effect of analgesics. Vet Surg 1991;20(3):222–5.
5. Morton DB, Griffiths PH. Guidelines on the recognition of pain, distress and discomfort in experimental animals and an hypothesis for assessment. Vet Rec 1985;116:431–6.
6. Smith JD, Allen SW, Quandt JE, et al. Indicators of postoperative pain in cats and correlation with clinical criteria. Am J Vet Res 1996;209:1674–8.
7. Katz J, Jackson M, Kavanagh B, et al. Acute pain after thoracic surgery predicts long-term post-thoracotomy pain. Clin J Pain 1996;12:50–5.
8. Attard AR, Corlett MJ, Kidner NJ, et al. Safety of early pain relief for acute abdominal pain. Br Med J 1992;305:554–6.

9. Brock N. Treating moderate and severe pain in small animals. Can Vet J 1995;36: 658–60.
10. Dohoo SE, Dohoo IR. Factors influencing the postoperative use of analgesics in dogs and cats by Canadian veterinarians. Can Vet J 1996;37:552–6.
11. Lascelles BD, Capner CA, Waterman-Pearson AE. Current British veterinary attitudes to perioperative analgesia for cats and small mammals. Vet Rec 1999; 145:601–4.
12. Watson AD, Nicholson A, Church DB, et al. Use of anti-inflammatory and analgesic drugs in dogs and cats. Aust Vet J 1996;74:203–10.
13. Machado CEG. Comparison of oxymorphone and hydromorphone in dogs: impact on isoflurane MAC and induction of anesthesia during hypovolemia [DVSc thesis]. University of Guelph 2002.
14. Lascelles BD, Waterman A. Analgesia in cats. In Pract 1997;19(4):203–13.
15. Wilcke JR. Idiosyncracies of drug metabolism in cats: effects on pharmacotherapeutics in feline practice. Vet Clin North Am Small Anim Pract 1984;14(6):1345–54.
16. Mathews KA. Non-steroidal anti-inflammatory analgesics: a review of current practice. Journal of Veterinary Emergency and Critical Care 2002;12(2):89–97.
17. Clutton RE. Cardiopulmonary disease. In: Seymour C, Gleed R, editors. Manual of small animal anaesthesia and analgesia. Cheltonham (PA): British Small Animal Veterinary Association; 1999. p. 155–81.
18. Waterman AE. Influence of premedication with xylazine on the distribution and metabolism of intramuscularly administered ketamine in cats. Res Vet Sci 1983; 35:285–90.
19. Clarke KW, Hall LW. A survey of anaesthesia in small animal practice: Association of Veterinary Anaesthesiologists/British Small Animal Veterinary Association Report. Journal of the Association of Veterinary Anaesthesiologists 1990;17:4–10.
20. Dyson DH, Maxie MG, Schnurr D. Morbidity and mortality associated with anesthetic management in small animal veterinary practice in Ontario. J Am Anim Hosp Assoc 1998;34:325–35.
21. Hamill JF, Bedofrd RF, Weaver DC, et al. Lidocaine before endotracheal intubation: intravenous or laryngotracheal? Anesthesiology 1981;55(5):578–81.
22. Sakabe T, Maekawa T, Ishikawa T. The effects of lidocaine on canine cerebral metabolism and circulation related to the electroencephalogram. Anesthesiology 1974;40:433–41.
23. White PF, Schlobohm RM, Pitts LH, et al. A randomized study of drugs for preventing increases in intracranial pressure during endotracheal suctioning. Anesthesiology 1982;57:242–4.
24. Milner QJ, Abdy S, Allen JG. Management of severe tracheal obstruction with helium/oxygen and a laryngeal mask airway. Anaesthesia 1997;52:1087–9.
25. Robinson EP, Fagella AM, Russell WL. Comparison of histamine release induced by morphine and oxymorphone administration in dogs. Am J Vet Res 1988;49: 1699–701.
26. Torske KE, Dyson DH. Epidural analgesia and anesthesia. Vet Clin North Am Small Anim Pract. 2000;30(4):859–74.
27. Wheeler AH, Aaron GW. Muscle pain due to injury. Curr Pain Headache Rep 2001;4:441–6.
28. Torske KE, Dyson DH, Conlon PD. Cardiovascular effects of epidurally administered oxymorphone and an oxymorphone-bupivacaine combination in halothane-anesthetized dogs. Am J Vet Res 1999;60:194–200.
29. Rouby JJ, Andreev A, Leger P, et al. Peripheral vascular effects of thiopental and propofol in humans with artificial hearts. Anesthesiology 1991;75:32–42.

30. Quandt JE, Rafee MR, Robinson EP. Butorphanol does not reduce the minimum alveolar concentration of halothane in dogs. Vet Surg 1994;23:156–9.
31. Nunes de Moraes A, Dyson DH, O'Grady MR, et al. Plasma concentrations and cardiovascular influence of lidocaine infusions during isoflurane anesthesia in healthy dogs and dogs with subaortic stenosis. Vet Surg 1998;27:486–97.
32. Hansen BD. Epidural catheter analgesia in dogs and cats: technique and review of 182 cases (1991–1999). Journal of Veterinary Emergency and Critical Care 2001;11(2):95–103.
33. Lamont LA, Tranquilli WJ, Mathews KA. Adjunctive analgesic therapy. Vet Clin North Am Small Anim Pract 2000;30(4):805–13.
34. Groudine SB, Fisher HA, Kaufman RP Jr, et al. Intravenous lidocaine speeds the return of bowel function, decreases postoperative pain and shortens hospital stay in patients undergoing radical retropubic prostatectomy. Anesth Analg 1998;86: 235–9.
35. Muir WW III. Drugs used to treat pain. In: Gaynor JS, Muir WW II, editors. Handbook of veterinary pain management. St. Louis (MO): Mosby; 2002. p. 142–63.
36. Field MJ, McLeary S, Hughes J. Gabapentin and pregabalin, but not morphine and amitriptyline, block both static and dynamic components of mechanical allodynia induced by streptozocin in the rat. Pain 1999;80:391–8.

Analgesia for the Critically Ill Dog or Cat: An Update

Bernie Hansen, DVM, MS

KEYWORDS

- Acute pain • Local anesthesia • Wound infusion
- Intravenous analgesia

Significant pain frequently accompanies acute illness[1] and is almost always present following surgery or trauma. This pain is considered acute in character and, as such, is intimately tied to the neurologic process of nociception. This feature is important for several clinically relevant reasons. First, acute pain contributes to the intensity of the postinjury stress response and, if poorly managed, may increase the risk of complications.[2–4] Nociception and the stress response to pain modify the immune response in complex ways that can produce immunosuppression. There is clinical evidence, at least in humans, that this sequela becomes most problematic in critical illness when the stress response is excessive and contributes to morbidity and mortality. Second, sustained nociception triggers the adaptive response of central sensitization. The subsequent development of hyperalgesia and allodynia intensifies pain and creates more challenges for the patient and the caregiver. Finally, acute pain usually responds, at least to some extent, to straightforward pharmacologic approaches, and drug therapy is an essential component of management of most patients that have significant acute pain. Anyone who has experience knows, however, that there is tremendous variation in patient response; some animals appear completely comfortable with modest drug therapy, whereas others that have similar conditions have distressing pain that is comparatively refractory to multiple drugs and all efforts at nonpharmacologic intervention.

Assessment of acute pain is beyond the scope of this review but serves as the basis for recognition of pain and evaluating patient response to therapy. Because injury and inflammation reliably produce nociception, pain is assumed to be present in animals that have these conditions, and at least some form of treatment should be considered regardless of clinical signs. Significant advancement toward the goals of including pain assessment in every physical examination (as in the Pain as a Vital Sign concept adopted by the International Veterinary Academy of Pain Management) and adoption of standardized assessment methods (as required by the American Animal Hospital Association for member hospitals) have occurred in the last 5 years.

Department of Clinical Sciences, North Carolina State University, College of Veterinary Medicine, 4700 Hillsborough Street, Raleigh, NC 27606, USA
E-mail address: bernie_hansen@ncsu.edu

Vet Clin Small Anim 38 (2008) 1353–1363
doi:10.1016/j.cvsm.2008.08.002 **vetsmall.theclinics.com**

Nonpharmacologic approaches to pain management remain the basis for all other therapy. Meticulous surgical technique limits tissue injury and postoperative nociception. Careful and compassionate nursing care must maintain hygiene, prevent thirst and hunger, properly position and cushion immobile patients, and support the metabolic processes of healing. Protecting naturally timid animals from excessive exposure to the clinic environment reduces the stress of the hospital experience, whereas engaging more energetic, gregarious animals serves to distract them from their pain. Family visits in the hospital keep the animal rooted in the knowledge that they have not lost their home. Physical therapy to prevent edema, thrombosis, and stiffening of joints and muscles is beneficial to many, particularly those that have chronic pain from osteoarthritis. We are only beginning to appreciate the value of physical rehabilitation therapy in animals following significant illness or injury, particularly in those that have major musculoskeletal injury and repair.

Opioids and nonsteroidal anti-inflammatory drugs are the two most important drug classes for acute pain management. For a more in-depth review of the use of these drugs in hospitalized patients, the reader is referred to the earlier version of this review (see the *Veterinary Clinics of North America* 2000) and the companion chapters in this issue. Two approaches that have seen increasing use in the companion animal ICU at North Carolina State University are presented in this review: the use of local anesthetics and the continuous-rate infusion of multiple agents.

LOCAL ANESTHETICS

Local anesthetics remain the only class of drug capable of completely blocking nociception from injury or surgery. Because of the efficacy of local anesthesia for intraoperative analgesia,[5–8] there has been considerable interest in expanding the role of these drugs for postoperative analgesia. Areas of interest include continuous intravenous (IV) infusions of lidocaine; continuous or intermittent infusion of local anesthetics into wounds, body cavities, and near nerves; regional analgesia with repeated epidural administration; and topical application of lidocaine.

Continuous nerve block with an infusion of drug remains the only available method to continuously block nociception. In theory, local anesthesia can provide complete analgesia of wounds. In practice, reaching this goal can be challenging. Many traumatic injuries produce damage that is too diffuse to allow a complete response to local anesthesia; however, the nature of many elective surgical procedures allows for the effective control of pain with local anesthetics applied before, during, or after the procedure.

Whereas splash blocks,[9,10] superficial infusion,[11] or single injections[5] of local anesthetics into wounds often fail to provide improved analgesia or provide only modest benefit, regional anesthesia (see the article by Lemke and Valverde found elsewhere in this issue) appears to provide substantial benefit.

In the author's experience, excellent postoperative anesthesia can often be obtained by performing a continuous nerve block or local wound infiltration by placing a fenestrated anesthetic delivery catheter into the surgical site before wound closure or near a nerve or nerve group that innervates the affected tissue. Although considerable clinical evaluation of continuous nerve blocks has been conducted in humans, comparatively little has been published regarding the technique in animals.

Precisely manufactured wound infusion catheters are available commercially (eg, veterinary perineural catheters, ReCathCo, Allison Park, Pennsylvania, www.recathco.com) or may be fashioned by hand using tubing such as 0.05-inch (outside diameter) polyethylene tubing. This sterile product may be purchased in individual 12-inch or 36-inch lengths (eg, Intramedic PE 90 polyethylene tubing, Becton-Dickenson, Franklin Lakes,

New Jersey, www.bd.com) or in bulk packages (100 feet) of nonsterile tubing (eg, Intramedic PE 90 Polyethylene Tubing [Non-Sterile], Becton-Dickenson). To fashion local anesthetic delivery catheters catheters out of polyethylene tubing, the following materials are needed:

1 Intramedic PE 90 polyethylene tubing (Becton-Dickenson)
1 insulin syringe with a 27- to 28-gauge needle
1 Luer adapter (Intramedic 20-gauge tubing adapter, Becton-Dickenson)
1 empty sterile 3-mL syringe
1 cigarette lighter
1 scissors
1 injection cap
64″ × 4″ gauze sponges or any other soft padded material
1 pair of examination gloves
1 syringe loaded with the agent of choice

If prepared in advance, the catheters can be made under clean conditions and then gas sterilized. If prepared at the time of surgery, all materials except the cigarette lighter (which is held by an assistant) must be sterile.

The catheter tubing may be cut into appropriate lengths (usually 12–36 inches). The cigarette lighter is used to flame the end of the catheter sufficiently to melt the plastic. When the catheter begins to melt, the operator pinches off the melted tip and draws it to a point, protecting fingers with the examination gloves, a gauze sponge, or both. A Luer adapter is firmly seated into the open end of the catheter, and a test injection of air is used to confirm that the seal at the tip is complete. If any air escapes the test injection, the tip is reheated and another attempt to seal it is made.

When sealed, the end of the catheter is rested on the sponge padding and the operator uses the insulin needle to perforate the tubing completely through both sides, beginning 5 mm proximal to the sealed tip and continuing every 5 to 10 mm up the desired length of tube. The purpose of the sponge padding is to prevent the needle tip from butting against the table work surface underneath and becoming dull. When the working length (or infusion surface—the total length of the portion of tube with perforations) exceeds 10 cm, the holes should be spaced approximately 10 mm apart to limit their total number. As each hole is placed, the catheter should be rotated 90° to prevent the holes from opening in the same plane. The length of the infusion surface of the catheter is determined by its desired use and location. If the goal is nerve block, and the catheter is to be implanted adjacent to (1) the brachial plexus, (2) a peripheral nerve (eg, a radial nerve block), or (3) the transected stump of a large nerve (eg, the sciatic and femoral nerves in a rear limb amputation), then the working surface need not be much longer than 5 cm. If the catheter is to be implanted into the long axis of a surgical wound, then it should be long enough to extend the length of the entire wound. At the time of packaging, the Luer adapter may be left on the catheter or may be removed and placed alongside the catheter in its package to facilitate catheter placement during surgery. A variety of lengths can be prepared and gas sterilized so that they are available for immediate use (**Table 1**).

Just before positioning the catheter in a patient, the device is primed with the anesthetic agent to be used. An injection cap with a Luer-Loc fitting may be connected to the catheter adapter. A common practice in the author's hospital is to connect the Luer adapter to a length of extension tubing that is, in turn, connected to a bacterial filter fitted with an injection cap. Regardless of the materials used, the entire system is purged with the local anesthetic agent of choice before placement into the patient. The most common agent used in the author's hospital is bupivacaine 0.25%. Using

Table 1
Wound infusion catheter lengths used frequently at the North Carolina State University veterinary teaching hospital

Catheter Tubing Length (cm)	Length of Infusion Surface (cm)
25	5
30	10
45	15
45	20
60	25
60	30
60	35
75	40

a sterile syringe, the drug is injected into the catheter with some force, and the operator observes the infusion surface to verify that droplets of the solution are present at every hole.

When the catheter is to be used as a perineural infusion device, it may be (1) placed by direct visualization of the nerve (eg, during limb amputation), (2) passed through a long needle that is advanced to the desired location by recognition of anatomic landmarks, or (3) advanced to the desired location through an IV catheter that was guided to the proper location by use of an electrical nerve stimulator. The use of electrical nerve stimulators was previously described by Mahler and Reece.[12] When the catheter is passed to the nerve through an IV catheter or needle, the Luer adapter, if attached, is temporarily removed from the proximal end of the tubing to allow the catheter or needle to be removed.

When using the catheter to infuse local anesthetic directly into the surgical wound, some principles regarding placement should be followed to optimize efficacy of the device. The author's clinical experience and practice on cadavers suggest that effective anesthesia is most likely to occur for tissues that lie within 2 cm of the catheter after the wound has been closed. Therefore, whenever possible, the catheter should be positioned into the deepest layer of the wound and include the most dorsal margin that contains proximal portions of the nerve axons that serve the wound area. The shape of the path that the catheter takes should bring the infusion surface into contact with as much tissue as possible. For irregular wounds, for example, the surgeon must lay the catheter in a serpentine path and loosely anchor the catheter at strategic points with a loop of absorbable suture. Any anchoring sutures must be loose enough to allow eventual withdrawal of the catheter. When a nerve is within the wound, a portion of the working surface of the catheter must be in close approximation to that tissue. When multiple tissue planes are present (eg, in a deep muscle incision in the pelvic limb), the catheter may need to wind its way across several tissue plane boundaries. More than one catheter may be needed to bring enough tissue into contact with local anesthetic. When exiting the catheter, the proximal end is tunneled subcutaneously and exits the skin through a separate stab incision that is created at least 3 cm from the surgical wound margin. Increasing the length of the subcutaneous tunnel increases the barrier to bacterial migration along the surface of the catheter. Following wound closure, the catheter at the exit site is anchored to the skin with 00 monofilament nylon suture or by enclosing it in a bilayer of 1-inch (2.54-cm) waterproof white tape and suturing the tape to the skin. If tape is not used, then the suture is passed through the skin under the catheter, and a square knot is placed to complete a loop that does not incorporate the catheter; two long ends are left to tie around the catheter in a series of knots that are snug but not so tight as to collapse it.

The first injection of local anesthetic should be administered before recovery from general anesthesia. Estimating the optimal volume of drug to be administered is often an educated guess based on the clinician's impression of the size, depth, and complexity of the wound. In some patients (eg, a large dog that has a total ear canal ablation), the ratio of volume needed to body size is relatively small, and a concentrated- form of anesthetic may be used. When the volume of infusate needed is judged to be large, however, 0.25% bupivacaine is often preferred over the 0.5% concentration because it provides nearly as intense anesthesia but with twice the volume to spread through the area. Either concentration needs to be administered at 4- to 6-hour intervals to maintain adequate anesthesia, so the clinician must calculate a volume that does not produce local anesthetic toxicity. In the case of bupivacaine, the total daily dose should probably not exceed 4 mg/kg in dogs[13,14] and 2 mg/kg in cats. The injection should be made with some force (5–20 psi) because slow injections under low pressure often yield erratic distribution of drug from the catheter. It is because of this erratic distribution that the author does not administer local anesthetics through these catheters as a slow continuous infusion despite the fact that continuous infusion with portable pumps accounts for a large proportion of the use of this technique in humans. The reasons for the erratic drug distribution are complex and currently under investigation by the North Carolina State University Comparative Pain Research Laboratory.

The second dose of bupivacaine should be administered at 4 hours. If the patient objects to the injection, then it should be immediately halted and the operator should wait 10 minutes for the injected proportion to numb the tissue in the immediate vicinity of the catheter. Discomfort is due to the "sting" (low pH) of the solution and the pressure entering the tissue. In many patients, the injection can be finished after this waiting period, with much less reaction.

Subsequent doses of drug are administered at 4- to 6-hour intervals and are modified according the patient's clinical signs. In most of the author's patients, the catheter is used for 1 to 3 days and then removed. Prior to removal of the device, the clinician allows at least 6 hours to pass from the time of the last injection to confirm that the patient is comfortable without the local anesthetic.

ANALGESIC DRUGS ADMINISTERED INTRAVENOUSLY BY CONTINUOUS-RATE INFUSION

For animals being treated with IV fluids that also require analgesic therapy, continuous infusion of analgesic drugs is convenient and often more effective than intermittent administration in response to patient signs. "Cookbook" formulations can be used for intraoperative fluid therapy and have the advantage of being made the same way and given at the same rate for every patient. Drug therapy can also be tailored to meet individual needs for postoperative or postinjury patients or animals that have other painful conditions such as pancreatitis, burns, severe dermatitis, and so forth. Drugs used most frequently in the North Carolina State University ICU are listed in **Table 2**.

All of these agents appear stable for several days in combination, and in any commonly used IV fluid.[15] When used within a few days, there is no need to protect the solution from light. When used in combination, the dosages for each of these drugs can be at the low end of the suggested range.

Table 2
Analgesic agents commonly used as continuous IV infusions

Drug	Species	Infusion Rate
Morphine	Canine	0.05–0.2 mg/kg/h
Hydromorphone	Canine	0.0125–0.05 mg/kg/h
Buprenorphine	Canine	2–4 μg/kg/h
	Feline	1–3 μg/kg/h
Fentanyl	Canine	2–6 μg/kg/h
	Feline	2–4 μg/kg/h
Lidocaine	Canine	2–4 mg/kg/h
Ketamine	Both	0.2–0.6 mg/kg/h
Medetomidine	Canine	1–3 μg/kg/h
	Feline	0.5–2 μg/kg/h

Opioids

Useful agents include hydromorphone and morphine in dogs, and fentanyl and buprenorphine in cats and small dogs. Hydromorphone should be avoided in cats due to the high incidence of drug-induced hyperthermia.[16,17] Morphine is an inexpensive choice for large dogs. Fentanyl is particularly useful when the clinician plans to transition the patient to a fentanyl patch. In that case, the infusion rate of fentanyl is adjusted to reach optimal effect before a patch is applied; the infusion is then tapered and discontinued over the next 8 to 24 hours while observing patient response. If the patient does well on the infusion but poorly when transitioned to the patch, failure of the patch should be suspected. A 25-μg patch provides approximately 10 μg/h of fentanyl to healthy cats, but delivery is highly variable.[18–20] For small cats, a 12.5-μg patch is available.

α_2-Adrenergic Agonists

The α_2-adrenergic agonists have marked sedative and analgesic properties that make them useful as preanesthetics and as analgesic adjuncts following surgery or injury. Commercially available drugs in this class include xylazine, medetomidine, and dexmedetomidine. Although xylazine is inexpensive and commonly used as part of preanesthetic protocols for relatively healthy animals, at the author's hospital, it is less effective as a sedative at low doses than the newer agents. Medetomidine consists of a racemic mixture of the *d*- and *l*- optical isomers; the inactive *l*- form is absent from dexmedetomidine, and this drug is twice as potent (not twice as efficacious) as the racemate.[21–23] All of these drugs have clear and profound cardiovascular effects. When administered to healthy dogs, medetomidine increases systemic vascular resistance and produces substantial reductions in heart rate and cardiac output. These effects are fully realized within seconds after IV bolus administration, and a dose of as little as 5 μg/kg IV has the full cardiovascular effect seen with higher dosages.[24] Nevertheless, the author has used continuous-rate infusions of medetomidine in dogs (and occasionally in cats) in an ICU environment for many years. The drug is particularly useful to assist sedation in vigorous, young animals following major elective surgical procedures. The patient must be hemodynamically stable and free of significant cardiac disease. In practice, the drug is administered IV as a continuous-rate infusion with no loading dose at an infusion rate of 1 to 3 μg/kg/h. Sedation ensues within an hour and generally peaks within 2 hours. The α_2-adrenergic agonists rarely suffice as sole analgesic therapy but appear to intensify the analgesia and sedation obtained from other drug classes.[25,26]

Lidocaine

Intravenous infusion of lidocaine provides some measure of analgesia, likely by a combination of mechanisms that includes reduction of ectopic activity by damaged primary afferent neurons.[27] The drug should not be administered to sick cats or cats under anesthesia because it causes significant cardiovascular depression in that species.[28] When local infusion of local anesthetics is being used, systemic administration should not be used, or the total dose must be calculated from both routes and the daily dosage not exceeded. Lidocaine 5% dermal patches are available in the United States (eg, Lidoderm, Endo Pharmaceuticals, Chadds Ford, Pennsylvania, www.lidoderm.com) and may be effective for painful superficial dermatologic conditions in dogs. Although some systemic absorption of lidocaine occurs in dogs following placement of the 700-mg 5% lidocaine patch, the concentration achieved is much lower than what is obtained by IV infusion and may be too low to provide meaningful systemic analgesia for acute pain.[29]

Ketamine

The role of ketamine in postinjury analgesia is presently unclear. Although the drug is a competitive *N*-methyl-D-aspartate receptor antagonist that has modest efficacy to inhibit central sensitization following injury, the results of clinical trials in human patients have been ambiguous.[30] Small studies addressing its use in veterinary patients suggest that there is some efficacy for analgesia and recovery of normal behaviors postoperatively.[31–33]

APPROACH

The use of standardized "recipes" for adding constant amounts of these drugs to IV fluids (eg, "morphine-lidocaine-ketamine") is an excellent method to provide a background of analgesia to patients during surgery and in the immediate perioperative period. In this system, everyone involved—doctors and staff—know they have to make the analgesic-fluid mix the same way, and hospital staff learn over time how animals respond to a particular approach. An advantage of this approach is that it becomes an easy way to incorporate analgesia therapy into a busy surgical practice with a low chance of making mistakes in preparation. Because of the wide variation in patient needs for analgesia, however, the author prefers to tailor drug infusion to meet individual patient needs during the first 1 to 3 days postoperatively in animals that require support with intravenous fluids.

A commonly employed treatment for patients in pain in the author's ICU that need sleep is to combine an opioid with lidocaine, ketamine, and medetomidine (for dogs) or with ketamine and medetomidine (for cats) (**Box 1**). This approach is particularly useful for vigorous postoperative patients that require sedation to sleep the night after surgery.

The most convenient method is to add any analgesic medications to fluids that are formulated to provide the maintenance needs for the patient. These are typically low-sodium fluids (eg, one-half or one-fourth strength saline, or commercial maintenance solutions with 40 mEq/L sodium) administered to maintain fluid homeostasis and at infusion rates that never change. Any additional fluid needs (eg, to make up for losses due to drainage, vomiting, diarrhea, polyuria, or excess evaporation) are met with a second fluid set run through the same IV catheter.

Box 1
Example of a tailored drug infusion plan

For this technique, plan on adding the drugs to a bag of fluids for which the administration rate will not change, which usually means picking a fluid and administration rate calculated to provide maintenance needs for water. For example, to calculate a drug plan for a 20-kg dog that is to receive morphine, lidocaine, ketamine, and medetomidine for the first 8 to 24 hours postoperatively, drug doses to consider might include

Morphine: 0.1 mg/kg/h × 20 kg = 2 mg/h

Lidocaine: 2.5 mg/kg/h × 20 kg = 50 mg/h

Ketamine: 0.1 mg/kg/h × 20 kg = 2 mg/h

Medetomidine: 2.0 μg/kg/h × 20 kg = 40 μg/h

The maintenance fluid administration rate for a dog this size lying quietly in a cage is roughly 800 mL/d or 33 mL/h. Therefore, a 1-L bag contains 1000/33 or 30 hour's worth of treatment, and to a 1-L bag one must add

Morphine: 2 mg/h × 30 hours = 60 mg = 4 mL

Lidocaine: 50 mg/h × 30 hours = 1500 mg = 75 mL

Ketamine: 2 mg/h × 30 hours = 60 mg = 0.6 mL

Medetomidine: 40 μg/h × 30 hours = 1200 μg = 1.2 mL

If the drugs are added to a 1-L bag of fluid, the final volume is greater than a liter—in this case 1081 mL. Therefore, 81 mL should be removed from the bag before addition of the medications.

Considerations regarding the use of continuous infusions include the following:

- Morphine (and to a lesser extent hydromorphone) tends to produce increased sedation and side effects when used at a dosage of >0.1 mg/kg/h (>0.05 mg/kg/h for hydromorphone) for more than 12 hours; therefore, the infusion rate must often be reduced by that time.
- Ketamine may provide some protection against central hypersensitivity at dosages too low to produce obvious clinical signs of ketamine treatment. In the author's experience, infusion rates of $\leq$0.2 mg/kg/h are less likely to produce the characteristic behavioral side effects of the drug.
- A reliable sign in cats of significant central effects of opioids is mydriasis. When pupils are dilated and are accompanied by signs of dysphoria, the infusion should be interrupted for 1 to 6 hours and restarted at a lower rate. Cats with dilated pupils should be kept in quiet, darkened cages whenever possible.
- The delay to peak sedation seen with a constant-rate infusion of α_2-adrenergic agonists is problematic if rapid sedation is required to address emergence delirium. In this case, a dose of 1 μg/mL may be diluted into 10 mL of saline and administered to the patient 1 mL (0.1 μg/kg) at a time, titrated to effect.
- Sedation and respiratory depression from opioids and medetomidine are much more likely when the animal is hypothermic. Caregivers should verify satisfactory recovery of consciousness and body temperature after surgery before sedation with these agents and provide heat support as needed.
- If sedation with any agent is excessive, the clinician should interrupt the infusion for up to a few hours and restart it at a lower rate or lower drug concentration.
- For cats and small dogs, 250-mL bags should be used or an in-line burette should be installed to meter the fluid. Putting all additives into such a container instead of a large bag limits waste and makes it easier to change the infusion mix.

- If additional fluids are needed, one should piggyback a separate bag and administration set onto the primary IV set at an injection port and administer as needed; the rate of the medicated fluid should not be changed.
- When first learning how to use drug infusions, one should start with lower dosages and gradually use higher infusion rates as the care team gains confidence and experience. The first few applications of the technique should be on patients whose infusion can begin before noon. Generally, by the time 4 to 6 hours have passed, drug effects and clinical signs will reach a plateau. After gaining confidence with this technique, some patients that receive fluids unattended overnight can be treated in this manner, assuming an electronic fluid pump is used and the drug effects reach a plateau by the end of the work day.
- Most postinjury and postoperative patients benefit from the addition of oral nonsteroidal anti-inflammatory drug therapy in addition to the infusion, providing there are no contraindications.
- As the patient recovers the ability to drink and as less drug is needed, the IV fluid rate can be slowed proportionately.

GABAPENTIN

Gabapentin is a structural analog of γ-aminobutyric acid introduced in 1993 as an anticonvulsant and later approved for treatment of the human chronic pain syndrome of postherpetic neuralgia. Its antinociceptive mechanism may be multifactorial but appears to include inhibition of neuronal voltage-dependent calcium channels, a process that reduces the release of excitatory neurotransmitters in nociceptive substrate of the spinal cord.[34] Although it is commonly used as an adjunct therapy for chronic pain in dogs and cats, there is growing interest in its use as an adjunct analgesic for the treatment of acute pain in veterinary patients because of recent trends in human medicine.[35] A common starting dose is 2 to 5 mg/kg twice a day, adjusted upward if needed or downward if sedation or ataxia develop. Gabapetin is started as soon as the animal tolerates oral medications while being treated concurrently with established drugs.

SUMMARY

Acute pain is a physiologically appropriate consequence of injury and inflammation but, in hospitalized patients, may increase complications from an exaggerated stress response. Because it is usually caused by nociception, drug therapy is often an effective component of patient management. Although the drugs used for analgesia have many potential side effects, when used properly and in combination, it is almost always possible to provide meaningful and safe analgesia to even critically ill patients.

REFERENCES

1. Wiese AJ, Muir WW III, Wittum TE. Characteristics of pain and response to analgesic treatment in dogs and cats examined at a veterinary teaching hospital emergency service. J Am Vet Med Assoc 2005;226(12):2004–9.
2. Chapman CR, Tuckett RP, Song CW. Pain and stress in a systems perspective: reciprocal neural, endocrine, and immune interactions. The Journal of Pain 2008;9(2):122–45.
3. Kehlet H, Dahl JB. Anaesthesia, surgery, and challenges in postoperative recovery. Lancet 2003;362(9399):1921–8.

4. Blanchard AR. Sedation and analgesia in intensive care. Medications attenuate stress response in critical illness. Postgrad Med 2002;111(2):59–60,63–4,67–70.
5. Savvas I, Papazoglou LG, Kazakos G, et al. Incisional block with bupivacaine for analgesia after celiotomy in dogs. J Am Anim Hosp Assoc 2008;44(2):60–6.
6. Almeida TF, Fantoni DT, Mastrocinque S, et al. Epidural anaesthesia with bupivacaine, bupivacaine and fentanyl, or bupivacaine and sufentanil during intravenous administration of propofol for ovariohysterectomy in dogs. J Am Vet Med Assoc 2007;230(1):45–51.
7. Novello L, Corletto F. Combined spinal-epidural anesthesia in a dog. Vet Surg 2006;35(2):191–7.
8. Kona-Boun JJ, Cuvelliez S, Troncy E. Evaluation of epidural administration of morphine or morphine and bupivacaine for postoperative analgesia after premedication with an opioid analgesic and orthopedic surgery in dogs. J Am Vet Med Assoc 2006;229(7):1103–12.
9. Buback JL, Boothe HW, Carroll GL, et al. Comparison of three methods for relief of pain after ear canal ablation in dogs. Vet Surg 1996;25(5):380–5.
10. Romans CW, Gordon WJ, Robinson DA, et al. Effect of postoperative analgesic protocol on limb function following onychectomy in cats. J Am Vet Med Assoc 2005;227(1):89–93.
11. Radlinsky MG, Mason DE, Roush JK, et al. Use of a continuous, local infusion of bupivacaine for postoperative analgesia in dogs undergoing total ear canal ablation. J Am Vet Med Assoc 2005;227(3):414–9.
12. Mahler SP, Reece JL. Electrical nerve stimulation to facilitate placement of an indwelling catheter for repeated brachial plexus block in a traumatized dog. Vet Anaesth Analg 2007;34(5):365–70.
13. Franquelo C, Toledo A, Manubens J, et al. Bupivacaine disposition and pharmacologic effects after intravenous and epidural administrations in dogs. Am J Vet Res 1995;56(8):1087–91.
14. Mazoit JX, Lambert C, Berdeaux A, et al. Pharmacokinetics of bupivacaine after short and prolonged infusions in conscious dogs. Anesth Analg 1988;67:961–6.
15. Trissel LA. Handbook on injectable drugs. 11 edition. Bethesda (MD): American Society of Health-System Pharmacists, Inc.; 2001.
16. Posner LP, Gleed RD, Erb HN, et al. Post-anesthetic hyperthermia in cats. Vet Anaesth Analg 2007;34(1):40–7.
17. Niedfeldt RL, Robertson SA. Postanesthetic hyperthermia in cats: a retrospective comparison between hydromorphone and buprenorphine. Vet Anaesth Analg 2006;33(6):381–9.
18. Hofmeister EH, Egger CM. Transdermal fentanyl patches in small animals. J Am Anim Hosp Assoc 2004;40(6):468–78.
19. Davidson CD, Pettifer GR, Henry JD Jr. Plasma fentanyl concentrations and analgesic effects during full or partial exposure to transdermal fentanyl patches in cats. J Am Vet Med Assoc 2004;224(5):700–5.
20. Egger CM, Glerum LE, Allen SW, et al. Plasma fentanyl concentrations in awake cats and cats undergoing anesthesia and ovariohysterectomy using transdermal administration. Vet Anaesth Analg 2003;30(4):229–36.
21. Slingsby LS, Taylor PM. Thermal antinociception after dexmedetomidine administration in cats: a dose-finding study. J Vet Pharmacol Ther 2008;31(2):135–42.
22. Granholm M, McKusick BC, Westerholm FC, et al. Evaluation of the clinical efficacy and safety of dexmedetomidine or medetomidine in cats and their reversal with atipamezole. Vet Anaesth Analg 2006;33(4):214–23.

23. Gomez-Villamandos RJ, Palacios C, Benitez A, et al. Dexmedetomidine or medetomidine premedication before propofol-desflurane anaesthesia in dogs. J Vet Pharmacol Ther 2006;29(3):157–63.
24. Pypendop BH, Verstegen JP. Hemodynamic effects of medetomidine in the dog: a dose titration study. Vet Surg 1998;27(6):612–22.
25. Hayashi K, Nishimura R, Yamaki A, et al. Comparison of sedative effects induced by medetomidine, medetomidine-midazolam and medetomidine-butorphanol in dogs. J Vet Med Sci 1994;56(5):951–6.
26. Grimm KA, Tranquilli WJ, Thurmon JC, et al. Duration of nonresponse to noxious stimulation after intramuscular administration of butorphanol, medetomidine, or a butorphanol-medetomidine combination during isoflurane administration in dogs. Am J Vet Res 2000;61:42–7.
27. Xiao WH, Bennett GJ. C-fiber spontaneous discharge evoked by chronic inflammation is suppressed by a long-term infusion of lidocaine yielding nanogram per milliliter plasma levels. Pain 2008;137(1):218–28.
28. Pypendop BH, Ilkiw JE. Assessment of the hemodynamic effects of lidocaine administered IV in isoflurane-anesthetized cats. Am J Vet Res 2005;66(4):661–8.
29. Ko J, Weil A, Maxwell L, et al. Plasma concentrations of lidocaine in dogs following lidocaine patch application. J Am Anim Hosp Assoc 2007;43(5):280–3.
30. Elia N, Tramer MR. Ketamine and postoperative pain—a quantitative systematic review of randomised trials. Pain 2005;113(1–2):61–70.
31. Sarrau S, Jourdan J, Dupuis-Soyris F, et al. Effects of postoperative ketamine infusion on pain control and feeding behaviour in bitches undergoing mastectomy. J Small Anim Pract 2007;48(12):670–6.
32. Wattananit S, Kalpravidh M. An assessment of epidural ketamine for hindlimb anesthesia in dogs. Thai Journal of Veterinary Medicine 2005;35(4):53–64.
33. Wagner AE, Walton JA, Hellyer PW, et al. Use of low doses of ketamine administered by constant rate infusion as an adjunct for postoperative analgesia in dogs. J Am Vet Med Assoc 2002;221(1):72–5.
34. Kong VK, Irwin MG. Gabapentin: a multimodal perioperative drug? Br J Anaesth 2007;99(6):775–86.
35. Huot MP, Chouinard P, Girard F, et al. Gabapentin does not reduce post-thoracotomy shoulder pain: a randomized, double-blind placebo-controlled study. Can J Anaesth 2008;55(6):337–43.

Neuropathic Pain in Dogs and Cats: If Only They Could Tell Us If They Hurt

Karol A. Mathews, DVM, DVSc

KEYWORDS

• Neuropathic pain • Dogs • Cats • Gabapentin
• Ketamine • Lidocaine

During the past 10 years, the physiology of nociceptive and inflammatory pain and its management have been taught to student veterinarians and animal health technicians. This topic has also been presented at many annual veterinary continuing education programs, wherein the focus of pain management has been predominantly associated with surgery and osteoarthritis in dogs and cats and, to a lesser degree, with traumatic and medical pain, but there has been little discussion on neuropathic pain as a primary focus. In the veterinary literature, textbooks and a few clinical reports present specific causes of neuropathic pain that is obvious and is presented under the specific aspects discussed in this article. Often, the clinical signs have been insidious and present for weeks to several months, with an obvious lesion difficult to find. Because pain in general can be difficult to recognize and isolate in many veterinary patients, neuropathic pain can be extremely difficult to identify unless we appreciate the occult nature of many of the predisposing causes.

The management of chronic pain, of which neuropathic pain is included, represents a major human public health issue. Because of the near-epidemic proportions of painful conditions in human beings, especially as the population ages, the need to improve pain outcomes is reflected by the congressional declaration of the present decade as the "Decade of Pain Control and Research," and the acknowledgment in January 2001 of pain as the "fifth vital sign" by the Joint Commission of Healthcare Organizations.[1] Harden states that "Increases in our understanding of the function of the neurologic system over the last few years have led to new insights into the mechanisms underlying pain symptoms, especially chronic and neuropathic pain. The rapidly evolving symptom- and mechanism-based approach to the treatment of neuropathic pain holds promise for improving the quality of life of our patients with neuropathic pain."[1]

Emergency and Critical Care Medicine, Department of Clinical Studies, Ontario Veterinary College, University of Guelph, Guelph, Ontario, N1G 2W1, Canada
E-mail address: kmathews@uoguelph.ca

Vet Clin Small Anim 38 (2008) 1365–1414
doi:10.1016/j.cvsm.2008.09.001 **vetsmall.theclinics.com**
0195-5616/08/$ – see front matter

The quest for relief from pain is pursued in human medicine because the existence of pain is known; the patient can verbalize his or her pain, what it feels like, where it is, and the relief he or she feels when treatment is appropriate. Because we all have experienced pain of various degrees and durations, it is an excellent topic for comparison and understanding with our veterinary patients. Because veterinary patients cannot tell us how painful they are, we, as veterinarians, have to understand what can cause pain, how pain manifests,[2,3] and how best to treat it. The purpose of this article is to raise awareness of the existence of neuropathic pain in our patients, in which pain may be a cause for behavioral changes (1) in the acute pain setting (at home or in the hospital); (2) at a later period after a traumatic or surgical experience; or (3) as the result of a chronic primary lesion affecting the (i) somatosensory and visceral peripheral nerve(s), (ii) the meninges, spine, spinal cord, and its nerve roots, or (iii) a lesion in the brain. Several alterations in sensory processing occur peripherally and centrally in the development of chronic neuropathic pain; however, two major events occur: (1) abnormal peripheral input and (2) abnormal central processing. The human clinical literature and the research literature are used as potential comparisons to the veterinary clinical setting.

The International Association for the Study of Pain (IASP) defines neuropathic pain as "pain initiated or caused by a primary lesion or dysfunction in the nervous system." This definition, however, is still unclear because the term *dysfunction* is nonspecific.[4] A proposed definition to clarify this is "pain arising as a direct consequence of diseases affecting the somatosensory system," with further clarification on the definition of "disease" that may be required.[4] How "normal," physiologic, or transient (words used for acute pain or true "nociceptive" pain) pain differs from neuropathic pain is in its origin. The sensory experience of nociceptive pain is attributable to immediate injury and tissue inflammation. It is a normal adaptive function of the nervous system signaling the type and location of the injury, and it is an awareness or warning to the individual experiencing this pain. The initiating lesion, and subsequent inflammatory process, initiate Aδ and C-fiber activity, causing sensitization, recruitment of silent nociceptors, and ionic channel and membrane receptor activation.[1,4] The origin of neuropathic pain, conversely, may be difficult to diagnose unless an obvious predisposing lesion or injury to the nervous system is easily identified.[4] Because this is a statement based on the human patient, one can definitely appreciate the difficulty in identifying such lesions in animals. Understanding the events that occur in the nervous system, originating from poorly managed acute pain, chronic pain, or primary lesions within the nervous system, is important because individual mechanisms causing pain are targets for therapeutic consideration. Some may be amenable to surgical therapy, whereas others require specific pharmaceutical intervention. Above all, by understanding these mechanisms, the means to prevent establishment of neuropathic pain is always pursued by meticulous surgical technique and using recommended current and future therapeutic measures.

A brief overview of "transient" and inflammatory pain transmission is important before discussing neuropathic pain, because severe noxious and inflammatory insults are also mediated by the same pathways, resulting in changes within the nervous system.[5] While making comparisons to our own experiences, it is interesting to note that although nociceptive processing is similar in human beings and domestic animals, based on anatomic differences in the ascending fiber densities of the spinothalamic tract, lower animals may have less refined stimulus characterization and localization capabilities, which may indicate an increased awareness of the adversive quality of the stimulus and autonomic responses.

PHYSIOLOGY AND PATHOPHYSIOLOGY

Peripheral Nervous System

The sensory nervous system is composed of two distinct classes of cells: glial cells and neurons. Glial cells nourish and support nerve cells. Neurons sense and conduct sensory information. The cell bodies of peripheral sensory nerves are located in the dorsal root ganglia of the dorsal root of the spinal nerves for nerves originating from lower than the head and in the trigeminal ganglia for nerves transmitting sensory information from the head (trigeminal, facial, glossopharyngeal, and vagus nerves).[6] In what might be considered a "comfortable state" (ie, in the absence of high-intensity sensory stimulation), the sensory afferent nerve fibers (slowly conducting unmyelinated C-fibers or rapidly conducting thinly myelinated Aδ fibers) are "silent," showing little or no spontaneous traffic.[6] Innocuous sensations or a low-intensity stimulus, such as touch or vibration, is transmitted from the periphery to the central nervous system (CNS) laminae III and IV of the dorsal horn by way of Aβ fibers (**Fig. 1**).[5,7] Normally Aβ fibers are not part of the pain pathway. Transient noxious stimuli (nociceptive

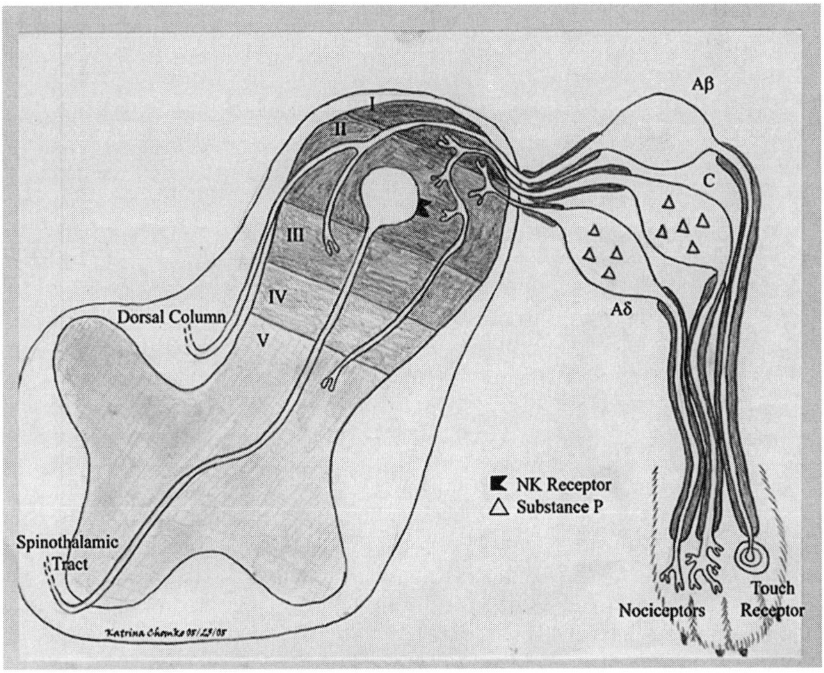

Fig. 1. Under normal conditions, innocuous sensations or a low-intensity stimulus, such as touch or vibration, is transmitted from the periphery to laminae III and IV of the dorsal horn by means of Aβ fibers; the signal is then relayed to the brain by way of the dorsal column somatosensory pathway. Noxious thermal or mechanical input (transduction), the protective nociceptive "first pain" experience, activates the Aδ fibers, which have small receptive fields, and functions as a warning and is protective to the animal. With increased intensity of the stimulus, C-fibers also conduct impulses along with Aδ fibers. C-fibers have a larger receptive field compared with Aδ fibers and are responsible for the "second pain" experience. The Aδ and C-fibers enter the dorsal horn of the spinal cord, wherein Aδ fibers solely and C-fibers predominantly terminate in laminae I and II. The Aδ and C-fiber ganglions express substance P (S-P), and the natural killer 1 (NK_1 [S-P]) receptors are expressed in the neurons of lamina II. The signal is then relayed to the brain by way of the spinothalamic tract.

pain) occurring in the periphery by a mechanical (eg, stepped on the toe, needle prick), thermal (eg, hot or cold object), or chemical stimulus evokes intensity-dependent increases in the rate of firing in rapidly conducting Aδ afferent fibers.[5] The Aδ fibers have small receptive fields and are activated by noxious thermal or mechanical input (transduction) (see **Fig. 1**). They conduct impulses (transmission) rapidly, and therefore are felt as the initial sensation of pain, or the "first pain," which has a sharp pricking quality and is localized and transient. This is a protective mechanism and acts as a warning to remove the body part from the stimulus.[7,8] With increased intensity of the stimulus, C-fibers also conduct impulses along with Aδ fibers. C-fibers are polymodal; may be activated by thermal, mechanical, or chemical stimuli; and constitute most cutaneous nociceptive innervation with larger receptive fields compared with Aδ fibers (see **Fig. 1**).[5,7] They are responsible for the "second pain," which is burning or throbbing.[8,9] The frequency of afferent traffic corresponds to the psychophysical report of pain sensation in human beings and the vigor of the escape response in animals.[10]

In the absence of tissue injury, termination of the afferent discharges occurs with cessation of the painful experience. When the stimulus results in tissue injury (inflammation), however, the C-fibers produce an ongoing afferent discharge that persists after the original insult has ceased and contributes to the ongoing second pain. Initially, this persistent discharge is facilitated by the injured tissue, whether skin, muscle, or viscera, resulting in infiltration of inflammatory cells that release chemical mediators and initiation of the arachidonic acid (AA) cascade by phospholipase-A_2 (PLA_2) and subsequent eicosanoid production.[11] It seems that the prominent role of this inflammatory process is to activate more silent nociceptors, which, in turn, release substance-P (S-P) (see **Fig. 1**), a pronociceptive peptide neurotransmitter.[5] Together, this increases the afferent input to the spinal cord, which is accompanied by an increased pain response for a given stimulus that would normally elicit less pain (hyperalgesia). This is referred to as peripheral sensitization.[12] This process also results in the pain experience spreading beyond the area of local injury; it is therefore "poorly localized" and described as a burning and throbbing sensation (secondary hyperalgesia).[12] Aδ and C-fibers have also been implicated in visceral nociciption.[13,14]

Central Nervous System

Processing of this nociceptive input at the level of the spinal cord occurs in the dorsal horn of the spinal cord. The Aδ and C-fibers enter the spinal cord by way of the dorsal roots of spinal nerves and synapse in specific laminae of the dorsal horn. Aδ fibers, solely, and C-fibers, predominantly, terminate in laminae I and II, from which location the the signal is then relayed, by way of the spinothalamic tract, to the brain (see **Fig. 1**).[5] Of importance in this process is the group of neurons called the wide-dynamic-range (WDR) neurons, which seem to be less sensitive to innocuous stimuli (Aβ input) but respond more vigorously to noxious stimulation.[9] These neurons receive input from somatic and visceral structures and are important in the expression of spinal facilitation of pain, or wind-up.[9] Repetitive firing of primary nociceptive afferents, such as occurs with inadequately treated pain of any cause, results in activation of WDR neurons and their release of glutamate into the synaptic cleft (**Fig. 2**).[9] Glutamate subsequently activates the *N*-methyl-D-aspartate (NMDA) receptors on the postsynaptic membrane. The NMDA receptors are only activated under conditions of persistent membrane depolarization. The glutamate receptor facilitates calcium conductance, resulting in up-regulation of receptors. S-P and brain-derived neurotrophic factor (BDNF) also participate in activating the intracellular signaling cascade, which increases the membrane's sensitivity to subsequent stimulation.[9] The reader is

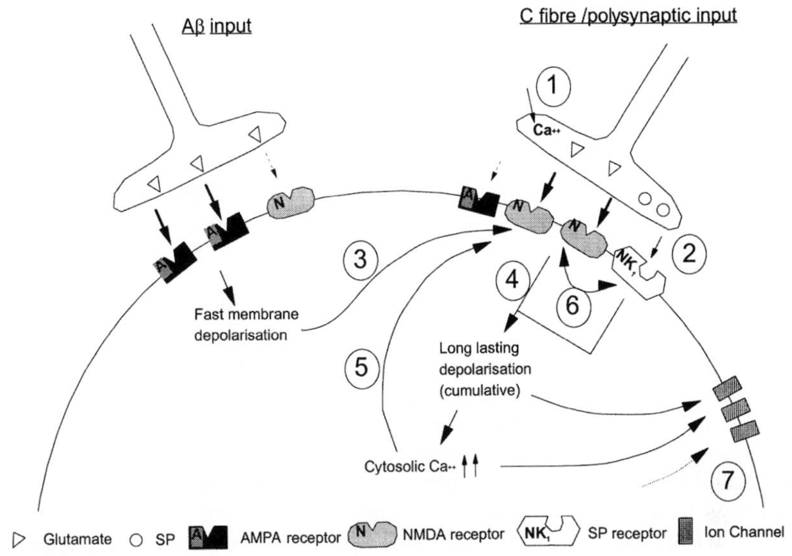

Fig. 2. Possible molecular mechanisms for the generation of wind-up. The diagram summarizes the mechanisms that may elicit wind-up. It represents a standard spinal neurone receiving monosynaptic input from mechanoreceptors and polysynaptic input from nociceptors, such as may occur in many deep dorsal and ventral horn neurones. Mechanisms are numbered from 1 to 7. Build-up of Ca^{2+} in the presynaptic terminal (1) leads to increased neurotransmitter release (2) of amino acids and S-P. (3) Activation of adenosine monophosphate acid (AMPA) receptors in the postsynaptic membrane causes fast membrane depolarization, which contributes to lifting the Mg^{2+} block of *N*-methyl-D-aspartate (NMDA) receptors. (4) Activation of NMDA receptors and natural killer-1 (NK_1) receptors generates a long-lasting cumulative depolarization. Cytosolic Ca^{2+} concentration increases as a result of Ca^{2+} entry through the NMDA ionophore; to a lesser extent, through some AMPA receptor channels; and through voltage-sensitive Ca^{2+} channels activated by depolarization. An elevated Ca^{2+} concentration (5) and the activation of NK_1 receptors by means of second-messenger systems (6) enhance the performance of NMDA receptors. (7) Finally, activation of NK_1 receptors, cumulative depolarizations, elevated cytosolic Ca^{2+}, and other factors regulate the behavior of membrane channels, which facilitates the production of action potentials and lead to wind-up. (*From* Herrero JF, Laird JMA, Lopez-Garcia JA. Wind-up of spinal cord neurones and pain sensation: much ado about something? Prog Neurobiol 2000;61(2):179; with permission.)

referred to articles by Herrero and colleagues[9] and Muir and Woolf[15] for a more in-depth review of the neurobiology of wind-up.

Of recent interest is the identification of a group of PLA_2 enzymes (group IVA $cPLA_2$ and group VI $iPLA_2$), constitutively expressed and active in the spinal cord, that have been implicated in centrally mediated hyperalgesia.[16] In addition to supplying substrate for the cyclooxygenase (COX) pathway, AA liberated by PLA_2 may play a role in augmenting nociception.[17] For example, AA potentiates NMDA receptor currents, and thus amplifies glutamate-mediated increases in intracellular calcium concentration by binding to sites on the NMDA receptor or by modifying the receptor's lipid environment. COX-1 and COX-2 are induced to participate in peripheral and central transmission of pain. Repetitive small afferent activity results in spinal release of prostaglandin E_2 and amino acids that serve to enhance transmitter release, leading to central sensitization.[18] Inhibition of COX by nonsteroidal anti-inflammatory drugs (NSAIDs) exerts a direct spinal action by blocking hyperalgesia induced by the activation of spinal glutamate and S-P receptors.[19] These findings demonstrate that the analgesic effects of NSAIDs can be dissociated from their anti-inflammatory actions. Spinal prostanoids are thus critical for the augmentation of pain processing at the spinal level.[19] Recently, spinal isoprostanes have been identified and shown to sensitize rat sensory neurons, producing a hyperalgesic state, thereby reducing mechanical and thermal withdrawal thresholds in rats.[20] Isoprostanes are a novel group of nonenzymatically generated AA metabolites formed directly in a non–COX-dependent manner by free radical oxidation of AA.[21]

The net effect of noxious sensory input is that high-frequency action potentials in the primary afferent neuron facilitate the second-order neurons to respond more vigorously to subsequent stimulation, a phenomenon termed *central sensitization*. This effect can last from hours to weeks, or even years (in certain situations, as is discussed in the section on neuropathic pain) after the causative event ends.[15,22]

The sensory input from the dorsal horn is transmitted through the ascending nociceptive pathways, and through the brain stem (medulla, pons, and midbrain), with contributions to the reticular activating system and the periaqueductal gray matter (PAG).[23] The PAG extends projections to the hypothalamus (initiating the neuroendocrine and autonomic responses) and the thalamus, providing an indirect alternative pathway for nociceptive sensory activity. Finally, the sensory activity from the thalamus reaches the cortex, in which it is perceived as pain. The perception of pain results in a normal behavioral response, such as withdrawal from the stimulus (nociceptive pain), and, depending on the circumstance and severity of the pain experienced, such as inflammatory or neuropathic pain, many other behavioral characteristics.[24] What is important to note is that although general anesthetics block the perception of pain (cortical component), the events in the dorsal horn are not blocked.[25] Whatever degree of wind-up that has been established during the surgical procedure continues to be experienced on recovery from general anesthesia. The sensory cortex can undergo considerable plasticity together with the changes that occur in subcortical structures; as such, supraspinal plasticity is believed to play a major role in shaping the pain experience.[26] The appropriate analgesics known to block the various steps along the nociceptive pathway to the thalamocortex can reduce the "memory" and establishment of chronic and neuropathic pain, and the reader is referred to the article by Lamont on multimodal pain management elsewhere in this issue for an in-depth discussion on this topic.

Endogenous Facilitatory Systems

In addition to descending inhibition of sensory input, descending excitatory or facilitatory influences from the brain stem or forebrain have been characterized.[27] Although descending inhibition is primarily involved in regulating suprathreshold responses to noxious stimuli, descending facilitation reduces the neuronal threshold to nociceptive stimulation. Descending facilitation has a general impact on spinal sensory transmission, and it induces sensory inputs from cutaneous and visceral organs.[28] One physiologic function of descending facilitation is to enhance an animal's ability to detect potential danger signals in the environment. Neurons in the rostral ventromedial medulla (RVM) not only respond to noxious stimuli but show "learning" type changes during repetitive noxious stimuli.[28] The RVM neurons undergo plastic changes during and fter tissue injury and inflammation. Descending facilitation is likely activated after injury, contributing to secondary hyperalgesia.[28]

Descending Inhibitory System

Whereas the ascending sensory pathways ensure delivery of the sensory activity, the descending modulatory pathways, or inhibitory systems, function to reduce the actual degree of pain perceived, acting as a "gate" to pain. Nociceptive inputs activate endogenous analgesic systems, which include structures within the thalamocortex, PAG, RVM, pons, and medullary and spinal cord dorsal horn.[27] The most important of these is the PAG, with its dense concentration of opioid peptides and receptors. A group of catecholaminergic nuclei in the pons, the locus ceruleus (LC), receives noradrenergic efferents from the PAG that descend to the spinal cord dorsal horn.[29] Activity of the LC is under the control of an α_2-autoreceptor and seems to contribute indirectly to analgesia at the level of the dorsal horn through these descending projections.[29,30] There is evidence that another nucleus (Kolliker Fuse) may be the primary source of descending noradrenergic fibers in the cat.[29] By activating descending inhibitory systems, painful information entering the CNS is significantly reduced. Thus, acute or physiologic pain is bearable, and it does not become chronic or pathologic pain.[27]

There are several transmitters and receptors at multiple sites within the descending inhibitory system.[29] The final site involved in the inhibitory pathway is the dorsal horn of the spinal cord. Substances identified in the dorsal horn neurons that serve to modulate nociceptive transmission are amino acids (γ-aminobutyric acid [GABA] and glycine), serotonin (5-hydroxytryptamine [5-HT]), norepinephrine (NE), and the endogenous opioid peptides (enkephalins, endorphins, and dynorphins).[31] The spinal cord opioid system acts presynaptically by blocking release of S-P and postsynaptically. Studies have shown that serotonin and NE contribute to antinociception in spinal pathways and supraspinal descending pathways, which are also disrupted in neuropathic pain.[31] A recent study suggested that after nerve injury, the tonically active noradrenergic inhibition of mechanically evoked spinal dorsal horn neuronal responses is lost.[32] This alteration in noradrenergic inhibitory control may be one of the many underlying mechanisms by which behavioral symptoms of hypersensitivity develop after nerve damage.[32] Although the dissection of the inhibitory system and its disruption continue to be investigated, it has been known for some time that a component of neuropathic pain and hyperalgesia is attributable to disruption of the normal endogenous inhibitory systems, such that the descending inhibitory system and the opioid system may become deficient at the spinal level.[33] For reviews in the veterinary literature, the reader is referred to articles by Muir and Woolf[15] and Lamont and colleagues.[34]

Summary of Events of Sensory Stimulation (Neuronal Plasticity)

1. The immediate (<1 second) reflexive and nociceptive responses associated with C-fiber input (activation)
2. The rapid (seconds) and progressive changes in excitability (wind-up)
3. The development of peripheral and central sensitivity (hours)
4. The activity-dependent alterations in intracellular signal molecules and gene expression that define a potentiated system (hours later)

All of these, in conjunction with disinhibition and Aβ-mediated pain, represent a series of neurobiologic events that are responsible for activation, modulation, and modification of the nervous system by sensory stimuli.[35]

NEUROPATHIC PAIN

In veterinary medicine, a major focus for assessing neurologic injury after surgery or trauma is commonly loss of motor and sensory function, or in certain illnesses, primarily a loss in motor function. In this setting, damage or disease of axons (axotomy) or myelin disrupts the ability to conduct nerve impulses, causing hypoesthesia and numbness (as described by human beings), in addition to potential loss of motor function. Because nerves are protoplasmic extensions of live cells, however, the neurons, respond actively to injury.[4] Surgery, trauma, and inflammatory states result in nociceptive input as previously described. Primary injury to nerves also confers pain. In rat models of peripheral nerve injury, the onset of ectopic action potential firing in the injured nerve corresponds to the onset of behavioral signs of pain, such as mechanical allodynia.[36]

The developing pain (neuropathy) is typically attributable to injury or disease that damages the axon or soma of sensory neurons or disrupts the myelin sheath that surrounds many axons (dysmyelination and demyelination).[37] Ectopic firing of these nerves tends to occur; in fact, some human patients with a neuropathic disorder report enhanced sensation at a certain level of tactile stimulus in areas normally hypoesthetic at rest.[5] Some human patients also experience paresthesias (tingling, prickling, burning), hyperesthesias (heightened sensation to a nociceptive stimulus), and dysesthesias (unpleasant or painful sensation) (**Box 1**).[5] The quality and pattern of altered sensitivity in neuropathic pain differ from transient or inflammatory pain. As an example, a cold stimulus, such as applying an ice pack to an acutely injured joint to reduce the inflammatory pain in the "normal" or "naive" painful individual, would be described as excruciating in a patient with neuropathic pain.[5] This difference in "experience" is thought to occur because of a reorganization of sensory transmission within the nervous system that occurs after nerve injury. Such changes include alterations in expression of neurotransmitters, neuromodulators, receptors, ion-channels (especially the tetrodotoxin-resistant [TTX-R] sodium channels),[38] and structural proteins. Some of these changes are involved in the reparative process, but others contribute to neuropathic pain. As an example, the Aβ-fibers may sprout into the laminae II region of the dorsal horn vacated by central terminals of C-fibers, wherein S-P and S-P (natural killer-1 [NK_1]) receptors are expressed (**Fig. 3**).[37] Alternatively, because of nerve injury, the disruption of the glial ensheathment allows the adjacent denuded axons to make contact, facilitating electrical (ephaptic) and chemical (by means of diffusible substances) cross-excitation. A cross-after-discharge can also occur, whereby normal A-fibers can activate C-fibers.[39] When light innocuous stimuli are applied to the area subserved by the nerve-injured area, the stimuli transmitted by the Aβ-fibers are processed in the dorsal horn as C-fiber sensory afferent stimuli with subsequent pain transmission (see **Fig. 3**).[5,40] During the healing process, there may also be a connection between the Aβ-fibers and the C-fibers. Therefore, the transmission of a normal innocuous "touch" stimulus elicited during transduction of the Aβ-fibers is coupled to the axon of the C-fiber. Subsequent transmission is then by means of the C-fiber, in which it is interpreted centrally as a noxious stimulus (allodynia) (see **Fig. 3**).[5]

Sensory-Sympathetic Coupling

Under physiologic conditions, primary afferent nerve endings are not sensitive to catecholamines and are functionally distinct from the efferent sympathetic nervous system.[5] Normally, sympathetic activity does not cause pain; nerve injury, however, can induce noradrenergic supersensitivity.[37,41] This sensory-sympathetic coupling

Box 1
Stimulus-evoked pain

Nociceptive

It is caused by an intense, noxious stimulus (sensory response) that threatens to damage normal tissue. It is also known as physiologic, because it is the body's normal defense mechanism, resulting in withdrawal (motor response) from the potentially external hostile environment.

Hyperalgesia (also called hyperpathia)

- An exaggerated pain response produced by a normally painful stimulus (eg, a pinprick).
- It can arise from peripheral or central mechanisms.

Peripherally

- Sensitization of primary afferent nociceptors (Aδ and C-fibers) occurs by inflammatory mediators, such as bradykinin, histamine, prostaglandins, and substance-P released from injured tissue. The stimulus in this area hurts more than a non-injured or inflamed area.
- Neuroma: a tangled mass of regenerating nervous tissue embedded in scar and connective tissue at the site of nerve injury. Neuromas accumulate or "uncover" pathologic and non-pathologic ion channels (eg, various sodium channels) and receptors (eg, norepinephrine) that result in foci of hyperexcitability and ectopic activity.

Centrally

- Sensitization: tissue injury triggers an increase in the excitability of neurons in the spinal cord generated by C-fiber activity. Any prolonged or massive input from C-nociceptors enhances the response of dorsal horn neurons to all subsequent afferent inputs. As a result, increased synaptic activity is seen at the dorsal horn of the spinal cord, leading to changes in their excitability. The receptive field of the dorsal horn also grows. This increased activity outlasts the original injury at the primary afferents leading to central sensitization. The concept of central sensitization involves the development of secondary hyperalgesia or allodynia. Secondary hyperalgesia results in an increased sensitivity to a stimulus that occurs beyond the area of injury or inflammation (ie, adjacent normal tissue).
- Central pain- pain experienced in the area of the body subserved by the lesion originating from a primary lesion of the CNS.

Allodynia

Pain produced by a stimulus that is not usually painful (eg, light touch), and may result from any of the following central mechanisms for stimulus-evoked pain:

- Central sensitization
- Reorganization or
- Loss of inhibitory controls.

Stimulus-independent or spontaneous pain

- Occurs without provocation, so symptoms can occur constantly or at any time.
- Paresthesias: abnormal sensation that is not unpleasant, such as tingling, prickling.
- Dysesthesias: unpleasant, usually burning sensation that can originate peripherally by way of ectopic impulses along the Aβ, Aδ and C-fibers, arising as spontaneous activity caused by processes, such as damaged ("leaky") sodium channels, that accumulate along affected nerves. Paroxysmal shooting or electrical pain and continuous burning pain probably occurs from ectopic or ephaptic discharges arising in any type of fiber or may occur as a result of reduced inhibitory input from the brain or spinal cord.

Data from Woolf CJ, Max MB. Mechanism-based pain diagnosis: issues for analgesic drug development. Anesthesiology 2001;95(1):241–9; and Woolf CJ. Dissecting out mechanisms responsible for peripheral neuropathic pain: implications for diagnosis and therapy. Life Sci 2004;74:2605–10.

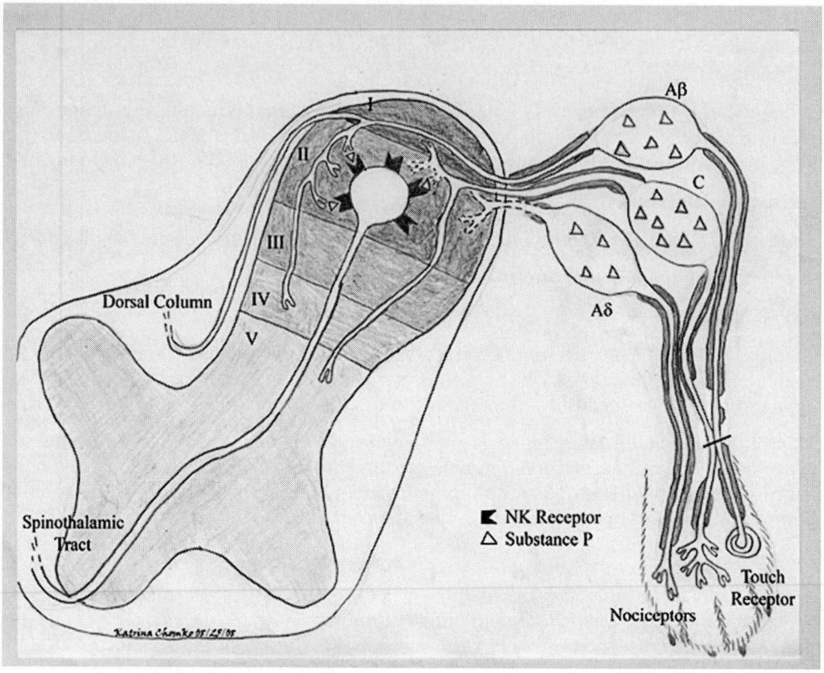

Fig. 3. Nerve injury–induced structural and neurochemical reorganization. After nerve injury, the transmission of a normal innocuous "touch" stimulus elicited during transduction of the Aβ fibers is coupled to the axon of the C-fiber. Subsequent transmission is then by means of the C-fiber, in which it is interpreted centrally as a noxious stimulus (allodynia). This reorganization may be attributable to: (1) the Aβ fibers may sprout into the laminae II region of the dorsal horn vacated by central terminals of C-fibers in which S-P and NK_1 (S-P) receptors are expressed; (2) nerve injury when the disruption of the glial ensheathment allows the adjacent denuded axons to make contact, facilitating electrical and chemical cross-excitation (a cross-after discharge can also occur, whereby normal A-fibers can activate C-fibers); or (3) during the healing process, there may also be a connection between the Aβ fibers and the C-fibers. With (1), (2), or (3), dorsal root ganglion neurons in Aβ fibers now express S-P and neurons in lamina II express a greater number of NK_1 receptors for pain transmission.

may contribute to stimulus-independent neuropathic pain in some human patients. Exogenous administration and endogenous release of NE increase the discharge of unmyelinated sprouts that have regenerated into a neuroma[42,43] After nerve damage in the rat, NE-containing sympathetic postganglionic fibers that normally innervate small blood vessels sprout, likely triggered by a neurotrophin, such as BDNF, and maintain nonsynaptic contact with sensory endings. In some instances, sympathetic sprouts encircle large-diameter dorsal root ganglia somata forming "baskets"[5]. Clinical evidence for a sympathetic contribution to neuropathic pain is supported by (1) patients with neuropathic pain often have accompanying signs, such as skin vasomotor activity and sweating; (2) neuropathic pain is often worsened by stimuli that evoke a sympathetic response, such as the startle response and emotional arousal; and (3) surgical destruction or pharmacologic blockade of the sympathetic outflow to the affected area often produces pain relief.[5] The effect of sympathetic blockade is not consistent, however, and in some patients, symptoms often recur within 6 months.[5] Neuropathic pain in animal models with L5 spinal nerve ligation, thought to be sympathetic dependent, was resistant to sympathectomy.[44] Even so, when conservative therapy fails, sympathetic blocks can be of benefit to some individuals and continue to be recommended for human patients.[45] Although noradrenergic supersensitivity would be extremely difficult to diagnose in veterinary patients, it is worthy of note should such signs manifest at some point after a triggering surgical or traumatic event.

Immune Response Mechanisms in Neuropathic Pain

Injury to nerves results in an inflammatory response at the site of nerve injury and in the CNS, which is similar to that occurring after damage to nonneural tissue. An excellent review on this topic presents evidence that inflammatory and immune mechanisms in the PNS and CNS play an important role in neuropathic pain.[11] It was found that infiltration of inflammatory cells, in addition to activation of resident immune cells in response to nervous system damage, leads to the subsequent production and secretion of various inflammatory mediators. These mediators were shown to promote neuroimmune activation and can sensitize primary afferent neurons and contribute to pain hypersensitivity. Also, the activated macrophages at the site of nerve injury produce proinflammatory substances, such as tumor necrosis factor-α (TNFα) and interleukin-1β (IL-1β), which are known to produce pain in experimental animals when given subcutaneously or applied directly to the nerve.[11]

Neuronal plasticity along the pathway for sensory transmission from the periphery through the spinal cord and in the cortex plays an important role in chronic pain, including inflammatory and neuropathic pain.[46] Recent studies indicate that microglia in the spinal cord are involved in neuropathic pain.[47,48] Activated microglia exert important functions, such as phagocytosis of cellular debris or neuronal signal processing, through communication with neurons, immune cells, and glial cells.[47] Activation of microglia occurs in most pathologic processes. The activation is accompanied by changes in morphology, up-regulation of immune surface antigens, and production of cytotoxic or neurotrophic molecues.[48] Spinal microglia are activated after peripheral nerve injury and may release many bioactive molecules, such as cytokines, chemokines, and neurotrophic factors (eg, BDNF), which then modulate the excitability of spinal neurons.[49] In addition to activation, increased density of microglia has been reported in the ipsilateral dorsal horn laminae I to III after peroneal nerve ligation in mice.[47] Anatomically, these areas are where primary sensory afferents innervating mechanoreceptors and nociceptors project (see **Fig. 1**). Therefore, the excitatory signals from the injured nerve to these spinal areas may be one of the primary factors triggering microglia activation.[47] Biochemical changes along the neuronal sensory pathway may be an additional cause for microglia activation.[50]

In the search for pharmacologic targets of chronic neurogenic pain, a recent finding is the role of the transient receptor potential (TRP) in neurogenic inflammation.[51] As previously mentioned, neurogenic inflammation is produced by overstimulation of peripheral nociceptor terminals by injury or inflammation of the tissues (peripheral sensitization). Small-diameter sensory neurons play a key role in the generation of neurogenic inflammation. There are several TRP receptors; however, cloning of the transient receptor potential vanilloid receptor 1 (TRPV1) has contributed significantly to the understanding of the molecular mechanisms involved in neurogenic inflammation. TRPV1 plays an integral role in the integration and modulation of various stimuli and nociceptor excitability, thus making it a true gateway for pain transduction.[51] In addition, TRPV1 is the end-point target of intracellular signaling pathways triggered by inflammatory mediators.[51] There is evidence for the involvement of this receptor in the etiology of peripheral and visceral inflammatory pain, such as inflammatory bowel disease (IBD), bladder inflammation, and cancer pain.[52] Worthy of note are the important and diverse physiologic functions played by the TRPV1 channel throughout the body. Targeting this receptor for analgesic purposes may be akin to targeting prostaglandins with the NSAID analgesics.

Descending Inhibitory Pathway

Various studies have identified the decreased efficacy of the descending inhibitory pathways in animals with neuropathic lesions.[33,53] These studies demonstrated reduced sensitivity to intrathecal or intravenous administration of morphine, indicating reduced opioid receptor function. In one study, after morphine administration, descending inhibition was almost 50% lower in neuropathic animals compared with normal controls[53] and those with arthritic pain.[54] Because descending inhibition normally acts as a spinal "gate" for sensory information, reduced inhibition increases the likelihood of the dorsal horn neuron firing spontaneously or more energetically to primary afferent input.[55] Of note, the decreased responsiveness to morphine could be prevented by pretreatment of the animals with an NMDA-receptor antagonist.[53,56] Although opioid receptors are less responsive in neuropathic pain, it seems that descending noradrenergic inhibition and increased sensitivity of spinal neurons to α_2-agonists may occur still with peripheral inflammation and nerve injury.[57] NE is released in the spinal dorsal horn by descending noradrenergic axons, which mainly originate from the LC and adjacent nuclei in the brain stem, and produces analgesia by stimulating α_2-adrenergic receptors.[58] NE and, to a lesser extent, serotonin (5-HT) are major components of the endogenous descending pain inhibitory system.[57] It has been suggested that chronic pain may partially result from altered or reduced levels of endogenous NE and serotonin activity at the spinal and supraspinal levels.[58] It is presumed that the NE and serotonin reuptake inhibitors (SRIs) attenuate pain by preventing presynaptic reuptake of NE and serotonin, resulting in increased postsynaptic levels and sustained activation of the descending pain inhibitory pathway.[58] This ultimately results in attenuation of neuronal hyperexcitability and alleviation of pain.

A study focusing on the spinal and supraspinal action of gabapentin demonstrated that gabapentin activates the descending noradrenergic system in a mouse nerve ligation model, as measured by increasing cerebrospinal fluid (CSF) NE levels.[59] In a follow-up human clinical study, oral gabapentin also significantly increased CSF NE concentration, when compared with the placebo group, after orthopedic or urogenital surgery in patients who had chronic pain. These findings indicate the responsiveness of the noradrenergic inhibitory system in neuropathic and chronic pain; however, this effect does not seem to be present when chronic pain is not established.[59]

Nerve injury may also disrupt the Aβ-fiber–mediated inhibition and the GABA-mediated inhibition of pain transmission neurons in the dorsal horn.[5,60] The loss of this activity may be within interneurons that ultimately releases the "brake" on central sensitization of dorsal horn neurons. The loss of this inhibitory process may contribute to spontaneous pain, hyperalgesia, or allodynia after nerve injury.[5,60]

Summary of Neuropathic Pain

Pain can be divided into three categories: physiologic, inflammatory, and neuropathic.[35,46,54,60]

1. Physiologic pain, such as the pain in response to a needle prick, serves to protect an animal from injury.
2. Inflammatory pain is caused as a consequence of tissue damage.

3. Neuropathic pain is a clinical syndrome of pain attributable to abnormal somatosensory processing in the PNS or CNS and may include spontaneous pain, paresthesia, dysthesia, allodynia, or hyperpathia (see **Box 1**). Neuropathic pain serves no beneficial purpose to the animal and can be regarded as a disease in itself. The pathophysiology of neuropathic pain is complex and incompletely understood. There are three pivotal phenomena intrinsic to the development of neuropathic pain:
   A. Central sensitization (ie, the process of "wind-up" and the resulting transcriptional changes in dorsal horn neurons leading to altered synaptic neurotransmitter levels and numbers of receptors)
   B. Central disinhibition (ie, an imbalance between the excitatory and inhibitory sides of the nervous system
   C. Phenotypic change of mechanoreceptive Aβ-fibers (light touching) to produce S-P, such that input from them is perceived as pain

BREAKTHROUGH PAIN

Breakthrough pain (BTP) is common in human patients who have cancer and in a variety of other problems causing pain. The reported incidence of BTP varies widely from 16% to 95% of those with persistent pain syndromes.[61] Such variability is likely attributable to lack of a clear consensus on the definition of BTP, but it is most commonly defined as an abrupt, short-lived, and intense pain that "breaks through" the around-the-clock analgesia that controls persistent pain.[61] The three subtypes of BTP are incident, idiopathic, and end-of-dose failure. BTP also is categorized as somatic, visceral, neuropathic, or mixed.[61] Appropriate assessment of the patient takes into consideration the source, severity, pattern, subtype, and cause of pain. Successful treatment is important because BTP has a profound impact on the patient's quality of life.[61]

BTP is easily recognized in the acute pain setting in hospitalized animals; however, veterinarians may be unaware of the occurrence of BTP in patients with persistent pain unless specific questions are asked of the client. Greater knowledge and awareness of BTP, especially when neuropathic pain may be occurring based on anatomic involvement of a lesion or history of previous events predisposing to neuropathic pain, should lead to recognition, diagnosis, and, ultimately, treatment of BTP in these patients.

DIAGNOSING NEUROPATHIC PAIN

Neuropathic pain may be difficult to diagnose in veterinary patients. Based on the various branches from the sensory pathways to subcortical areas in the brain, the "emotional" aspects of pain, in addition to the sensation of pain, are experienced, which alters the animal's "personality." A change in behavior, such as "dullness" or occasional aggression, may be noted by the owner in addition to obvious signs of pain. A comparison can be made to the human clinical and research setting as a potential resource for recognizing, diagnosing, and treating neuropathic pain in veterinary patients.

Neuropathic pain is frequently associated with chronic pain; however, it also occurs in the acute setting before surgery when associated with trauma or a neoplastic or inflammatory condition encroaching on neural tissue or after surgery when transient or persistent iatrogenic injury has occurred. In the acute setting in human medicine, patients noted to be at risk for progression to persistent pain include those with severe pain and those with injury to any part of the PNS or CNS.[62] The importance of being aware of the animals "at-risk" for development of chronic neuropathic pain in the acute setting is to ensure that appropriate intervention is instituted before, during, or after surgery to prevent such a debilitating situation, which may be difficult to diagnose once established at a later date.

In the human setting, the diagnosis of neuropathic pain may be based solely on history and examination findings as judged by an experienced clinician. This requires five of eight features suggestive of neuropathic pain:[62]

1. History consistent with nerve injury
2. Pain within but not necessarily confined to an area of sensory deficit
3. Pain in the absence of ongoing tissue damage
4. Character of pain: burning, pulsing, shooting, or stabbing
5. Paroxysmal or spontaneous pain
6. Associated dysesthesias
7. Allodynia, secondary hyperalgesia, or hyperpathia
8. Associated autonomic features

Obviously, it is difficult to apply all these features to veterinary patients, but a select few can be applied. The investigators who conducted one study believe that clinical vigilance, with regard to history taking and sensory examination, remains the key factor in the diagnosis of neuropathic pain in the acute setting (**Box 2**).[62] This would certainly be applicable to veterinary medicine. In addition to the eight points listed previously, the possibility of neuropathic pain was considered when "unexpected" levels of pain were present for the trauma or surgical procedure time course after surgery or after trauma. In situations in which the diagnosis of neuropathic pain was uncertain, a positive response to blinded intravenous lidocaine (0.5-mg/kg bolus, then 3 mg/kg) given over 20 minutes and a "placebo" of the same volume of saline administered over the same duration was used to assess a change in the pain severity score in human patients.[62] A positive response to lidocaine was seen as an overall reduction in the visual rating scale (VRS) of greater than 50% and also a change in VRS at least twice that of the placebo (saline). In this study group, trauma (43.1%) and surgery (27.5%) were the leading causes of neuropathic pain. Most members of the trauma group were victims of motor vehicle accidents (including four traumatic amputations), with some patients who had sporting injuries and one patient who had received burns. The surgical group included patients having had gynecologic surgery, laparotomy, or thoracotomy and those with ischemic limbs after vascular surgery. A total of 29.4% of cases were classified in the "other" causes group. These included patients with neuropathic pain after intercostal catheter insertion; patients with compartment syndrome secondary to coagulopathy, acute cancer pain, spontaneous spinal abscess, or vasculitis; and other patients with no precipitating cause identified.[62] From the patient population identified with acute neuropathic pain in this study, we can definitely make the assumption that there is the potential for this to occur in veterinary patients.

When assessing pain in animals, it is important to interact with them to assess their response to you and to establish if, and how much, pain is detected when moving. It is obvious from personal experience that our "injured or ill part" frequently hurts more when we move but may be minimally painful at rest. Movement-evoked pain in the postoperative period may alert the clinician to the potential for nerve entrapment if there is an exaggerated vocal and behavioral response for the given stimulus or absolute reluctance to move, although most of these animals tend to appear extremely painful at rest also.[24] Another test of evoked pain is pressing around the surgical wound to assess the presence of mechanical hyperalgesia, which may be disproportional to that expected when neuropathic pain exists. It is interesting to note that assessing pain at rest and then with evoked stimuli, or if BTP or incident pain should occur, can be

Box 2
Simple tests for the assessment of stimulus-evoked neuropathic pain in humans

The tests are performed on normal (uninjured) skin. The description of the sensation is included to give the reader an impression of what a cat and dog may also experience when tested. Tests using temperature or stroking stimuli would require a shaved area which could be performed once an area of involvement was identified using the pinprick or pressure tests.

Allodynia

Manual light pressure of the skin

Normally non-painful but elicits a dull, burning pain in the affected area when compared to an unaffected area

Light manual pinprick with a sharpened wooden stick or stiff von Frey hair

Sharp superficial pain elicited in the affected area but not in the unaffected area

Stroking skin with a brush, gauze, or cotton applicator

Sharp, burning, superficial pain in affected area but not in the unaffected area

Manual light pressure at the joints

Deep pain is elicited at the joints of the affected area but not in the unaffected area

Thermal cold

Contact of the skin with objects at 20°C is painful, often burning, temperature sensation in affected area but the unaffected area

Thermal warm

Contact of the skin with objects at 40°C is a painful, burning temperature sensation in the affected area but not the unaffected area

Hyperalgesia

Manual pinprick of the skin with a safety pin

Sharp superficial pain that is normally painful but the stimulus produces a more exaggerated response in the affected area compared to the unaffected area

Thermal cold

Contact of the skin with coolants such as acetone or cold metal is normally painful, often a burning, temperature sensation which produces a more exaggerated response on the affected area when compared to the unaffected area

Thermal heat

Contact the skin with objects at 46°C

Painful burning temperature sensation

Algometer

$A\delta$ and C-fibre activity arising from nociceptors and $A\beta$ fiber activity arising from mechanoreceptors

The response is a lower threshold and tolerance, or suprathreshold response to stimuli

Data from Harden RN. Chronic neuropathic pain. Mechanisms, diagnosis, and treatment. Neurologist 2005;11(2):11–22.

confusing when conducting pain studies and assessing various therapeutic modalities. Recent trials in human medicine suggest that pain assessment at rest should be assessed separately from several types of evoked pain.[26] This is an important point to consider in veterinary medicine, wherein descriptors for assessing pain should be included in each scoring system and "at rest" and "stimulus-evoked" components should be introduced. The algometer and thermal tests have been used in some veterinary studies as objective measures for stimulus-evoked assessment of pain.

Neuropathic pain scales are published in human medicine. The Neuropathic Pain Scale[63] and the Leeds assesment of neuropathic symptoms and signs (LANSS) Pain Scale[64] are used in human medicine in an attempt to gain greater precision in the description and diagnosis of neuropathic pain. Both scales are validated against the "gold standard" of the clinician's diagnosis in classic neuropathic pain states, which tends to be associated with chronic pain conditions. Neither scale has been assessed in human postoperative and posttrauma settings, wherein a mixed presentation of nociceptive and neuropathic pain is the norm.[62] When chronic neuropathic pain is experienced, however, these scales are valuable in localizing the lesion based on history of illness or injury and descriptions of pain experienced.[63,64] Because the descriptions (eg, dull, aching, burning versus sharp, lancinating) are used to diagnose the type of neuropathic pain in human patients, these scales are of no value in veterinary patients. Client observation of behavior may identify sharp, lancinating, and ectopic firing pain; however, this may coexist with constant dull, burning, and aching pain.

In human medicine, the prevalence of chronic pain is high within the community; however, it is reported that neuropathic pain may only occur in 1% to 3% of patients seen in pain clinics.[62] Although this may seem to be a small number, the pain experienced by these patients is severe to excruciating and uses a large percentage of the clinics' time resources.[62] In veterinary medicine, pain severity and precise localization can be difficult to assess;[65] however, with recent history, physical examination with attention to detail, and experience, pain assessment can be made in most cases. Chronic neuropathic pain, however, may be difficult to suspect because the presenting signs may be subtle and client observations may be vague. A veterinary study investigating the prevalence and characteristics of pain among dogs and cats examined as outpatients at a veterinary teaching hospital identified a slightly higher prevalence of neuropathic pain (dogs [8%] and cats [7%]) than occurs in human beings.[66] In this study, a total of 1153 dogs and 652 cats were examined as outpatients at The Ohio State University Teaching Hospital during 2002. Of these, 231 (20%) dogs and 92 (14%) cats had evidence of pain. The characteristics of pain were recorded from the examination of these patients. The categories of pain were as follows:

1. Inflammatory (pain considered to be initiated by chemical inflammatory mediators released by tissue damage)
2. Neuropathic (defined as pain caused or initiated by a primary lesion or dysfunction in the PNS or CNS). Pain was then further categorized as:
   A. Primary hyperalgesia (peripheral sensitization) was considered to exist when the animal responded adversely to light touch directly on the area of the body from which the pain originated (ie, the area of primary hyperalgesia).
   B. Secondary hyperalgesia (central sensitization) was considered to exist when the animal responded adversely to light touch to an uninjured area surrounding the area of primary hyperalgesia.
   C. Allodynia (pain elicited from noninjured tissues by nonnoxious stimuli) was considered to exist when the animal responded adversely to light touch applied to normal (noninjured) tissues distant from the area of primary hyperalgesia.

D. Hyposensitivity (an apparently reduced pain response when pain would have been expected to be present because of tissue or nerve injury) was considered to exist when a dog or cat with obvious tissue or nerve damage demonstrated reduced or no signs of pain during physical examination.

The findings were as follows: 82% of dogs and 83% of cats demonstrated a primary hyperalgesic response; 17% of dogs and 15% of cats demonstrated a secondary hyperalgesic response; and hyposensitivity was noted in 2% of cats and dogs. The mechanism assessed to cause pain was inflammatory in 76% of cats and dogs and neuropathic in 8% of dogs and 7% of cats, with inflammatory and neuropathic pain identified in 16% of dogs and 17% of cats. The presence of pain was noted to last for less than 7 days in most animals, with 11% of dogs and 13% of cats experiencing pain for longer than 1 month but less than 1 year and 6% of dogs and 1% of cats experiencing pain for longer than 1 year.[66] As a comparison, a slightly higher rate of neuropathic pain was diagnosed in the emergency setting of the same hospital, using similar criteria.[67] In this study of 179 dogs and 60 cats examined during 2003, neuropathic pain alone was identified in 9% of dogs and 3% of cats and combined neuropathic and inflammatory pain was identified in 23% of cats and dogs. Hyposensitivity was diagnosed in none of these animals. There were no individual patient case histories given on specific behavior patterns, potential causes, or development of neuropathic pain.

Some conditions are well known to cause neuropathic pain in cats and dogs, but the major challenge is the recognition of the not so well-known, or previously unreported, conditions that cause neuropathic pain.

In addition to history taking and neurologic examination, electrodiagnostic testing is used in the overall neurologic assessment in human patients.[68] Electrodiagnostic methods are available for veterinary patients,[69,70] and the reader is referred to these texts for an in-depth discussion on potential utility and findings in detecting neuropathic pain. Although sensory nerve and dorsal nerve root conduction studies do not specifically evaluate nociceptive fibers, detailed evaluation of the sensory peripheral nervous system (PNS) by means of sensory nerve action potential studies and conduction, along with dorsal nerve root and dorsal horn studies using cord dorsum potential analysis, can provide a wealth of information on the involvement of the peripheral sensory nervous system as a whole (Paul Cuddon, personal communication, 2008).[69] This has been demonstrated in the evaluation of feline diabetic neuropathy.[71]

NEUROPATHIC PAIN–ASSOCIATED CONDITIONS

Neuropathic Pain Associated with Trauma: Accidental and Surgical

Intraoperative considerations for the prevention of neuropathic pain

Specific details are described for surgical procedures on peripheral nerves in veterinary surgical texts.[72] Caution is mentioned to identify and handle neural tissue at the surgical site carefully; however, there often is not the same emphasis for many surgical procedures in which neural tissue may be inadvertently incorporated in the surgical procedure. Because nerve ligation is a model for the study of neuropathic pain, it may be prudent to identify neural tissue and ensure that this is not incorporated in ligatures at any surgical site to prevent the potential for development of neuropathic pain that may be difficult to identify and treat at a later date. Should transection or excessive manipulation or traction of neural tissue be necessary, application of a lidocaine and bupivacaine mixture to neural tissue at least 5 minutes before handling is recommended. Lidocaine confers its effect earlier than bupivacaine, with bupivacaine having a longer duration of effect. Overall, gentle handling of tissue to reduce the inflammatory response is essential.

Inguinal hernia repair

Inguinal hernia repair is a relatively common procedure in veterinary medicine. The potential for nerve injury during the repair may be similar to that for human patients. In a prospective study of 315 human patients undergoing inguinal hernia repair, patients were seen for follow-up at 6, 12, and 24 months and were assessed for the presence of pain, numbness, paresthesia, and recurrence.[73] At 1 year, 62.9% of patients had groin or inguinal pain and 11.9% of patients had moderate to severe pain. Two hundred seventy-six patients were seen at 2 years after surgery; of these patients, 53.6% had pain and 10.6% continued to report moderate to severe pain. The predictors for long-term postoperative pain in this study were lack of preoperative bulge at the hernia site and the presence of numbness in the surgical area after surgery. Three distinct types of chronic pain were identified. The most common and most severe pain was somatic, localized to the common ligamentous insertion to the pubic tubercle. The second type of pain was neuropathic and was referable to the ilioinguinal or genitofemoral nerve distribution. This was likely attributable to injury to the genitofemoral nerves, at surgery or subsequently by encroachment of scar tissue. The third type of pain was visceral ejaculatory pain. Twenty-four percent of patients had postoperative numbness at 2 years. Numbness was most common in the distribution of cutaneous branches of the ilioinguinal and iliohypogastric nerves.[73] The conclusions of this study were to consider surgical strategies to reduce associated long-term painful experiences. Again, an association of numbness and pain may occur in veterinary patients, and such assessment would be beneficial during follow-up examination. Perineal hernia repair is also a standard procedure in veterinary patients with the potential for neuropathic pain to occur.

Pelvic fractures

Pelvic fractures occur with some frequency in veterinary medicine, and it would be a reasonable assumption that complications in our patients might parallel those in human patients. A high incidence of chronic pain (48.4%) was found in a follow-up study of 161 human patients at a median of 5.6 years after pelvic fracture repair.[74] Most of these patients had a combination of somatic nociceptive, visceral nociceptive, and neuropathic pain, along with a high incidence of other complications. One complication noted related to leg dysfunction, which was significantly higher in the group with chronic pain than in the group without chronic pain (62.8% versus 20.5%). A lower health-related quality of life was also seen when compared with patients without chronic pain.[74] No comment was made as to whether the primary injury, surgical repair, or progressive scarring and neural reorganization contributed to outcome.

When assessing complications associated with motor function in veterinary patients, a sensory examination (see **Box 2**)[66] or electrodiagnostics[69] to identify the potential of established neuropathic pain to be a cause of, or to be coexistent with, motor deficits may identify a neuropathic pain component. Pelvic fractures and repair may result in nerve injury to the femoral nerve and cauda equina. The cauda equina lies within the lumbosacral canal and is composed of the seventh lumbar (L7), sacral, and coccygeal nerve roots. Injury of these roots causes deficits of sciatic, pudendal, pelvic, perineal, and caudal rectal nerve function. Motor dysfunction is readily recognized in these injuries in veterinary patients; however, sensory dysfunction, such as subtle hypoesthesia (which may reflect hyperalgesia depending on the stimulus) or hyperesthesia, may not consistently be evaluated. When present, this may suggest the presence of persistent or intermittent neuropathic pain.

Pudendal nerve entrapment

Pudendal nerve entrapment is a potential problem after perineal hernia repair or pelvic or sacral trauma. The injury may happen during trauma or the surgical procedure, or at some later point should the nerve become entrapped in a postsurgical or traumatic fibrous scar. Pudendal nerve entrapment is a cause for chronic disabling perineal pain (anorectal or urogenital, especially when sitting); urinary hesitancy, frequency, or urgency; constipation or painful bowel movements; and sexual dysfunction in men and women.[75] The diagnosis of pudendal nerve entrapment was based on clinical factors, neurophysiologic studies, and response to pudendal nerve infiltrations. The neurophysiologic testing included bilateral pudendal nerve distal motor latency tests and electromyography (EMG) in pudendal nerve innervated muscles.[75] Acute injury was defined as acute denervation with increased insertional activity or fibrillations. Chronic injury was defined as chronic neurogenic change illustrated by complex repetitive discharges, increased compound muscle action potential (CMAP) amplitude, long duration motor units, and CMAP polyphasia.[75] Patients refractory to conservative management underwent surgical decompression. After surgical decompression, 60% of patients were classified as responders based on one of the following three criteria: a greater than 50% reduction in visual analog score (VAS), a greater than 50% improvement in global assessment of pain, or a greater than 50% improvement in function and quality of life.[75] Pudendal nerve entrapment may be suspected in dogs and cats when there is a historical event compatible with entrapment for which the owner describes similar findings to those occurring in human beings and if pain can be elicited on rectal or vaginal examination, lifting of the tail, or when forced to sit. Pain on rectal examination can commonly be elicited in dogs with cauda equina syndrome. Electrodiagnostic testing would be a valuable tool to confirm clinical suspicion.[69]

Limb nerve entrapment

Iatrogenic nerve entrapment is a complication of surgical limb procedures but most notably occurs during limb fracture repair. A case report describing neuropathic pain in a cat after sciatic nerve entrapment during femoral fracture repair[76] underscores the importance of vigilance and awareness required to recognize this complication. The day after repair, deep pain was absent in this cat but severe pain was present on manipulation of the coxofemoral joint. Corticosteroid therapy was instituted for 48 hours with no improvement. Hind limb amputation was performed because of lack of function. At 38 days after amputation, the cat was presented again because of continually progressive behavioral changes of hiding, inappropriate urination, and shaking of the stump. This was treated as a primary urinary tract problem; in addition, amitriptyline was prescribed. The urinary clinical signs did improve; however, shaking of the stump and difficulty in walking and standing gradually worsened. On repeat presentation at 60 days after amputation, pain could not be elicited at the hip joint or stump of this cat. Neuropathic pain was suspected, however. Treatment with morphine, lidocaine, and ketamine was instituted until the signs of pain resolved. The duration of treatment was 37 hours: ramping up to effect over 18 hours, with a gradual reduction during the remaining 19 hours (details given in the section on treatment using ketamine). After this, the cat seemed to be pain-free and was discharged home on amitriptyline at a dosage of 10 mg every 12 hours for 21 days. At 10 months, the cat still seemed to be free of pain.[76] This case illustrates the presence of neuropathic pain even when hypoesthesia was present and when there was evidence for central pain. Frequently, amputation is performed because of motor nerve injury; however, it is important to identify the exact level of the lesion to ensure that the nerve injury is relieved so as to prevent ongoing or potential future development of neuropathic pain.

Another potential cause for nerve entrapment is that attributable to heterotopic calcification associated with hematoma formation at a site of trauma. Heterotopic calcification, otherwise known as heterotopic osteochondrofibrosis, has been identified in von Willebrand–depleted Doberman pinschers.[77] A mass composed of osseous, chodrous, or fibrous tissue, or a combination thereof, formed in or around the muscles of the hip in these dogs. The mass severely limited the coxofemoral joint range of motion, especially when the joint was extended. Trauma was associated in two cases. Similar ossification attributable to injury, hematoma, and unstable fractures may entrap a peripheral nerve, potentially resulting in delayed neuropathic pain.

Amputation

Phantom limb pain is a known syndrome in human patients, but it also may occur in veterinary patients. The cause may be attributable to peripheral sensitization as a result of spontaneous activity from sprouting regenerating nerve endings or neuroma formation that gives rise to secondary changes in otherwise silenced small dorsal root ganglia cells, central sensitization, or cortical reorganization.[37,41] There has been an association of severity of preamputation pain with postamputation phantom pain. Prevention of phantom pain by preoperative epidural analgesia and postoperative local anesthesia, however, resulted in variable responses.[78] There seems to be no consistent effective treatment. Many therapies, including surgical exploration, tricyclic antidepressants (TCAs), sodium channel blockers, topical capsaicin, and gabapentin, all used with efficacy in other neuropathic states, may be ineffective or unproved in controlled studies of phantom limb pain.[78] Interestingly, neuropathic pain occurs in 60% of human patients after limb amputation but usually not until 1 year after surgery. This highlights the ongoing changes occurring in the PNS and CNS established by a precipitating event before experiencing neuropathic pain in some patients and conditions. Phantom limb pain is rarely reported in veterinary medicine.[76] Potential clinical signs, other than those occurring in nerve entrapment noted previously, may be chewing at the stump, intermittent unprovoked crying, or "jumping up or away" indicating lancinating pain attributable to ectopic firing.

Lumbosacral lesions

A common cause for neuropathic pain in dogs is degenerative lumbosacral stenosis or the cauda equina syndrome. Many other terms have been used to describe this syndrome, which is attributable to soft tissue and bony changes, possibly in conjunction with abnormal motion of the lumbosacral joint impinging on the nerve roots or vasculature of the cauda equina.[79] There are many causes for lumbosacral lesions (degenerative lumbosacral stenosis [the most common disease of the cauda equina in large-breed dogs], idiopathic stenosis, discospondylitis, trauma, neoplasia, inflammatory disease, vascular compromise, and congenital abnormalities), and they are discussed in detail elsewhere.[79] A full description of the physical examination to identify subtle abnormalities is well described and beyond the scope of this article;[79] however, inclusion of a rectal examination and palpation of the lumbosacral joint with manipulation of the tail is one of many maneuvers to include in the neurologic examination.[79] A thorough focused neurologic examination in dogs exhibiting signs of pain, as described for human patients with pudendal entrapment, dysesthesias, or motor dysfunction secondary to sciatic or caudal rectal nerve compression, is important because results of diagnostic imaging may be misleading. A study evaluating the severity of clinical signs (lumbosacral pain, paresis, lameness, urinary and fecal incontinence, and dysesthesias) to severity of cauda equina compression using diagnostic imaging revealed a lack of correlation.[80] Although correlation of clinical signs and diagnostic imaging was poor, the investigators recommended pursuing MRI because it is invaluable in accurately identifying the underlying disease process and giving the surgeon in-depth preoperative knowledge of the site and extent of the lesion. In dogs with minimal MRI changes, the investigators commented that cauda equina neuritis may be the cause of pain. Cauda equina neuritis has been described in dogs in which marked interstitial and perivascular infiltration with mononuclear cells, axonal degeneration, and demyelination was present.[81]

Spinal cord injury

Spinal cord injury (SCI) may be attributable to trauma, ischemia, hemorrhage, or extradural compression (eg, intervertebral disc extrusion resulting in persistent or intermittent somatic or visceral neuropathic pain). Several problem-based conditions discussed may also apply to lesions associated with SCI.

Intervertebral disc herniation

One of the most common causes of neuropathic pain is intervertebral disc herniation. Dogs and cats are almost always painful on presentation (or exhibit pain during the neurologic examination), some excruciatingly so. The occurrence of acute cervical disc extrusions was reported to occur at C2 to C3, C3 to C4, and C4 to C5 in decreasing frequency in one study[82] and with the same frequency in another.[83] Signs of pain are low head and neck carriage, neck guarding, stilted and cautious gait, and spasms of cervical spinal muscles. Pain can also be identified if the animal is lame. Radicular pain (root signature or referred pain) is observed with impingement of nerve roots C5 to C8, with a frequency up to 50%.[84] Pain may also be elicited during the neurologic examination with manipulation of the affected limb. Surgical treatment is recommended because conservative management using corticosteroids, muscle relaxants, and cage rest has a high recurrence rate.[85] The reason given for this is the presence of a large amount of disc material present in the spinal canal and difficulty with total immobilization of the cervical region. Based on the pathophysiology of neuropathic pain, and the experience of this for the individual, it would be inhumane not to treat the patient with moderate to excruciating pain adequately. By reducing the pain, however, the animal tends to move the cervical region more, potentially compromising neurologic function further. Relieving the pain by surgical treatment is paramount in the author's opinion. The pain may not be relieved in some cases, however, when extruded disc material is still present and impinging on nerve roots. Occasionally, re-exploration is required when the pain is excruciating and nonresponsive to multimodal analgesic therapy.

Thoracolumbar intervertebral disc disease (IVDD) also results in pain and neurologic dysfunction of varying degree in cats and dogs.[85] Spinal hyperesthesia, kyphosis, and reluctance to walk are obvious signs of pain and may occur without neurologic deficits in a percentage of cases.[86] Despite the lack of motor neurologic dysfunction, these dogs can have substantial spinal cord compression as seen on diagnostic imaging. Another report indicated that 64% of dogs had back pain and paresis.[87] If recurrence of clinical signs occurs after surgical treatment, it may be related to a second disc extrusion; cicatrix formation at the previous surgery site; or hyperesthesia resulting from surgical manipulation, residual hemorrhage, or disc material.[88] As with cervical disc disease, pain management is extremely important to avoid continuing acute pain and establishment of chronic neuropathic pain. The reader is referred to an article by Coates[85] for a review of conservative versus surgical treatment and recurrence rates of thoracolumbar IVDD.

Thoracolumbar IVDD in cats does occur but at a much lower rate than in dogs, and it is reported in older and younger (<5 years of age) cats. Similar diagnostic and surgical techniques are recommended in cats as in dogs.

Fibrocartilaginous Embolic Myelopathy

Fibrocartilaginous embolic myelopathy (FCEM) is noted to be painful on acute disc extrusion because the owners note a yelp followed by the neurologic deficits. Pain may also be elicited on presentation, but pain is reported to subside abruptly in most dogs. (The reader is referred to an article by Dewey[89] for further information on this topic.) It is not unexpected for dogs with FCEM to remain extremely painful for several days, however, requiring constant analgesic administration titrated to effect (observation of the author and Neurology Service at the Ontario Veterinary College). This may be attributable to secondary hemorrhage or release of vasoactive substances at the site of ischemia (Paul Cuddon, personal communication, 2008) or to associated epaxial muscle tear at the site of extrusion (observation of Neurology Service at the Ontario Veterinary College). Based on these observations, pain assessment and management must be considered in dogs or cats that have FCEM.

Discospondylitis and Vertebral Osteomyelitis

Discospondylitis and vertebral osteomyelitis are most commonly reported in medium- to large-breed dogs but may occur in any dog or cat.[90] The most common presenting sign is mild to severe spinal pain. This may or may not be associated with neurologic deficits or fever.[90] Because any bacterial or fungal organism may be the causative agent, a definitive diagnosis should be attempted with culture and sensitivity testing performed on aspirates from the affected area and blood cultures. Because the diagnostic yield from blood cultures in veterinary medicine is low in general, aspirates from the lesion are recommended. Cytologic examination of the aspirate should be performed immediately as an aid in selection of empiric therapy before receiving the antibiogram, which may take several days. Suggested antimicrobial drugs can be found an the article by Thomas.[90]

Potential Sources of Neck and Back Pain in Cats and Dogs

The previous sections provide examples of the more common clinical conditions causing neuropathic neck and back pain in cats and dogs; however, there several others that should be considered. The reader is referred to an article by Webb[91] for a review on this topic.

Polyradiculoneuritis

Polyradiculoneuritis is most commonly associated with motor nerve and ventral nerve root and ventral horn motor dysfunction, although a milder but significant dorsal nerve root and dorsal root ganglial inflammation can result in hyperesthesia with touch and manipulation. This is made worse by the fact that the animal cannot withdraw from the stimulus. Electrophysiologic studies in dogs with acute polyradiculoneuritis did reveal a sensory dysfunction in some affected dogs (Paul Cuddon, personal communication, 2008).[92] Physiotherapy, a recommended management for these dogs, can be extremely uncomfortable. It is important for the caregiver to be cognizant of this when treating these patients and to consider adding some form of pain management, especially in the first several days of the disease.

Vascular Innervation as a Cause of Spinal Pain

Myelinated fibers of spinal cord blood vessels in dogs and cats may function in sensory innervation. It may be that innervation of blood vessels shares pathways with nerves that supply other structures in the bony vertebral canal and also contribute to pain development in this area.[93]

PRIMARY LESIONS OF THE PERIPHERAL OR CENTRAL NERVOUS SYSTEM

Peripheral Nervous System

A fairly common yet sometimes difficult lesion to identify initially is a tumor involving the PNS. Malignant peripheral nerve sheath tumors (MPNSTs), previously called schwannomas or neurofibromas, are a primary cause of chronic neurogenic lameness in dogs[94] and cats.[95] When a source for limb pain and lameness cannot be identified in the thoracic or pelvic limbs, an MPNST should be considered. Ultrasonographic examination and fine-needle aspiration (US-FNA) of an identifiable mass are frequently diagnostic.[96–98] Because there are potential limitations to obtaining a definitive diagnosis using US-FNA as the result of an extremely proximal location of the mass, lack of tumor identification on US, or false-negative results of nondiagnostic aspirates of the mass, this technique should not necessarily be seen as a single diagnostic tool but as being complementary to CT and MRI, which allow evaluation of proximal nerve structures and the spinal cord.[99] When limb dysfunction occurs, potentially attributable to motor and sensory dysfunction (hyperesthesia or hypoesthesia), and amputation is the suggested treatment, it is essential that the primary lesion also be removed. This may require a hemilaminectomy should the tumor extend into, or beyond, the proximal nerve roots.[74] Leaving the tumor would continue to cause chronic pain and result in an extremely poor quality of life.

Masses within subcutaneous tissue[100] and within muscle with local invasion of neural tissue can present similar to nerve sheath tumors.[101–103]

There are many other neurologic conditions causing lameness in dogs and cats, the discussion of which is beyond the scope of this article; however, the reader is referred to a review on the topic by McDonnell and colleagues.[94]

Diabetic Neuropathy

Diabetes mellitus is a well-recognized cause for neuropathic pain in human beings. Dogs and cats also can develop a neuropathy associated with this endocrinopathy, although cats have a much more dramatic clinical presentation when compared with dogs, whose neuropathy is often subclinical. Despite the subclinical nature of canine diabetic neuropathy, peripheral sensory nerve conduction slowing was described in one report.[104] The small number of early reports of diabetic-associated neuropathy in cats concentrated on the clinically obvious motor dysfunction, consisting of a palmigrade and plantigrade stance and gait and a generalized weakness, with no mention of peripheral sensory abnormalities.[105] More recently, however, an extensive electrophysiologic, biochemical, and histologic study performed on feline diabetic neuropathy definitively demonstrated equal involvement of sensory and motor nerves in these cats, with the sensory dysfunction involving the most proximal dorsal (sensory) nerve roots and the entire length of the peripheral sensory nerves in the thoracic and pelvic limbs.[71] It is the presence of this sensory neuropathy and radiculopathy that may explain the observation that many cats with diabetes exhibit an aversion to being petted and cuddled and are commonly "cranky and aloof." Many of these cats also resent having their paws touched, reminiscent of people who have a "diabetic hand and foot" (Dr. Paul Cuddon, personal communication, Colorado State University). When these behaviors are observed in dogs or cats, a trial of amitriptyline is suggested to see if behavioral patterns improve.

Central Pain Syndrome

Tumors of the central nervous system

In human beings, tumors involving pathways subserving somatic sensibilities of pain and temperature, such as the dorsal horn; the spinothalamic, spinoreticular, and spinomesencephalic tracts; and the cerebral cortex, can result in pain. The area of pain experienced is that subserved by the location and the pathway involving the neoplastic process. This is referred to as central pain.[106] In people, the highest incidence of these tumors is within the spinal cord, lower brain stem, and ventroposterior thalamus.[106] Hemihyperesthesia and hyperresponsiveness resembling the central pain syndrome in human beings have been reported in a dog with a forebrain oligodendroglioma.[107] This 4-year-old boxer dog presented with alterations in behavior, mentation, and circling, but the most notable clinical finding was right-sided hemihyperesthesia and hyperresponsiveness. Exaggerated responses, such as flinching, jumping away from the stimulus, and biting, were elicited by nonnoxious stimuli, such as a light pinprick and pinching of the skin, applied to various areas on the right side of the body. The clinical impression was that the dog was experiencing a significant amount of pain during the examination. Similar stimuli applied to the left side did not elicit a response. Although the lesion in this case was highly suspicious for a brain tumor because of the altered mentation and circling, the recognition of hyperesthesia required a careful and methodical examination. Spinal cord lesions causing central pain may be more subtle, nonspecific, and more difficult to diagnose unless a similar examination is performed.

Congenital/developmental lesions

A Chiari-like malformation with syringomyelia (also known as syringohydromyelia) is a cause for central pain syndrome associated with moderate to severe neuropathic pain in human beings and dogs.[108] This seems to be a genetic disorder in Cavalier King Charles spaniels and is characterized by a mismatch between the caudal fossa volume and its contents (the cerebellum and caudal brain stem).[108] Because of obstruction of normal CSF movement through the foramen magnum by means of the normal outflow pathways, syringomyelia, a fluid-filled cavitation, and dilation of the central canal within the spinal cord result. The behavior exhibited by affected dogs is suggestive of neuropathic pain because it has the characteristics of allodynia, or dysesthesia. For example, dogs seem to dislike touch to certain areas of skin and may be unable to tolerate grooming or a neck collar. Signs may be unilateral, such as scratching on one side only at rest and while walking, and often without making skin contact.[108] For details on diagnostic findings and therapeutic suggestions, the reader is referred to articles by Rusbridge and Jeffery[108] and Rusbridge.[109]

The examples of central pain presented here highlight the importance of history taking with respect to obvious or subtle changes in behavior. Questions must be asked relating to potential behavior elicited by the cat or dog, extrapolated from the human experience (eg, crawling insects, itchiness), such as "scratching motion without touching the skin," continually biting or attacking an area on the body, frequently turning (looking) at the same area, or yelping for no reason (lancinating pain). The physical and neurologic examination and the diagnostic modalities presented here can be considered for all patients that are suspected of having central pain syndrome.

Vasculitis

Vasculitis associated with the meninges and spinal cord can be a cause for central pain. The recommended diagnostic tests, however, differ from those previously discussed because of the inflammatory nature of these diseases. Vasculitis has been identified as a cause of neuropathic pain in beagle dogs, and has been termed "beagle pain syndrome." This pain syndrome is associated with a generalized vasculitis, perivasculitis, and vascular thrombosis. The small- to medium-sized muscular arteries in many organs, including the cervical meninges, are consistently involved. The clinical signs, laboratory abnormalities, and vascular lesions suggest that the condition is immune mediated and may serve as a naturally occurring animal model of human immune system–mediated vasculitides, such as polyarteritis nodosa, infantile polyarteritis, and Kawasaki disease. Neuropathic pain is reported in some of these human conditions.[110,111] There are many other diseases that produce inflammation of the meninges, especially involving the cervical region, resulting in varying severity of cervical pain. These include granulomatous meningoencephalomyelitis (GME), aseptic meningitis, and breed-associated aseptic meningitis seen in such breeds as the Bernese Mountain dog.

NEUROPATHIC PAIN OF VISCERAL ORIGIN

The evidence for neuropathic pain of visceral origin is presented in the section on the individual clinical syndrome, in which veterinary and human illnesses are compared.

Feline Interstitial Cystitis

Feline interstitial cystitis (FIC) is a well-recognized problem in cats and is an example of visceral inflammation resulting in neurogenic pain, which also occurs in human beings.[112] Human patients who have interstitial cystitis (IC) have bladder pain and urinary urgency. Studies in cats with IC have demonstrated abnormalities in the bladder, sensory neurons, CNS, and sympathetic efferent neurons.[113] These cats have decreased excretion of glycosaminoglycan (GAG), increased bladder permeability, and neurogenic inflammation. The reduced protection of bladder uroepithelium by lowered GAG levels may facilitate increased contact of urine with the primary afferent nerve terminals innervating the bladder, resulting in a local release of neurotransmitters and neurogenic inflammation. S-P is increased in the urinary bladders of people and cats with IC.[114] High-affinity S-P receptors have also been identified in the bladders of cats with FIC.[114] Experimentally induced cystitis in rats produces neurogenic sensory and reflex changes similar to those seen in human patients who have cystitis.[115] Inflammation of the bladder activates A-δ and C-fiber mechanosensitive afferents with significant recruitment of "silent" afferents. The silent afferents are mechanically insensitive afferent neurons that develop mechanosensitivity during inflammatory states. The afferent fiber barrage generated from the inflamed bladder is believed to result in a slowly developing, and maintained, increase in the excitability of spinal cord dorsal horn neurons producing central sensitization.[115] Treatment in human beings consists of pentosan polysulfate sodium, which is primarily thought to be effective through GAG layer replacement, amitriptyline, muscle relaxants, and alpha-blockers. For pain management, gabapentin, hydrocodone, and opioids have proved to be helpful.[112,116] Amitriptyline is recommended for cats diagnosed with FIC.[117]

Gastrointestinal System

There are indications that central sensitization may contribute to a secondary pain hypersensitivity in the gastrointestinal tract in a way that resembles secondary hyperalgesia in the skin.[118–120] The following are illnesses that cause neuropathic pain in human beings and potentially could produce the same pain syndromes in cats and dogs.

Visceral Pain Associated with Spinal Cord Injury

Human beings with SCI resulting in partial to complete paraplegia or partial to complete tetraplegia may experience visceral pain without identifiable gastrointestinal, genitourinary, or pelvic abnormalities that could account for visceral pain symptoms.[121] The mechanisms of this are unknown. Theories put forth are that visceral pain may be caused by (1) a continuous slow fiber discharge caused by unrecognized alterations in visceral function, (2) a phenomenon occurring at the sympathetic chain ganglia, or (3) a distortion of the afferent impulses from the viscera crossing the zone of injury in the spinal cord.[121] Another theory proposed is that the neurologic mechanisms of visceral pain are different from those in somatic pain and that brief acute visceral pain may initially be triggered by the activation of high-threshold afferent impulses.[121] Visceral pain seems to have a substantially delayed time of onset, with the average onset time after SCI being 4.2 years. Although the number of persons with visceral pain is less than the number of persons with musculoskeletal or neuropathic pain, visceral pain was the pain most often described as severe or excruciating.[121] A question veterinarians may ask is "does visceral pain occur after SCI in our patients, and how would we know?"

Inflammatory Bowel Disease

Idiopathic IBD is frequently diagnosed in dogs and cats[122] but occurs more frequently in cats.[123,124] From a neuropathic perspective, IBD is similar to other conditions of persistent afferent barrage to the dorsal horn. As with the urinary bladder, true "nociceptors" may be "disguised" within the mechanoreceptors that have a low or high threshold for response and encode for the intensity of the stimulus in the gastrointestinal tract.[125] Both classes of mechanoreceptors are capable of processing and transmitting sensory input in the noxious range. Also, low- and high-threshold mechanoreceptors are capable of becoming sensitized in the presence of inflammation.[125] The presence of silent fibers and their recruitment during inflammatory conditions has also been documented.[115,118] Therefore, visceral afferent fibers innervating the gastrointestinal tract are capable of changing their behavior during organ inflammation to increase the peripheral barrage into the spinal cord, giving rise to visceral pain and hyperalgesia.[119,122] In situations in which cats that have IBD and are being treated with an appropriate dose of corticosteroids still appear uncomfortable to the owner, the author has recommended amitriptyline. Anecdotal reports from veterinarians indicating noticeable improvement in behavior suggest that a potential neuropathic component exists.

Pancreatitis/Pancreatic Pain

Abdominal pain is a key feature of acute and chronic pancreatitis in dogs and human beings but not consistently so in cats. There is evidence that pain in chronic pancreatitis and pancreatic cancer is triggered by pancreatic neuropathy.[126] Damage to intrapancreatic nerves seems to support the maintenance and exacerbation of neuropathic pain in people. In chronic pancreatitis, intrapancreatic nerves are invaded by immune cells. This observation led to the hypothesis that neuroimmune interactions play a role in the pathogenesis of chronic pancreatitis and the accompanying abdominal pain syndrome. Similarly, pancreatic cancer cells infiltrate the perineurium of local extrapancreatic nerves, which may partially explain the severe pain experienced by human patients. In recent years, the involvement of a variety of neurotrophins and neuropeptides in the pathogenesis of pancreatic pain was discovered.[126] In another human study, electrical stimulation of the gastrointestinal tract with concurrent recordings using an electroencephalogram showed that pain in chronic pancreatitis leads to changes in cortical projections of the nociceptive system.[127] Similar findings have been described in somatic pain disorders, including neuropathic pain.[127] Potentially these mechanisms exist in cats and dogs, explaining the apparent severe to excruciating pain experienced in some animals with repeated episodes of pancreatitis.

TREATMENT

Several animal models of neuropathic pain are used to assess individual and combination pharmacologic therapies. The therapies discussed are those that have been tested using these models. The peripheral mononeuropathy models receive ligation, partial ligation, and transection of various peripheral nerves to simulate the common human clinical setting. These include nerve root injuries or plexus avulsion injuries resulting in thermal and mechanical hyperalgesia, cold allodynia, and tactile allodynia.[128–130] These models also resemble peripheral nerve injuries in cats and dogs. Central neuropathic models of pain have been created by ischemia of the spinal cord, which correlates to the ischemic, traumatic, or radiation injuries in the human clinical setting.[131] Based on the response to various analgesic drugs, these models offer guidelines for treatment of neuropathic pain in human patients, which may also be extended to veterinary patients.

Neuropathic pain cannot be adequately managed with a single pharmacologic class unless tapering from a multimodal regimen. Severe pain requires several classes of medications and procedures. A recent report on pain management in the human trauma patient reported that with aggressive pain management, the military has decreased acute and chronic pain conditions.[132] The individual medications discussed here are intended to be administered in conjunction with those from a different class in an attempt to block the various mechanisms involved in sensory transmission. Before, and often during, any surgical procedure, various different analgesics and analgesic modalities can be used to reduce the inciting nociceptive afferent impulse. Many of these can be continued after surgery to reduce peripheral and central sensitization (the reader is referred to the articles by Lamont, Lemke and Creighton, Valverde, and Dyson elsewhere in this issue and an article by Lemke and Dawson[133] on local and regional analgesia).

Stimulus-Evoked Pain

Movement-evoked pain can be difficult to manage, especially when associated with nerve involvement. When increasing dosages of analgesics are given to stop movement-evoked pain, the patient may experience the adverse effects of the analgesic when at rest (ie, dysphoria, panting with opioids). Because movement is essential for a rapid recovery, local delivery of local anesthetics (ie, intrapleural, intra-articular, amputation site) or administration of two or more classes of analgesics (ie, multimodal therapy) is recommended. Other examples of stimulus-evoked pain could be related to pressing around the surgical wound to assess the presence of mechanical hyperalgesia. In one study, low-dose ketamine infusion reduced the intensity of mechanical hyperalgesia around the surgical wound for 24 hours after surgery.[134] Similarly with postoperative dental pain, a research analgesic had little effect on pain at rest but was quite effective in reducing pain on opening the mouth.[135] Managing pain in situations other than when the patient is at rest can be challenging, requiring analgesic protocols and procedures specifically prepared for the individual patient and the associated problem.

Breakthrough Pain

Breakthrough pain (BTP) can definitely be associated with neuropathic pain. This may occur in the postoperative setting or intermittently at home in animals on chronic pain medication for cancer or neuropathic pain. As described by human patients, this pain is severe or excruciating and of rapid onset, which can disable or even immobilize the patient.[136] Should this occur in the hospital, intravenous administration of an opioid is the primary treatment. The analgesic protocol should be reassessed for duration and dose of the prescribed medication and to ensure that there is no underlying problem causing this pain. If the pain seems to be severe, this may be an indication of a neuropathic component. Careful observation as to the cause of BTP is required. If a single analgesic agent is being used, consider the addition of other analgesics of a different class (the reader is referred to the articles by Lamont and Robertson elsewhere in this issue).

When BTP occurs at home, a careful history is required to obtain clues about the cause and pattern of BTP. Opioid analgesics are the primary treatment (eg, tramadol, oxycodone); however, it may be difficult to administer oral medication when animals exhibit excruciating pain. If this cannot be controlled, parenteral administration has to be considered. Fentanyl buccal tablets seem to be effective in human patients for breakthrough of neuropathic pain;[137] however, no veterinary studies as to efficacy are available. The dose or dosing frequency of an around-the-clock analgesic should be adjusted for patients with end-of-dose BTP. Short-acting oral opioids are useful when given preemptively in human patients with predictable incident BTP, whereas rapid-onset transmucosal lipophilic opioids (eg, fentanyl buccal tablet) are most effective for patients with unpredictable incident or idiopathic BTP. In addition to pharmacologic therapy, nonpharmacologic strategies are often helpful in alleviating pain and anxiety and should be considered on an individual patient basis as a supplement to pharmacologic intervention for BTP.

Pain management must be considered throughout the hospital stay, and a plan should be formulated based on the severity of injury, the invasiveness of the surgical procedure (controlled injury), the anatomic area of surgery (assumed descending order of discomfort: oral cavity, rectum/vagina/testicles/penis, thorax, abdomen, and limbs), the definite or potential involvement of neural tissue, and pain experienced before surgery.

The Hospitalized Patient: Acute Pain Management

Opiates/Opioids

Opiates/opioids are frequently used to manage pain in veterinary patients. Opioids bind to opioid receptors peripherally and centrally. Peripherally, they prevent neurotransmitter release and nociceptor sensitization, especially in inflammatory tissue. Centrally, opioids modulate afferent input into the substantia gelatinosa of the dorsal horn, wherein the C-fibers terminate, and in cortical areas that blunt the perception of pain.[138] Because opiates have a specific effect on C-fiber input and not on Aβ-fibers, in which tactile allodynia (Aβ-stimulus) is a component of the pain syndrome, opioids may not be beneficial. Therefore, the effectiveness of the opioids depends on the underlying mechanism causing the pain. As previously mentioned, opioid receptors in the descending pathway may be reduced or inactivated in neuropathic pain; therefore, their efficacy is frequently inadequate when used alone. Of interest, the closer the nervous system lesion is to the CNS, the less effective the opiates are.[139] For example, peripheral nerve injuries tend to respond better to opioid therapy than nerve root injuries, which respond better than spinal cord injuries. Because neuropathic pain is not as responsive as nonneuropathic conditions to opioids, titration of the dose to effect, which may be beyond the maximum recommended in textbooks, while avoiding side effects, is suggested for human patients.[139] Notable side effects in dogs and cats are dysphoria, panting, respiratory depression, inappropriate antidiuretic hormone secretion with oliguria and edema, urinary retention, nausea and vomiting, inability to ambulate, and ileus as an infrequent finding. Frequently used systemic opioids are fentanyl, morphine, and hydromorphone. Should side effects occur, switching to another opioid is recommended because higher dosages may be better tolerated in any individual given a different opioid.[139] It is the author's experience that fentanyl seems to have fewer side effects than morphine and hydromorphone at higher dosages, especially in cats. The shorter half-life of fentanyl also makes it the best choice in patients with CNS pain because withdrawal for assessment is more easily planned. With the understanding that opioids may be ineffectual in some neuropathic pain states, it may be unwise to increase the dose to that which results in noticeable side effects. Nausea and vomiting raise intracranial pressure (ICP), and thus would be a concern in patients who have head injuries. Cortical depression may mask increasing ICP and delay administration of hypertonic saline or mannitol therapy. Also, peripheral neurologic signs may seem to be worse because bladder emptying and limb motion beyond the area of spinal injury are significantly decreased with opioid use. As an example, the author has noted continual lack of voluntary bladder emptying in cats with sacrococcygeal injuries while on opiate analgesia. With a 1-mL/min titration of diluted naloxone at 0.1 mL naloxone (0.4 mg/mL) diluted in 10 mL saline to ensure that analgesia is not totally reversed, while gently palpating the urinary bladder to initiate voluntary micturition, it is possible to reverse the inhibitory effects of the opiate on detrusor function should this be a factor. Detrusor dysfunction may occur after systemic or epidural use of opiates, regardless of the cause of pain, usually in the postoperative setting. The author frequently uses the naloxone titration technique to reverse the side effects of opioids, especially if the patient is dysphoric. In larger animals, a mixture of naloxone, 0.25 mL (0.4 mg/mL), diluted in saline, 10 mL, is used for titration. Once the side effects are reversed and a "pleasant" state of rest is achieved, or the patient is aware and can respond during the neurologic assessment, titration is halted. A frustrating situation for criticalists and neurologists is the requirement for withdrawal from analgesics before neurologic examination. It is suggested that an appointment be made for the neurologic assessment, which is strictly adhered to so that withdrawal of the analgesics can be planned, therefore avoiding long periods when the patient is without analgesic therapy.

Methadone is probably the preferred opioid to manage neuropathic pain because in addition to its opioid analgesic properties, it is an NMDA receptor antagonist and SRI.[132] The prolonged half-life of methadone in human beings with drug accumulation and delayed onset of adverse effects[132] does not occur in dogs at doses up to 1 mg/kg administered parenterally.[140] Oral methadone is not absorbed in dogs, however.[141] Buprenorphine may also be suitable for moderate pain, but increasing the dose to greater than that recommended has no advantage because of the ceiling effect (the reader is referred to the article by Robertson elsewhere in this issue).

Based on the actions of opiates, it is recommended that they be included in a multimodal regimen to manage neuropathic pain rather than as a single agent.

N-methyl-D-aspartate receptor antagonists

The NMDA receptor is located on postsynaptic neurons in the dorsal horn. It has various binding sites that regulate its activity, which include glutamate, magnesium, glycine, and polyamine binding sites. Nerve injury causes an increase in spinal glutamate, which opens the NMDA ionophore channel, causing an influx of calcium and resulting in a cascade effect leading to spinal wind-up. The channel may be blocked by the NMDA receptor antagonists, such as ketamine, amantadine, and dextromethorphan. In animal models of neuropathic pain, the allodynic and hyperalgesic states were sensitive to NMDA receptor antagonists. Ketamine is a commonly used anesthetic and analgesic agent in veterinary medicine. Amantadine is a drug recently introduced for chronic pain management in veterinary medicine. Recent studies in dogs, however, report that dextromethorphan is not absorbed in this species,[142] and it is therefore not recommended for chronic neuropathic pain.

Ketamine

Ketamine is the most commonly used NMDA receptor antagonist in veterinary medicine. Its use is increasing for postoperative and other acute pain management situations in human medicine, including severe trauma.[132,143,144] Ketamine binds noncompetitively to the phencyclidine site of the NMDA receptor and to the σ-opioid receptor, resulting in intense analgesia and prevention of wind-up.[132] The combination of ketamine and a benzodiazepine or ketamine and morphine has been shown to be beneficial in human patients.[145] Dosages as low as 2.5 μg/kg/min or less have reduced opioid requirements in postoperative human patients. There are similar reports on the use of low-dose ketamine in the veterinary literature. These reports include pre- and intraoperative use;[146–148] pre- and postoperative use;[149] or, pre-, intra-, and postoperative use in dogs.[150] In one study assessing the efficacy of ketamine (0.5 mg/kg administered intravenously as a bolus before surgery, 10 μg/kg/min during surgery, and 2 μg/kg/min for 18 hours after surgery) for amputation pain, in which neuropathic pain is certainly a concern, an improvement in postoperative pain scores was noted over a 3-day duration when compared with an opioid-alone regimen.[150] Another study, however, compared two doses of ketamine (loading dose of 150 μg/kg with a constant rate infusion [CRI] of 2 μg/kg/min versus a 700-μg/kg loading dose and CRI of 10 μg/kg/min) on feeding behavior in bitches after mastectomy and noted that the higher dose of ketamine resulted in improved patient feeding behavior.[151] It is the experience of the author and her colleagues at the Ontario Veterinary College that low doses of ketamine (<0.5 mg/kg intravenous loading dose and <1.0 mg/kg/h CRI), even in combination with opiates, with or without lidocaine or with or without NSAIDs, are frequently inadequate to manage severe pain in dogs and cats with multiple and massive bite wounds, severe pancreatitis, multiple orthopedic injuries after surgery, and postoperative cauda equina syndrome or cervical disc herniation as examples. Most of these cases have a component of neuropathic and inflammatory pain. A point to consider when comparing doses with those used in human patients is the fact that a typical intravenous anesthetic induction dose for ketamine in human patients is 0.6 to 2.1 mg/kg, whereas a dose of 5 to 10 mg/kg is generally recommended in dogs. Because the anesthetic induction dose of ketamine is approximately five times higher in dogs compared with people, there is the potential that a higher "low-dose" for analgesia may be required in cats and dogs, which is the author's observation. As an example of potential requirements, a dog with severe refractory cauda equina pain before surgical correction required an intravenous titrated dose of ketamine of 4 mg/kg to manage the violent postoperative behavior. This was followed by a 4-mg/kg CRI (in combination with morphine) for several hours to maintain "sleep" overnight. The ketamine CRI was slowly reduced over 16 hours to assess analgesic requirements and avoid the hyperalgesic state. After this, the dog seemed to be comfortable and demonstrated normal behavior and appetite on a reduced dose of morphine. An NSAID could not be administered because of previous administration of corticosteroids.

The 6-kg cat with neuropathic pain associated with hind limb amputation reported previously[76] received medetomidine at a dose of 100 μg to induce anesthesia, morphine at a dose of 1.5 mg, and ketamine at a dose of 20 mg given intramuscularly. A CRI of lactated Ringer's solution containing morphine at a dose of 0.06 mg/mL, lidocaine at a dose of 0.24 mg/mL, and ketamine at a dose of 0.06 mg/mL of solution was established. The initial infusion was started at 5:00 PM at a rate of 5 mL/h. This was increased to 11 mL/h the next morning at 8:00 AM, was increased to 18 mL/h at 9:00 AM, was increased further to 24 mL/h at 10:00 AM, and was then decreased at 11:00 AM to 11 mL/h when the cat began to show signs of excessive sedation. The infusion was continued for a further 19 hours for a total of 36 hours. Amitriptyline at a dosage of 10 mg administered orally every 12 hours was continued for 21 days. This treatment led to resolution of the neuropathic pain the cat had experienced for 60 days after amputation.[76] Similar acute treatment strategies are reported in human patients who have reflex sympathetic dystrophy.

When considering analgesic therapy, it is also prudent to be aware of potential adverse effects, especially in critically ill or traumatized patients. Reports in the literature have documented concerns for increased ICP with ketamine administration; however, this was documented in subjects in which the P_{CO_2} was not controlled[152,153] When the P_{CO_2} was held constant, an increased ICP did not occur during ketamine administration.[154] It has also been shown that ketamine does not directly dilate cerebral vessels, which potentially increases ICP.[154] In fact, when combined with a benzodiazepine, ketamine attenuated the increasing ICP in patients with an already increased ICP.[155,156] Ketamine demonstrated no adverse effects on cerebral hemodynamics in patients that had head trauma and, in fact, reduced the ICP.[157] The adverse effects on the cardiovascular system of analgesic doses of ketamine have also been questioned.[132] When comparing total intravenous anesthesia using a propofol-ketamine combination with an inhalation-opioid technique in coronary artery surgery in human patients, it was found that there was a reduced need for inotrope support in the patients receiving ketamine and that there was also a reduced incidence of myocardial infarction.[157] Because pain in head-injured dogs and cats can be difficult to manage, especially when there are other neurologic and orthopedic injuries, low-dose ketamine may be a potential addition to the multimodal analgesic regimen. Beginning with a low dose initially with frequent assessment is required, however, because there are no treatment strategy reports in the veterinary literature using ketamine for pain management in dogs and cats that have head injuries.

Sodium channel blockers

Sodium channels are responsible for the voltage-dependent sodium flux that serves to depolarize the excitable membrane.[139] After nerve injury, there is up-regulation of distinct types of TTX-insensitive, or TTX-R sodium channels in the neuroma, including C-afferent neurons and small-diameter dorsal root ganglion neurons that may serve as ectopic generator sites. The reader is referred to the articles by Lamont elsewhere in this issue for further discussion on this topic. This channel is blocked by local anesthetic agents at plasma concentrations that do not produce an afferent conduction block.[158] The TTX-sensitive (S) sodium channels are preferentially expressed in large and medium dorsal root ganglion neurons and are reported to be four times more sensitive than TTX-R sodium channels to lidocaine therapy.

Lidocaine

Systemically administered lidocaine has been shown to be effective in the treatment of several neuropathic pain disorders at doses that do not produce anesthesia or slow cardiac conduction. This class 1B antiarrhythmic provides analgesia separate from the direct local anesthetic properties. When administered systemically, lidocaine blocks the ectopic afferent neural activity at the NMDA receptor within the dorsal horn.[132] Several veterinary studies have shown benefit of lidocaine infusions during anesthesia in dogs.[159,160] One veterinary study reports lidocaine at a 1.0-mg/kg intravenous bolus followed by a 0.025-mg/kg/min intravenous CRI administered during and after surgery having similar efficacy to morphine at a 0.15-mg/kg intravenous bolus followed by a 0.1-mg/kg/h intravenous CRI.[161] No veterinary studies have evaluated lidocaine's analgesic efficacy when used alone in neuropathic pain states; however, a case report included lidocaine with morphine and ketamine to treat neuropathic pain in a cat.[76] Infusions of lidocaine have led to a significant improvement in human patients experiencing chronic neuropathic pain.[162] Based on the different sensitivity of lidocaine on the TTX-R and TTX-S sodium channels, the response to lidocaine therapy varies depending on the neural lesion and sodium channel involvement.[163] In human medicine, patients report that the pain associated with spontaneous ectopic discharges seems to be responsive to lidocaine therapy in most instances; however, this type of pain may also be mediated by α-adrenergic receptor sensitization, which may not respond to lidocaine.[163] Also, not all neuropathic pain symptoms in human beings are underlined by ectopic discharges; therefore, this type of pain may respond differently to lidocaine therapy.[163] The clinical importance of this is that when neuropathic pain is suspected in dogs and cats, lack of lidocaine responsiveness should not be interpreted as the nonexistence of neuropathic pain but that the underlying mechanism is not primarily involving the TTX-S sodium channel. Lidocaine infusions have been evaluated in cats with no apparent benefit when used alone[164] and may be associated with adverse effects in this species. The reader is referred to the articles by Lamont and Robertson elsewhere in this issue for further information.

Tocainide, mexiletine, and flecainide

These agents are analogues of lidocaine and have also been shown to relieve neuropathic pain in some human patients.[165] Again, there are no veterinary reports on analgesic efficacy in dogs or cats with neuropathic pain; however, mexiletine is used chronically in dogs with cardiac arrhythmias.[166]

α_2-Receptor agonists

The α_2-receptor is coupled through G-proteins to hyperpolarize spinal projection neurons and to inhibit transmitter release from small primary afferents. Spinally administered α_2-agonists have been shown to reverse the dysesthetic and allodynic components of pain states observed after peripheral nerve injury in rats and human beings.[165,167] The α_2-agonists function in the inhibitory pathway by binding receptors in the LC, which receives efferent noradrenergic axons from the PAG; the noradrenergic axons then extend to the spinal cord. Activation in the LC seems to contribute to analgesia indirectly at the level of the dorsal horn through these descending projections.[165,167] Several studies have shown a benefit of clonidine, an α_2-agonist, in reducing pain scores and opioid use for a variety of human painful states.[168] Medetomidine is the most commonly used α_2-agonist in veterinary medicine in North

America; however, dexmedetomidine is also approved for use in veterinary patients in other parts of the world (the reader is referred to the articles by Lamont elsewhere in this issue for an in-depth discussion on α_2-agonist agents in veterinary medicine and an article by Sinclair[169] for a review of the clinical use of medetomidine in small animal practice). Medetomidine may be administered by means of several routes, including the epidural, intra-articular, perineural, and parenteral routes, alone or in combination with several other medications. As an example of its use in neuropathic pain in the dog, the author has administered medetomidine (1–3 μg/kg/h) in addition to fentanyl at a low dosage (3–4 μg/kg/h) and corticosteroids for management of the severe pain associated with meningitis. Intra- and postoperative pain management for intervertebral disc herniation is another example for α_2-agonist administration to otherwise healthy dogs.

Regional analgesia

There are significant benefits to the use of regional analgesia, epidural analgesia, or continuous peripheral nerve blocks (CPNBs).[170] Regional analgesia improved pain control, improved outcomes, and produced greater satisfaction in human patients.[171] CPNBs are being used more frequently in human medicine, in which greater satisfaction is reported compared with systemic analgesia.[132] Of interest is the use of CPNBs in veterinary medicine. The local anesthetic agent can be delivered as a continuous infusion or as an intermittent bolus. There are no reports in the veterinary literature as to the efficacy of this technique; however, the main technical problem with all the available multiple-hole delivery tubes tested as a slow rate continuous infusion is the poor dispersion of the local anesthetic, resulting in erratic results (please see the article by Hansen elsewhere in this issue). For bolus infusion, however, in which a sufficient pressure can be generated to deliver the local anesthetic through the tubing, the dispersion into the wound seems to be uniform (please see the article by Hansen elsewhere in this issue). For cavitary (eg, joints, pleural space) analgesia, the continuous infusion through an open-ended tube may work satisfactorily. This technique can be also be used with ambulatory infusers (and various ambulatory infusion systems, Mila International Inc., Erlanger, Kentucky) in dogs on an outpatient basis after joint surgery. There must be strict adherence to aseptic technique in placement and maintenance of the catheters and in the dosing of lidocaine. Although the benefits of local analgesia far outweigh the potential risks, these risk factors must also be considered. In human medicine, the major risks for this technique are local anesthetic toxicity and nerve injury; however, phrenic nerve blockade, inadvertent epidural or subarachnoid spread, infection, and hematoma have also been reported to occur infrequently.[132] The reader is referred to more in-depth discussions on veterinary application of nerve blocks[133] and epidural analgesia (see the article by Valverde in this issue) and to a recent review on applications and outcomes in human medicine.[132]

Nonsteroidal anti-inflammatory analgesics

The NSAIDs are widely used in human and veterinary medicine for acute and chronic pain management. The NSAIDs variably target COX-1 and COX-2, or specifically COX-2, to manage osteoarthritic pain while sparing the constitutive functions of COX-1. Although COX-1 is mainly recognized for its constitutive functions, it is induced to participate in some pathologic states, such as transmission of pain peripherally and centrally, and may also generate prostaglandins at sites of inflammation. COX-2 is also induced, especially in inflammatory conditions like osteoarthritis, and functions in central and peripheral pain transmission. COX-2, however, has several important constitutive functions, especially in the gastrointestinal tract and kidney.

COX-3, characterized as generated from COX-1, is expressed in the brain and brain microvasculature and has been proposed to be a target of the analgesics/antipyretics acetaminophen and dipyrone. The NSAIDs act peripherally at sites of inflammation but also have direct spinal cord action by blocking hyperalgesia induced by the activation of spinal glutamate and S-P receptors.[19] These findings demonstrate that the analgesic effects of NSAIDs can be dissociated from their anti-inflammatory actions in the periphery. Spinal prostanoids are thus critical for the augmentation of pain processing at the spinal cord level.[19] The NSAIDs have been shown to be effective analgesics for moderate to severe pain in cats and dogs. No veterinary studies specifically assessing the efficacy of managing neuropathic pain have been reported, however. When neuropathic pain is assumed to be present, such as with limb amputation and crushing injuries, the addition of a parenterally administered NSAID to an opioid improves analgesia and pain scores compared with an opioid alone (Karol Mathews, DVM, DVSc, unpublished data, 2001). Of interest, inhibition of COX-2 has been shown to benefit recovery after injury to the brain or spinal cord in laboratory animals.[172] The proposed mechanism is that the CNS injury increases COX-2 expression. Prolonged elevation of COX-2 contributes to inflammation, programmed cell death, free radical–mediated tissue damage, and alterations in cellular metabolism. The action of COX-2 inhibitors decreases synthesis of prostanoids and free radicals. Because of this dominant metabolic reaction, however, COX-2 inhibition results in shunting of AA away from the COX pathway down alternate enzymatic pathways (eg, cytochrome P450 epoxygenase), resulting in the synthesis of potentially neuroprotective eicosanoids.[172] Strauss[172] proposed that COX-2 inhibition blocks delayed cell death and neuroinflammation. Although the role of NSAIDs may prove to be of benefit in CNS injury in laboratory animals, the benefits in the clinical setting have yet to be confirmed. Prior to NSAID therapy, the individual patient must be identified for potential adverse effects and the absolute contraindication for coadministration with corticosteroids.

Gabapentin

Gabapentin is an antiepileptic agent. The analgesic effect is attributable to gabapentin's ability to bind with the high-affinity $\alpha_2\delta$-subunits of voltage-dependent calcium channels, blocking calcium currents at the spinal and supraspinal levels and blocking maintenance of spinal cord central sensitization.[173–175] It is suggested that gabapentin activates the descending noradrenergic system and induces spinal NE release, which subsequently produces analgesia by means of spinal α_2-adrenoceptor stimulation. Recently, gabapentin has also been recommended for acute postoperative pain in human patients, in whom the most benefit seems to be when chronic pain is present.[59,176] Further studies confirm gabapentin's supraspinal analgesic action in activating the descending noradrenergic system after peripheral nerve injury in rats.[177]

These studies indicate that perioperative administration of gabapentin to animals with nerve injury may reduce the potential establishment of, or ongoing, neuropathic pain. It is the author's observation that gabapentin has reduced the pain in dogs and cats experiencing refractory neuropathic pain secondary to cervical or thoracolumbar intervertebral disc disease or pelvic trauma. Initially, gabapentin is administered in combination with an opioid and an NSAID; however, gradually, these analgesics may be tapered and gabapentin remains as the sole method of analgesia. There is an extremely wide dose range for gabapentin, and it should be given to effect. The dose-limiting side effect is usually sedation. Frequently, some animals need several weeks to months for resolution of their pain, potentially requiring a lifetime of medication. Careful lowering of the drug dosage is recommended to assess the dosing requirement. Initially, eliminating the middle dose in the three times daily treatment regimen is suggested to assess the ongoing requirement. Because dosing to effect is the method by which the appropriate dose is selected, once this effect is reached, treatment twice daily rather than three times daily may suffice. Gabapentin is excreted by the kidneys, and animals with renal insufficiency may require less frequent dosing because of slower elimination. Tapering of the dose is important because stopping the drug abruptly may lead to rebound pain that may be severe. The author's method of dosing is to start with 10 mg/kg administered orally every 8 hours in dogs and 5 mg/kg administered orally in cats and to ramp up or taper down to effect (dose range: 5–25 mg/kg). There may be a potential advantage to commencing gabapentin before any surgical procedure involving the PNS and CNS.

Gabapentin is also used in human patients for management of neuropathic pain associated with diabetes, cancer, and primary nerve compression.[139]

Acupuncture

Because neuropathic pain is difficult to manage with pharmaceutical agents, there is a growing interest in the use of acupuncture as an adjunct to a multimodal pharmaceutical regimen. For the past 12 years at least, the National Institutes of Health have listed pain management as an indication for acupuncture therapy. There is a sound physiologic mechanism for the analgesic effects of acupuncture.[178,179] Acupuncture is the stimulating of specific anatomic points in the body to produce therapeutic or analgesic effects. Placement of fine-gauge needles may decrease muscle spasms when inserted into trigger points. Placement of needles at specific acupuncture points can induce the release of a variety of neurotransmitters, which can affect the processing of sensory input, including blockade of C-fiber input and amplification of the inhibitory system, as previously discussed. Proper needle placement, with administration of various frequencies of electrical stimulation, releases endorphins, serotonin, and NE. Another benefit of acupuncture therapy is that there are no associated adverse effects, such as those that may occur with any pharmaceutical agent. Based on sound physiologic evidence for the benefit of acupuncture in acute and chronic pain states, the details of which are given in the section on chronic pain management, acupuncture is highly recommended in the management of neuropathic pain.

Chronic Pain Management

Opiates/Opioids

As in the acute setting, opioids can be used in the chronic pain state. The opioids most frequently used in veterinary medicine for chronic pain management are the fentanyl patch, oxycodone, sustained-release morphine (with the greatest potential side effects), and tramadol (a synthetic codeine analogue that is a weak μ-receptor agonist). Although methadone may be taken orally in people, it is not absorbed orally in dogs, and is therefore not recommended for oral administration in this species.[140,141]

Rarely should opioids be used alone for neuropathic pain; however, in severe pain, a high dose of an opiate, in addition to other drugs, may be necessary. Should pain seem to worsen with increasing doses of an opioid, however, opioid-induced hyperalgesia (OIH) should be considered. Experimental evidence in human patients suggests that opioid tolerance and OIH do occur within 1 month of continuing opioid use. Some investigators thus indicate that these findings might limit the clinical utility of opioids in controlling chronic pain.[180] This is a point to consider in veterinary patients because there may be the potential for opioid tolerance to occur; therefore, pain should not necessarily be interpreted as worsening of the underlying condition. A recent review identified OIH to occur in rats, mice, and human beings after acute or chronic administration of opioids.[181]

Tramadol

Tramadol is a synthetic codeine analogue that is a weak μ-receptor agonist. Of interest, when managing neuropathic pain, tramadol inhibits neuronal reuptake of NE and serotonin, in addition to possibly facilitating their release.[182,183] It is thought that these effects on central catecholaminergic (descending inhibitory) pathways contribute significantly to the drug's analgesic efficacy.[183] These effects may be an advantage in animals that have neuropathic pain. Tramadol is recommended for the management of acute and chronic pain of moderate intensity associated with a variety of conditions, including neuropathic pain in human patients.[184] There are no reports in the veterinary literature assessing the efficacy of tramadol in neuropathic pain. One study, however, reported comparable analgesia in dogs when they were administered preoperative tramadol at a dose of 2 mg/kg or morphine at a dose of 0.2 mg/kg for pain management after ovariohysterectomy for pyometra.[185] In North America, only oral formulations of tramadol are commercially available (the reader is referred to the article by Lamont elsewhere in this issue). In the United States, tramadol is available in various tablet strengths, in an extended-release formulation, and in combination with acetaminophen (the reader is referred to the article by Lamont elsewhere in this issue). Only the extended-release preparation and the combination with acetaminophen are currently available in Canada (the reader is referred to the article by Lamont elsewhere in this issue) in the noncompounded formulations. Tramadol is commonly prepared by a local compounding pharmacy, however. At the Ontario Veterinary College, 5-mg, 10-mg, 25-mg, 50-mg, and 100-mg capsules and a 5-mg/mL suspension are prepared from tramadol powder. A recent study reported a pharmacokinetic study of a tramadol solution prepared from the pure dry powder and administered intravenously to dogs.[186] Using doses of 1 mg/kg, 2 mg/kg, and 4 mg/kg, the elimination half-life ranged from 1.5 to 2 hours and the active metabolite was detected only in low amounts. In this small group of dogs, intravenous tramadol administration seemed safe, with increasing sedation noted with increasing dose.[186] These investigators suggest that further investigation using larger numbers of dogs of various breeds is warranted. The oral dosing guidelines at this time are based on extrapolation from human patients in addition to clinical experience with animal patients. KuKanich and Papich[187] reported that a simulated oral dosing regimen of 5 mg/kg every 6 hours in dogs resulted in plasma concentrations of tramadol and its principal metabolite that were consistent with levels associated with analgesia in people. Based on current information, a starting dosage range of 1 to 5 mg/kg administered orally every 6 to 8 hours for cancer pain, 1 to 2 mg/kg administered every 8 to 12 hours for osteoarthritis in dogs (increasing to effect), and 1 to 2 mg/kg administered every 12 to 24 hours for cats is recommended. Because dysphoria has been a common side effect in cats, dose recommendations for this species are more conservative. As with any medication for managing pain, titration of the dose is required to minimize sedation or dysphoria in cats and dogs. Dosing guidelines for the extended-release formulations are more difficult to estimate; at this time, there are no published pharmacokinetic data in dogs or cats to guide recommendations for this formulation (the reader is referred to the article by Lamont elsewhere in this issue). Combination products, such as those combined with an NSAID (eg, tramadol, acetaminophen), are not recommended because the NSAID has a dose-limiting requirement that restricts the dosing of tramadol or any other opioid-NSAID combination. An NSAID of choice can be administered separately from the tramadol or any other opioid. Acetaminophen is toxic to cats; thus, this combination product should never be used in this species.

Common side effects associated with tramadol administration include sedation and dysphoria, especially in cats. It has also been reported to decrease the seizure threshold in certain human patients.[188] Because of its inhibitory effect on serotonin uptake, tramadol should not be used in patients that may have received monoaminoxidase inhibitors, such as selegiline (Anipryl).

Gabapentin

In addition to its use in surgical or traumatic neurologic conditions, gabapentin is used in human patients for management of neuropathic pain associated with diabetes, cancer, and primary nerve compression.[139] The reader is referred to the section on acute pain management for details.

Pregabalin

Pregabalin has a similar pharmacologic profile as gabapentin and is used to manage neuropathic pain in human patients.[177,189] Pregabalin seems to cause less mental confusion and sedative side effects than those reported with gabapentin. A dosage for pregabalin has not been established for veterinary patients. Pregabalin is much more expensive than gabapentin.

Amantadine

Amantadine is an oral NMDA receptor antagonist with activity similar to that of ketamine.[190] The only study reporting the chronic use of amantadine in the veterinary literature showed improved activity and lameness scores in refractory canine osteoarthritic pain when used in combination with meloxicam compared with meloxicam alone.[191] The dosage of amantadine used in this randomized, blind, placebo-controlled study was 3 to 5 mg/kg administered orally every 24 hours; however, a starting dosage of 3 mg/kg administered orally every 24 hours is suggested. Meloxicam was administered at a standard dose of a 0.2 mg/kg orally administered loading dose, followed by a dosage of 0.1 mg/kg administered orally every 24 hours thereafter. This study gives hope to the potential benefit of amantadine in managing chronic neuropathic pain similar to that of ketamine in the acute pain setting. In the United States and Canada, amantadine is available commercially as 100-mg capsules and as 10-mg/mL oral syrup. A 100-mg tablet formulation is also available in the United States (the reader is referred to the article by Lamont elsewhere in this issue).

Dextromethorphan

Dextromethorphan is an oral NMDA receptor antagonist and has been recommended for management of neuropathic pain in human beings. Unfortunately, however, dextromethorphan is not absorbed when given to dogs by the oral route, and is therefore not recommended in this species.[192]

Tricyclic antidepressants

Imipramine and amitriptyline are two commonly recommended TCAs for veterinary patients. The TCAs block the reuptake of catecholamines, thereby enhancing adrenergic transmission.[139] In addition, amitriptyline serves as an NMDA receptor antagonist. The TCAs may be effective adjunctive analgesics for a range of neuropathic conditions or can be used alone in IBD and FIC.[117] In people, the analgesic effects of these drugs seem to occur at lower than antidepressant doses.[139] When other traditional analgesics have failed to achieve complete analgesia, the addition of imipramine or amitriptyline may prove successful in managing refractory chronic pain. These products may be distasteful and may require some creative method of administration. Although it has been reported that it can take 2 to 4 weeks for these drugs to achieve maximal effectiveness, in the author's experience, clinical improvement occurs within 48 hours of amitriptyline administration when combined with other analgesics or when used in combination with corticosteroids for feline IBD and continues to improve further over time. In FIC, however, no improvement was observed after 7 days of administration of amitriptyline at a dosage of 10 mg per cat administered every 24 hours.[193] The recommended dosage of amitriptyline for dogs is 1 to 2 mg/kg administered orally every 12 to 24 hours; for cats, the recommended dosage is 2.5 to 12.5 mg per cat administered orally every 24 hours. The dosage of imipramine for dogs is 0.5 to 1 mg/kg administered orally every 8 hours; for cats, the recommended dosage is 2.5 to 5 mg per cat administered orally every 12 hours.

Lidocaine dermal patches

Lidocaine 5% dermal patches (Lidoderm patch, Endo Pharmaceuticals, Chadd Ford, Pennsylvania) are frequently used in human patients with neuropathic pain attributable to a variety of causes. The low systemic concentrations achieved by transdermal lidocaine application suggest that efficacy is achieved by means of blockade of PNS rather than CNS sodium channels.[194] Successful results with the application of this patch have been obtained in children who have intractable and disabling neuropathic pain originating at and around the site of previous surgical procedures. These sites were identified at a nephrectomy scar, laminectomy scar, an inguinal area scar from a cardiac catheterization procedure, and a laparotomy scar in which surgical involvement of a nerve was suspected.[195] Worthy of note is that these procedures, and many others in which nerve entrapment may occur, are performed in cats and dogs.

Pharmacokinetic studies of the lidocaine patch in dogs found that lidocaine peak levels occurred at 9.5 to 12 hours after patch application, reached steady-state concentrations between 24 and 48 hours, and decreased dramatically at 60 hours after application. Low plasma lidocaine concentrations remained for 6 hours after patch removal.[196,197] No analgesic efficacy studies have been reported in dogs or cats.

Lamotrigine

Lamotrigine is an anticonvulsant and is the oral sodium channel antagonist of choice in human patients with chronic neuropathic pain. Dosing requires a slow titration to 400 mg/d.[139] Lamotrigine is not suitable for use in dogs because the plasma elimination half-life is only 2 to 3 hours (compared with 22–24 hours in human beings) and its metabolite has cardioactive properties that may have significant cardiovascular depressant effects.[52]

Acupuncture

Acupuncture has been used for centuries as a primary or complimentary treatment modality for the treatment of acute and chronic pain states in human patients. Acupuncture has more recently become a widely accepted treatment for pain in veterinary medicine. The relief of pain by acupuncture can be explained neurophysiologically by neuromodulatory actions at the local, regional (segmental), and CNS (suprasegmental) levels. Specific acupuncture points are rich in neurovascular endings. Because a specific region of the body is served by the same myelotome (specific spinal cord segment), sensory cutaneous stimulation by means of acupuncture needle placement causes functional reflex reactions to the muscles, muscle vessels, and the ligaments that receive sensory or motor innervation from that same myelotome. In addition, acupuncture is thought to block pain signals from reaching the spinal cord ascending nociceptive pathways and the thalamocortex by a mechanism called the "gate theory." Acupuncture primarily stimulates proprioceptors in skin and muscle, which send impulses to the dorsal horn of the spinal cord by way of heavily myelinated Aβ and 1A sensory nerves, with a rapid conduction velocity. Pain is carried to the spinal cord by way of thinly myelinated Aδ and unmyelinated C-fibers, which have a much slower conduction velocity. Because proprioceptive impulses reach the spinal cord first, they cause blockade of Aδ and C-fiber input by the prior release of endogenous opiates (endorphins). In addition, mechanical stimulation of somatic and visceral "fields" by acupuncture needle placement has been shown to decrease the spontaneous and noxious evoked activity of most dorsal horn neurons, including WDR cells, high-threshold cells, and high-threshold inhibitory cells, reducing the perception of pain. At the suprasegmental spinal cord and brain level, there is strong evidence to indicate that acupuncture exerts its analgesic effect by means of modulation of the descending pain control system, consisting of three parts, above the level of the dorsal horn of the spinal cord. These are the pontine system (nucleus raphe magnus), the mesencephalic system (PAG and periventricular gray system), and the cortical/diencephalic system. Each system uses different endogenous opioid peptides, which are all stimulated by means of acupuncture and electroacupuncture. The long-term analgesic effect of acupuncture has been suggested to be related to the activation of a serotonergic and metencephalinergic neurologic circuit in the mid-diencephalon, resulting in continuous inhibition of nociceptive stimuli, in addition to being related to longer lasting peripheral activation of low-threshold muscular mechanoreceptors, increasing the activity of large-diameter heavily myelinated nerve fibers and resulting in blockade of Aδ and C-fiber input into the spinal cord[178] (Paul Cuddon, personal communication, 2008).

FUTURE THERAPEUTIC MODALITIES

Vanilloid Receptor-1 Antagonists

The identification and cloning of the TRPV1 represented a significant step in the understanding of the molecular mechanisms underlying the transduction of noxious chemical and thermal stimuli by peripheral nociceptors.[198] The TRPV1 channel activity is potentiated by proinflammatory agents, a phenomenon that is thought to underlie the peripheral sensitization of nociceptors that leads to thermal hyperalgesia. The validation of the TRPV1 receptor as a key therapeutic target for pain management has resulted in the development of orally active antagonists. Because of the many physiologic roles of this receptor, the real challenge is to develop effective antagonists involved in pain transduction but to preserve the physiologic activity of TRPV1 receptors.[198] The TRPV1 receptor is also expressed in the CNS, and it seems to play an important role in pain mediated by central sensitization. The TRPV1 antagonists currently being investigated effectively reduce thermal hyperalgesia and mechanical allodynia associated with inflammatory and osteoarthritic pain in research models. With identification of peripheral and central roles of the TRPV1 receptor, the future potential of TRPV1 antagonists as analgesics for neuropathic pain may be a consideration.

Serotonin and Norepinephrine Reuptake Inhibitors

As the descending inhibitory system seems to be dysfunctional in neuropathic pain states, SRI and norepinephrine reuptake inhibitor (NRI) mixed compounds are being investigated for analgesic efficacy. Recently, duloxetine, a mixed SRI and NRI with potency at both transporters, was the first reuptake inhibitor approved for the treatment of diabetic neuropathy.[199] Published preclinical data evaluating this compound in neuropathic and inflammatory models of pain have demonstrated analgesic activity.[199] In a more recent study investigating the SRI and NRIs, the investigators suggest that compounds with affinity for NE and serotonin reuptake inhibition may be beneficial for the treatment of neuropathic pain, whereas compounds with greater affinity for NE reuptake inhibition may be more beneficial for the treatment of visceral pain.[31]

As these agents gain more popularity in human medicine as being effective in treating neuropathic pain, they may also become available for veterinary investigation.

SUMMARY

Cats and dogs share a nervous system similar to that of human beings. They also encounter similar surgical, traumatic, inflammatory, and metabolic conditions. Because human beings experience neuropathic pain associated with these and other pathologic situations, it would seem reasonable to assume that cats and dogs share this experience. Neuropathic pain is difficult to diagnose in veterinary patients because they are unable to verbalize their pain. By assuming that neuropathic pain may exist based on the history of events that each patient has experienced, a focused client history and neurologic examination may identify a lesion resulting in persistent or spontaneous pain. Should neuropathic pain be diagnosed, it is important to identify the particular cause responsible for generating a particular pain because this represents the first anatomic target for treatment. Although it is impossible to discriminate burning from prickling and lancinating from stabbing in veterinary patients, behavioral patterns described by owners may assist with lesion localization. Once neuropathic pain is diagnosed, a trial analgesic or acupuncture session(s) should be prescribed with instructions for owners to observe behavior. Dosing of the analgesic can be titrated to the patient's needs while avoiding adverse effects. When a particular analgesic may be ineffectual, an alternate class should be tried. As research into the neurobiologic mechanisms of neuropathic pain continues, specific therapies for its management should eventually appear in the human clinical setting and should subsequently be investigated for veterinary clinical use.

ACKNOWLEDGMENTS

The author is extremely grateful to Dr. Paul Cuddon, Colorado State University, for his contribution on electrodiagnostics (especially its application to cats with diabetic neuropathy), the physiologic action of acupuncture, and his critical review of this manuscript.

REFERENCES

1. Harden RN. Chronic neuropathic pain. Mechanisms, diagnosis, and treatment. Neurologist 2005;11(2):11–22.
2. Morton DB, Griffiths PHM. Guidelines on the recognition of pain, distress and discomfort in experimental animals and an hypothesis for assessment. Vet Rec 1985;116:431–6.
3. Lascelles BDX. Advances in the control of pain in animals. Vet Annu 1996;36:1–15.
4. Niv D, Devor M. Refractory neuropathic pain: the nature and extent of the problem. Pain Pract 2006;6(1):3–9.
5. Taylor BK. Pathophysiologic mechanisms of neuropathic pain. Curr Pain Headache Rep 2001;5:151–61.
6. Doubell TP, Mannion RJ, Woolf CJ. The dorsal horn: state dependent sensory processing, plasticity and generation of pain. In: Wall PD, Melzack R, editors. Textbook of pain. 4th edition. Philadelphia: Churchill Livingstone Inc; 1999. p. 165–82.

7. Byers MR, Bonica JJ. Peripheral pain mechanisms and nociceptor plasticity. In: Loeser JD, Butler SH, Chapman CR, et al, editors. Bonica's management of pain. 3rd edition. Philadelphia: Lipincott Williams & Wilkins; 2001. p. 26–72.
8. Price DD. Characteristics of second pain and flexion reflexes indicative of prolonged central summation. Exp Neurol 1972;37:371–91.
9. Herrero JF, Laird JMA, Lopez-Garcia. Wind-up of spinal cord neurones and pain sensation: much ado about something. Progr Neurobiol 2000;61:169–203.
10. Raja SN, Meyer RA, Campbell JN. Peripheral mechanisms of somatic pain. Anesthesiology 1988;68:571–90.
11. Moalem G, Tracey DJ. Immune and inflammatory mechanisms in neuropathic pain. Brain Research Review 2006;S51:240–64.
12. Handwerker HO, Reeh PW. Nociceptors: chemo pain and inflammation. Pain Res Manag 1991;4:59–70.
13. Kumazawa T. Primitivism and plasticity of pain-implication of polymodal receptors. Neurosci Res 1998;32:9–31.
14. McMahon SB, Koltzenburg DN. Visceral pain. Br J Anaesth 1995;75:132–44.
15. Muir WW III, Woolf CJ. Mechanisms of pain and their therapeutic implications. J Am Vet Med Assoc 2001;219(10):1346–56.
16. Killermann Lucas K, Svensson CI, Hua X-Y, et al. Spinal phospholipase A2 in inflammatory hyperalgesia: role of group IVA cPLA2. Br J Pharmacol 2005;144(7): 940–52.
17. Menschikowski M, Hagelgans A, Siegert G. Secretory phospholipase A2 of group IIA: is it an offensive or a defensive player during atherosclerosis and other inflammatory diseases? Prostag Other Lipid Mediat 2006;79:1–33.
18. Malmberg AB, Yaksh TL. Cyclooxygenase inhibition and spinal release of prostaglandin E2 and amino acids evoked by paw formalin injection: a microdialysis study in unanesthetized rats. J Neurosci 1995;15:2768–76.
19. Malmberg AB, Yaksh TL. Hyperalgesia mediated by spinal glutamate or substance P receptor blocked by spinal cyclo-oxygenase inhibition. Science 1992;257:1276–9.
20. Evans AR, Junger H, Southall MD, et al. Isoprostanes, novel eicosanoids that produce nociception and sensitize rat sensory neurons. J Pharmacol Exp Ther 2000;293:912–20.
21. Cook JA, Fan H, Halushka PV. Prostaglandins, thromboxanes, leukotrienes, and other products of arachidonic acid. In: Fink MP, Abraham E, Vincent JL, et al, editors. Textbook of emergency and critical care. 5th edition. Philadelphia: Elsevier Saunders; 2005. p. 219–26.
22. Woolf CJ. Excitability changes in central neurons following peripheral damage; role of central sensitization in the pathogenesis of pain. In: Willis WD Jr, editor. Hyperalgesia and allodynia. New York: Raven Press; 1992. p. 221–43.
23. Craig AD, Dostrovsky JO. Processing of nociceptive information at supraspinal levels. In: Yaksh TL, Lynch C III, Zapol WM, editors. Anesthesia: biologic foundations. Philadelphia: Lippincott-Raven; 1997. p. 625–42.
24. Mathews KA. Pain assessment and general approach to management. Appendix: descriptive pain assessment scale. Vet Clin North Am Small Anim Pract 2000;30(4):753.
25. Hellyer PW, Robertson SA, Fails AD. Pain and its management. In: Tranquilli WJ, Thurmon JC, Grimm KA, editors. Lumb & Jones' veterinary anesthesia and analgesia. 4th edition. Ames (IA): Blackwell Publishing; 2007. p. 31–57.
26. Woolf CJ, Max MB. Mechanism-based pain diagnosis: issues for analgesic drug development. Anesthesiology 2001;95(1):241–9.

27. Zhuo M. Cellular and synaptic insights into physiological and pathological pain. Can J Neurol Sci 2005;32:27–36.
28. Zhuo M, Gebhart GF. Modulation of noxious and non-noxious spinal mechanical transmission from the rostral medial medulla in the rat. J Neurophysiol 2002; 88(6):2928–41.
29. Stamford JA. Descending control of pain. Br J Anaesth 1995;75:217–27.
30. Budai D, Harasawa I, Fields HL. Midbrain periaqueductal gray (PAG) inhibits nociceptive inputs to sacral dorsal horn nociceptive neurons through alpha2-adrenergic receptors. J Neurophysiol 1998;80:2244–54.
31. Leventhal L, Smith V, Hornby, et al. Differential and synergistic effects of selective norepinephrine and serotonin reuptake inhibitors in rodent models of pain. J Pharmacol Exp Ther 2007;320:1178–85.
32. Rahman W, D'Mello R, Dickenson AH. Peripheral nerve injury-induced changes in spinal alpha(2)-adrenoceptor-mediated modulation of mechanically evoked dorsal horn neuronal responses. Pain 2008;9(4):350–9.
33. Zimmermann M. Pathobiology of neuropathic pain. Eur J Pharmacol 2001;429: 23–37.
34. Lamont LA, Tranquilli WJ, Grimm KA. Physiology of pain. Vet Clin North Am Small Anim Pract 2000;30(4):703–28.
35. Woolf CJ, Salter MW. Neuronal plasticity: increasing the gain in pain. Science 2000;288:1765–8.
36. Liu CN, Wall PD, Ben-Dor E, et al. Tactile allodynia in the absence of C-fiber activation: altered firing properties of DRG neurons following spinal nerve injury. Pain 2000;85:503–21.
37. Woolf CJ, Shortland P, Coggeshall RE. Peripheral nerve injury triggers central sprouting of myelinated afferents. Nature 1992;355:75–7.
38. Novakvic SD, Tzoumaka E, McGivern JG, et al. Distribution of the tetrodotoxin-resistant sodium channel PN3 in rat sensory neurons in normal and neuropathic conditions. J Neurosci 1998;18:2174–87.
39. Amir R, Devor M. Functional cross-excitation between afferent A- and C-neurons in dorsal root ganglia. Neuroscience 2000;95:189–95.
40. Doubell TP, Mannion RJ, Woolf CJ. The dorsal horn: state-dependent sensory processing, plasticity and the generation of pain. In: Wall PD, Melzack R, editors. Textbook of pain. Edinburgh (UK): Churchill Livingstone; 1999. p. 165–81.
41. McLachlan EM, Janig W, Devor M, et al. Peripheral nerve root injury triggers noradrenergic sprouting within dorsal root ganglia. Nature 1993;363:543–5.
42. Chabal C, Jacobson L, Russell LC, et al. Pain response to perineuronal injection of normal saline, epinephrine and lidocaine in humans. Pain 1992;49:9–12.
43. Sato J, Perl ER. Adrenergic excitation of cutaneous pain receptors induced by peripheral nerve injury. Science 1991;251:1608–10.
44. Ringkamp M, Eschenfelder S, Grethel EJ, et al. Lumbar sympathectomy failed to reverse mechanical allodynia and hyperalgesia-like behaviour in rats with L5 spinal nerve injury. Pain 1999;79:143–53.
45. Day M. Sympathetic blocks: the evidence. Pain Pract 2008;8(2):98–109.
46. Costigan M, Woolf CJ. Pain: molecular mechanisms. Pain 2000;(Suppl 3):35–44.
47. Keller AF, Beggs S, Salter MW, et al. Transformation of the output of spinal lamina I neurons after nerve injury and microglia stimulation underlying neuropathic pain. Mol Pain 2007;3:27.
48. Bruce-Keller AJ. Microglial-neuronal interactions in synaptic damage and recovery. J Neurosci Res 1999;58:191–201.

49. Kempermann G, Neumann H. Neuroscience. Microglia: the enemy within? Science 2003;302:1689–90.
50. Zhang F, Vadakkan KI, Kim SS. Selective activation of microglia in spinal cord but not higher cortical regions following nerve injury in adult mouse. Mol Pain 2008;4:15–31.
51. Planells-Cases R, Garcia-Sanz N, Morenilla-Palao C. Functional aspects and mechanisms of TRPV1 involvement in neurogenic inflammation that leads to thermal hyperalgesia. Pflugers Arch 2005;451(1):151–9.
52. Messeguer A, Planells-Cases R, Ferrer-Montiel A. Physiology and pharmacology of the vanilloid receptor. Curr Neuropharmacol 2006;4(1):1–15.
53. Mayer DJ, Mao J, Price DD. The development of morphine tolerance and dependence is associated with translocation of protein kinase C. Pain 1995;61:365–74.
54. Lombard MC, Besson JM. Attempts to gauge the relative importance of pre- and postsynaptic effects of morphine on the transmission of noxious messages in the dorsal horn of the rat spinal cord. Pain 1989;37(3):335–45.
55. Woolf CJ, Mannion RJ. Neuropathic pain: aetiology, symptoms, mechanisms, and management. Lancet 1999;353:1959–64.
56. Attal N, Bouhassira D. Mechanisms of pain in peripheral neuropathy. Acta Neurol Scand 1999;100(Suppl 173):12–24.
57. Tanabe M, Takasu K, Kasuya N, et al. Role of descending noradrenergic system and spinal alpha2-adrenergic receptors in the effects of gabapentin on thermal and mechanical nociception after partial nerve injury in the mouse. Br J Pharmacol 2005;144:703–14.
58. Ren J, Ruda R. Descending modulation in persistent pain: an update. Pain 2002; 100(1–2):1–6.
59. Hayashida K, DeGoes S, Curry R, et al. Gabapentin activates spinal noradrenergic activity in rats and humans and reduces hypersensitivity after surgery. Anesthesiology 2007;106(3):557–62.
60. Woolf CJ. Dissecting out mechanisms responsible for peripheral neuropathic pain: implications for diagnosis and therapy. Life Sci 2004;74:2605–10.
61. Payne R. Recognition and diagnosis of breakthrough pain. Pain Med 2007; 8(Suppl 1):S3–7.
62. Hayes C, Browne S, Lantry G, et al. Neuropathic pain in the acute pain service: a prospective survey. Acute Pain 2002;4:45–8.
63. Galer BS, Jensen MP. Development and preliminary validation of a pain measure specific to neuropathic pain: the neuropathic pain scale. Neurology 1997;48:332–7.
64. Bennett M. The LANNS pain scale: the Leeds assessment of neuropathic symptoms and signs. Pain 2001;92:147–57.
65. Anil SS, Anil L, Deen J. Challenges of pain assessment in domestic animals. J Am Vet Med Assoc 2002;220(3):313–9.
66. Muir WW III, Wiese AJ, Wittum TE. Prevalence and characteristics of pain in dogs and cats examined as outpatients at a veterinary teaching hospital. J Am Vet Med Assoc 2004;224:1459–63.
67. Wiese AJ, Muir WW III, et al. Characteristics of pain and response to analgesic treatment in dogs and cats examined at a veterinary teaching hospital emergency service. J Am Vet Med Assoc 2005;226:2004–9.
68. Konen A. Measurement of nerve dysfunction in neuropathic pain. Curr Rev Pain 2000;4:388–94.
69. Cuddon PA, Murray M, Kraus K. Electrodiagnosis. In: Slatter D, editor. Textbook of small animal surgery. 3rd edition. Philadelphia: Saunders; 2003. p. 1108–18.

70. Cuddon PA. Electrophysiology in neuromuscular disease. Vet Clinics North Am Small Anim Pract 2002;32(1):31–62.
71. Mizisin AP, Shelton GD, Burgess ML, et al. Neurological complications associated with spontaneously occurring feline diabetes mellitus. J Neuropathol Exp Neurol 2002;61(10):872–4.
72. Rodkey WG, Sharp NJH. Surgery of the peripheral nervous system. In: Slatter D, editor. Textbook of small animal surgery. 3rd edition. Philadelphia: Saunders; 2003. p. 1218–26.
73. Cunningham J, Temple WJ, Mitchell P, et al. Cooperative hernia study. Pain in the postrepair patient. Ann Surg 1996;224(5):598–602.
74. Meyhoff CS, Thomsen CH, Rasmussen LS, et al. High incidence of chronic pain following surgery for pelvic fracture. Clin J Pain 2006;22:167–72.
75. Popeney C, Ansell A, Renney K. Pudendal entrapment as an etiology of chronic perineal pain: diagnosis and treatment. Neurol Urodyn 2007;26(6):820–7.
76. O'Hagan BJ. Neuropathic pain in a cat post-amputation. Aust Vet J 2006;84: 83–6.
77. Dueland RT, Wagner SD, Parker RB. von Willebrand heterotopic osteochondrofibrosis in Doberman pinschers: five cases (1980–1987). J Am Vet Med Assoc 1990;197(3):383–8.
78. Nikolajsen L, Jensen TS. Phantom limb pain. Curr Rev Pain 2000;4(2):166–70.
79. De Risio L, Thomas WB, Sharp NJH. Degenerative sacral stenosis. Vet Clin North Am Small Anim Pract 2000;301:111–32.
80. Mayhew PD, Kapatkinn AS, Wortman JA, et al. Association of cauda equina compression on magnetic resonance images and clinical signs in dogs with degenerative lumbosacral stenosis. J Am Anim Hosp Assoc 2002;38:555–62.
81. Griffiths IR. Polyradiculoneuritis in two dogs presenting as neuritis of the cauda equina. Vet Rec 1983;112:360–1.
82. Hoerlein BF. Intervertebral disc disease. In: Canine neurology: diagnosis and treatment. Philadelphia: WB Saunders; 1978. p. 470–560.
83. Morgan PW, Parent J, Holmberg DL. Cervical pain secondary to intervertebral disc disease in dogs: radiographic findings and surgical implications. Prog Vet Neurol 1993;4:76–80.
84. Seim HB III, Prata RG. Ventral decompression for treatment of cervical disk disease in the dog: a review of 54 cases. J Am Anim Hosp Assoc 1982;18:233–40.
85. Coates JR. Intervertebral disk disease. Vet Clin North Am Small Anim Pract 2000;30(1):77–110.
86. Sukhiani HR, Parent JM, Atilola MA, et al. Intervertebral disk disease in dogs with signs of back pain alone: 25 cases (1986–1993). J Am Vet Med Assoc 1996;209:1275–9.
87. Brown NO, Helphrey ML, Prata RG. Thoracolumbar disk disease in the dog: a retrospective analysis of 187 cases. J Am Anim Hosp Assoc 1977;13:665–72.
88. Funquist B. Decompressive laminectomy for thoraco-lumbar disc protrusion in the dog. Acta Vet Scand 1970;11:445–51.
89. Dewey CW. Myelopathies: disorders of the spinal cord. In: A practical guide to canine and feline neurology. Ames (IA): Blackwell; 2003. p. 321–3.
90. Thomas WB. Diskospondylitis and other vertebral infections. Vet Clin North Am Small Anim Pract 2000;30(1):169–82.
91. Webb AA. Potential sources of neck and back pain in clinical conditions in cats and dogs. Vet J 2003;165:193–213.
92. Cuddon PA. Electrophysiologic assessment of acute polyradiculoneuropathy in dogs: comparison with Guillain-Barré syndrome in people. J Vet Intern Med 1998;12:294–303.

93. Heavner JE, Coates PW, Racz G, et al. Myelinated fibres of spinal cord blood vessels—sensory innervation? Curr Rev Pain 2000;4(5):353–5.
94. McDonnell JJ, Platt SR, Clayton LA. Neurologic conditions causing lameness in companion animals. Vet Clin North Am Small Anim Pract 2001;31:17–38.
95. Okada M, Kitagawa M, Shibuya H, et al. Malignant peripheral nerve sheath tumor arising from the spinal canal in a cat. J Vet med Sci 2007;69(6):683–6.
96. Platt SR, Graham J, Chrisman CL, et al. Magnetic resonance imaging and ultrasonography in the diagnosis of a malignant peripheral nerve sheath tumor in a dog. Vet Radiol Ultrasound 1999;40:367–71.
97. Rose S, Long C, Knipe M, et al. Ultrasonographic evaluation of brachial plexus tumors in five dogs. Vet Radiol Ultrasound 2005;46(6):514–7.
98. da Costa RC, Parent JM, Dobson H, et al. Ultrasound-guided fine needle aspiration in the diagnosis of peripheral nerve sheath tumors in 4 dogs. Can Vet J 2008;49(1):77–81.
99. Kraft S, Ehrhart EJ, Gall D, et al. Magnetic resonance imaging characteristics of peripheral nerve sheath tumors of the canine brachial plexus in 18 dogs. Vet Radiol Ultrasound 2007;48(1):1–7.
100. Tremblay N, Lanevschi A, Dore M, et al. Of all the nerve! A subcutaneous forelimb mass on a cat. Vet Clin Pathol 2005;34(4):417–20.
101. Montoliu P, Pumarola, Zamora A, et al. Femoral mononeuropathy caused by a malignant sarcoma: two case reports. Vet J 2007 Sep 20.
102. Jones JC, Rossmeis JH, Waldron DR, et al. Retroperitoneal hemangiosarcoma causing chronic hindlimb lameness. Vet Comp Orthop Trauma 2007;20(4): 335–9.
103. Vasilopulos RJ, Mackin AJ, Jennings D, et al. What is your neurologic diagnosis? Vet Med Today J Am Vet Med Assoc 2002;221(10):1397–9.
104. Steiss JE, Orsher AN, Bowen JM. Electrodiagnostic analysis of peripheral neuropathy in dogs with diabetes mellitus. J Vet Res 1981;12(12):2061–4.
105. Kramek BA, Moise S, Cooper B, et al. Neuropathy associated with diabetes mellitus in the cat. J AmVet Med Assoc 1984;184(1):42–5.
106. Bovie J. Central pain. In: Wall PD, Melzack R, editors. Textbook of pain. 3rd edition. New York: Churchill Livingstone; 1994. p. 871–902.
107. Holland CT, Charles JA, Smith SH, et al. Hemihyperesthesia and hyper-responsiveness resembling central pain syndrome in a dog with a forebrain oligodendroglioma. Aust Vet J 2000;78(10):676–80.
108. Rusbridge C, Jeffery ND. Pathophysiology and treatment of neuropathic pain associated with syringomyelia. Vet J 2008;175:164–72.
109. Rusbridge C. Chiari-like malformation with syringomyelia in the cavalier King Charles spaniel: long-term outcome after surgical management. Vet Surg 2007;36(5):396–405.
110. Snyder PW, Kazacos EA, Scott-Moncrieff, et al. Pathologic features of naturally occurring juvenile polyarteritis in beagle dogs. Vet Pathol 1995;32(4):337–45.
111. Albassam MA, Houston BJ, Greaves P, et al. Polyarteritis in a beagle. J Am Vet Med Assoc 1989;194(11):1595–7.
112. Buffington CA. Visceral pain in humans: lessons from animals. Curr Pain Headache Rep 2001;4:44–51.
113. Buffington CAT, Chew DJ, Woodworth BE. Feline interstitial cystitis. J Am Vet Med Assoc 1999;215:682–7.
114. Buffington CAT, Wolfe SA. High affinity binding sites for [3H] substance P in urinary bladders of cats with interstitial cystitis. J Urol 2000;163:1112–5.
115. Joshi SK, Gebhart GF. Visceral pain. Curr Rev Pain 2000;4(6):499–506.

116. Phatak S, Foster HE Jr. The management of interstitial cystitis: an update. Nat Clin Pract Urol 2006;3(1):45–53.
117. Chew DJ, Buffington CA, Kendell MS, et al. Amitriptyline treatment for severe recurrent idiopathic cystitis in cats. J Am Vet Med Assoc 1998;213:1282–6.
118. Gebhart GF. Peripheral contributions to visceral hyperalgesia. Can J Gastroenterol 1999;13(Suppl. A):37A–41.
119. Gebhart GF. Pathobiology of visceral pain: molecular mechanisms and therapeutic implications. IV. Visceral afferent contributions to the pathobiology of visceral pain. Am J Physiol Gastrointest Liver Physiol 2000;278:G834–8.
120. Moshiree B, Zhou Q, Price DD, et al. Central sensitisation in visceral pain disorders. Gut 2006;55:905–8.
121. Kogos SC Jr, Richards JS, Baños JH, et al. Visceral pain and life quality in persons with spinal cord injury: a brief report. J Spinal Cord Med 2005;28(4):333–7.
122. Jergens AF, Moore FM, Haynes JS, et al. Idiopathic inflammatory bowel disease in dogs and cats: 84 cases (1987–1990). J Am Vet Med Assoc 1992;201(10):1603–8.
123. Tams TR. Feline inflammatory bowel disease. Vet Clin North Am Small Anim Pract 1993;23(3):569–86.
124. Jergens AE. Managing the refractory case of feline IBD. J Feline Med Surg 2003;5(1):47–50.
125. Sengupta JN, Gebhart GF. Mechanosensitive afferent fibers in the gastrointestinal and lower urinary tracts. In: Gebhart GF, editor. Visceral pain. Seattle (WA): IASP Press; 1995. p. 75–98.
126. Ceyhan GO, Michalski CW, Demir IE, et al. Pancreatic pain. Best Pract Res Clin Gastroenterol 2008;22(1):31–44.
127. Dimcevski G, Sami SA, Funch-Jensen P, et al. Pain in chronic pancreatitis: the role of reorganization in the central nervous system. Gastroenterology 2007; 132(4):1546–56.
128. Kim SH, Chung JM. An experimental model for peripheral neuropathy produced by segmental spinal nerve ligation in the rat. Pain 1992;50:355–63.
129. Bennett GJ, Xie YK. A peripheral mononeuropathy in rat that produces disorders of pain sensation like those seen in man. Pain 1988;33:87–107.
130. Shir Y, Seltzer Z. A-fibres mediate mechanical hyperesthesia and allodynia and C-fibres mediate thermal hyperalgesia in a new model of causalgia from pain disorders in rats. Neurosci Lett 1990;115:62–7.
131. Hao JX, Xu XJ, Aldskogius H. Photochemically induced transient spinal ischemia induces behavioral hypersensitivity to mechanical and cold stimuli, but not to noxious-heat stimuli, in the rat. Exp Neurol 1992;118:187–94.
132. Malchow RJ, Black IH. The evolution of pain management in the critically ill trauma patient: emerging concepts from global war on terrorism. Crit Care Med 2008;36(Suppl):S345–57.
133. Lemke KA, Dawson SD. Local and regional anesthesia. Vet Clin North Am Small Anim Pract 2000;30(4):839–57.
134. Stubhaug A, Breivik H, Eide PK, et al. Mapping of punctuate hyperalgesia around a surgical incision demonstrates that ketamine is a powerful suppressor of central sensitization to pain following surgery. Acta Anaesthesiol Scand 1997; 41:1124–32.
135. Gilron I, Max MB, Lee G, et al. Effects of the AMPA/kainate antagonist LY293558 on spontaneous and evoked postoperative pain. Clin Pharmacol Ther 2000;68: 320–7.
136. McCarberg BH. The treatment of breakthrough pain. Pain Med 2007;8(Suppl 1): S8–13.

137. Simpson DM, Messina J, Hale M. Fentanyl buccal tablet for the relief of breakthrough pain in opioid-tolerant adult patients with chronic neuropathic pain: a multicenter, randomized, double-blind, placebo-controlled study. Clin Ther 2007;29(4):588–601.
138. Sacerdote P, Limiroli E, Gaspani L. Experimental evidence for immunomodulatory effects of opioids. Adv Exp Med Biol 2003;521:106–16.
139. Wallace MS. Pharmacologic treatment of neuropathic pain. Curr Pain Headache Rep 2001;5:138–50.
140. KuKanich B, Lascelles BD X, Papich MG. Validation of a high-pressure liquid chromatography and fluorescence polarization immunoassay for the determination of methadone in canine plasma. Ther Drug Monit 2005;27(3):389–92.
141. Kukanich B, Lascelles BD, Aman AM, et al. The effects of inhibiting cytochrome P450 3A, p-glycoprotein, and gastric acid secretion on the oral bioavailability of methadone in dogs. J Vet Pharmacol Ther 2005;28(5):461–6.
142. Kukanich B, Papich MG. Plasma profile and pharmacokinetics of dextromethorphan after intravenous and oral administration in healthy dogs. J Vet Pharmacol Ther 2004;27(5):337–41.
143. Correll GE, Maleki J, Gracely EJ, et al. Subanesthetic ketamine infusion therapy: a retrospective analysis of a novel therapeutic approach to complex regional pain syndrome. Pain Med 2004;5:263–75.
144. Galinski M, Dolveck F, Combes X, et al. Management of severe acute pain in emergency settings: ketamine reduces morphine consumption. Am J Emerg Med 2007;25:385–90.
145. Sveticic GMD, Gentilini AMSPD, Eichenberger UMD, et al. Combinations of morphine with ketamine for patient-controlled analgesia: a new optimization method. Anesthesiology 2003;98:1195–205.
146. Muir WW III, Wiese AJ, March PA. Effects of morphine, lidocaine, ketamine, and morphine-lidocaine-ketamine drug combination on minimum alveolar concentration in dogs anesthetized with isoflurane. Am J Vet Res 2003;64:1155–60.
147. Solano AM, Pypendop BH, Boscan PL, et al. Effect of intravenous administration of ketamine on the minimum alveolar concentration of isoflurane in anesthetized dogs. Am J Vet Res 2006;67:21–5.
148. Pascoe PJ, Ilkiw JE, Craig C, et al. The effects of ketamine on the minimum alveolar concentration of isoflurane in cats. Vet Anaesth Analg 2007;34:31–9.
149. Slingsby LS, Waterman-Pearson AE. The post-operative analgesic effects of ketamine after canine ovariohysterectomy—a comparison between pre- or post-operative administration. Res Vet Sci 2000;69:147–52.
150. Wagner AE, Walton JA, Hellyer PW, et al. Use of low doses of ketamine administered by constant rate infusion as an adjunct for postoperative analgesia in dogs. J Am Vet Med Assoc 2002;221:72–5.
151. Sarrau S, Jourdan J, Dupuis-Soyris F, et al. Effects of postoperative ketamine infusion on pain control and feeding behaviour in bitches undergoing mastectomy. J Small Anim Pract 2007.
152. Wyte SR, Shapiro HM, Turner P, et al. Ketamine-induced intracranial hypertension. Anesthesiology 1972;36:174–6.
153. Takeshita H, Okuda Y, Sari A. The effects of ketamine on cerebral circulation and metabolism in man. Anesthesiology 1972;36:69–75.
154. Schwedler M, Miletich DJ, Albrecht RF. Cerebral blood flow and metabolism following ketamine administration. Can Anaesth Soc J 1982;29(3):222–6.
155. Himmelseher S, Durieux ME. Revising a dogma: ketamine for patients with neurological injury? Anesth Analg 2005;101:524–34.

156. Albanese J, Arnaud S, Rey M, et al. Ketamine decreases intracranial pressure and electroencephalographic activity in traumatic brain injury patients during propofol sedation. Anesthesiology 1997;87:1328–34.
157. Botero CA, Smith CE, Holbrook C, et al. Total intravenous anesthesia with a propofol-ketamine combination during coronary artery surgery. J Cardiothorac Vasc Anesth 2000;14:409–15.
158. Devor M, Wall PD, Catalan N. Systemic lidocaine silences ectopic neuroma and DRG discharge without blocking nerve conduction. Pain 1992;48:261–8.
159. Nunes de Moraes A, Dyson DH, O'Grady MR, et al. Plasma concentrations and cardiovascular influence of lidocaine infusions during isoflurane anesthesia in healthy dogs and dogs with subaortic stenosis. Vet Surg 1998;27:486–97.
160. Valverde A, Doherty TJ, Hernandez J, et al. Effect of lidocaine on the minimum alveolar concentration of isoflurane in dogs. Vet Anaesth Analg 2004;31:264–71.
161. Smith LJ, Bentley E, Shih A, et al. Systemic lidocaine infusion as an analgesic for intraocular surgery in dogs: a pilot study. Vet Anaesth Analg 2004;31:53–63.
162. Challapalli V, Tremont-Lukats IW, McNicol ED, et al. Systemic administration of local anesthetic agents to relieve neuropathic pain. Cochrane Database Syst Rev 2005;19(4):CD003345.
163. Mao J, Chen LL. Systemic lidocaine for neuropathic pain relief. Pain 2000;87:7–17.
164. Pypendop BH, Ilkiw JE, Robertson SA. Effects of intravenous administration of lidocaine on the thermal threshold in cats. Am J Vet Res 2006;67:16–20.
165. Yaksh TL, Pogrel JW, Lee YW, et al. Reversal of nerve-ligation induced allodynia by spinal alpha 2 adrenoreceptor agonists. J Pharmacol Exp Ther 1995;272:207–14.
166. Meurs KM, Spier AW, Wright NA, et al. Comparison of the effects of four antiarrhythmic treatments for familial ventricular arrhythmias in boxers. J Am Vet Med Assoc 2002;221(4):522–7.
167. Rauck RL, Eisenach JC, Jackson K, et al. Epidural clonidine treatment for refractory reflex sympathetic dystrophy. Anesthesiology 1993;79(6):1163–9.
168. Reuben SS, Ekman EF. Preventing the development of chronic pain after orthopedic surgery with preventative multimodal analgesic techniques. J Bone Joint Surg Am 2007;89:1343–58.
169. Sinclair MD. A review of the physiological effects of alpha2-agonists related to the clinical use of medetomidine in small animal practice. Can Vet J 2003;44:885–97.
170. Ong BY, Arneja A, Ong EW. Effects of anesthesia on pain after lower-limb amputation. J Clin Anesth 2006;18:600–4.
171. Schulz-Stubner S, Boezart A, Hata JS. Regional analgesia in the critically ill. Crit Care Med 2005;33:1400–7.
172. Strauss KI. Antiinflammatory and neuroprotective actions of COX-2 inhibitors in injured brain. Brain Behav Immun 2008;22:285–98.
173. Felix R. Voltage-dependent calcium channel alpha2delta axillary subunit; structure, function and regulation. Recept Channels 1999;6:351–62.
174. Takeuchi Y, Takasu K, Honda M, et al. Neurochemical evidence that supraspinally administered gabapentin activates the descending noradrenergic system after peripheral nerve injury. Eur J Pharmacol 2007;556(1–3):69–74.
175. Takasu K, Honda M, Ono H, et al. Spinal alpha(2)-adrenergic and muscarinic receptors and the NO release cascade mediate supraspinally produced effectiveness of gabapentin at decreasing mechanical hypersensitivity in mice after partial nerve injury. Br J Pharmacol 2006;148(2):233–44.

176. Seib RK, Paul JE. Preoperative gabapentin for postoperative analgesia: a meta-analysis. Can J Anaesth 2006;53:461–9.
177. Tanabe M, Takasu K, Takeuchi Y, et al. Pain relief by gabapentin and pregabalin via supraspinal mechanisms after peripheral nerve injury. J Neurosci Res 2008 [Epub ahead of print].
178. Karavis M. The neurophysiology of acupuncture: a viewpoint. Acupunct Med 1997;15(1):33–42.
179. Gaynor JS. Acupuncture for management of pain. Vet Clin North Am Small Anim Pract 2000;30(4):875–84.
180. Chu LF, Clark DJ, Angst MS. Opioid tolerance and hyperalgesia in chronic pain patients after one month of oral morphine therapy: a preliminary prospective study. J Pain 2006;7(1):43–8.
181. Bichot S, Troncy E. Improving opioid use considering possible opioid-induced hyperalgesia in veterinary medicine. International Veterinary Academy of Pain Management and Université de Montreal Congress 2007, November 1–3, 2007, Montral, Quebec, Canada Proceedings. p. 339.
182. Dayer P, Desmeules J, Collart L. Pharmacology of tramadol. Drugs 1997; 53(Suppl 2):18–24.
183. Desmeules JA, Piguet V, Collart L, et al. Contribution of monoaminergic modulation to the analgesic effect of tramadol. Br J Clin Pharmacol 1996;41:7–12.
184. Arbaiza D, Vidal O. Tramadol in the treatment of neuropathic cancer pain: a double-blind, placebo-controlled study. Clin Drug Investig 2007;27:75–83.
185. Mastrocinque S, Fantoni D. A comparison of pre-operative tramadol and morphine for the control of early post-operative pain in canine ovariohysterectomy. Vet Anaesth Analg 2003;30:220–8.
186. McMillan CJ, Livingston A, Clark CR, et al. Pharmacokinetics of intravenous tramadol in dogs. Can J Vet Res 2008;72:325–31.
187. KuKanich B, Papich MG. Pharmacokinetics of tramadol and the metabolite O-desmethyltramadol in dogs. J Vet Pharmacol Ther 2004;27:239–46.
188. Gardner JS, Blough D, Drinkard CR, et al. Tramadol and seizures: a surveillance study in a managed care population. Pharmacotherapy 2000;20:1423–31.
189. Field MJ, Cox PJ, Stott E, et al. Identification of the alpha2-delta-1 subunit of voltage-dependent calcium channels as a molecular target for pain mediating the analgesic actions of pregabalin. Proc Natl Acad Sci U S A 2006;103: 17537–42.
190. Blanpied TA, Clarke RJ, Johnson JW. Amantadine inhibits NMDA receptors by accelerating channel closure during channel block. J Neurosci 2005;25: 3312–22.
191. Lascelles BDX, Gaynor J, Smith ES, et al. Evaluation of amantadine in a multimodal analgesic regimen for the alleviation of refractory canine osteoarthritis pain. J Vet Intern Med 2008;22(1):53–9.
192. Kraijer M, Fink-Gremmels J, Nickel RF. The short-term clinical efficacy of amitriptyline in the management of idiopathic feline lower urinary tract disease: a controlled clinical study. J Feline Med Surg 2003;5(3):191–6.
193. Brochu RM, Dick IE, Tarpley JW. Block of peripheral nerve sodium channels selectively inhibits features of neuropathic pain in rats. Mol Pharmacol 2006;69: 823–32.
194. Nayak S, Cunliffe M. Lidocaine 5% patch for localized chronic neuropathic pain in adolescents: report of five cases. Pediatric Anesth 2008;18:554–8.
195. Weiland L, Croubels S, Baert K, et al. Pharmacokinetics of a lidocaine patch 5% in dogs. J Vet Med 2006;53:34–9.

196. Ko J, Weil A, Maxwell L, et al. Plasma concentrations of lidocaine in dogs following lidocaine patch application. J Am Anim Hosp Assoc 2007;43:280–3.
197. Sisson A. Current experiences with anticonvulsants in dogs and cats. In: Proceedings of the 15th American College of Veterinary Internal Medicine Forum. Lake Buena Vista, Fl; 1997. p. 596–8.
198. Cui M, Honore P, Zhong C, et al. TRPV1 receptors in the CNS play a key role in broad-spectrum analgesia of TRPV1 antagonists. J Neurosci 2006;26(37):9385–93.
199. Jones CK, Peters SC, Shannon HE. Efficacy of Duloxetine, a potent and balanced serotonergic and noradrenergic reuptake inhibitor, in inflammatory and acute pain models in rodents. J Pharmacol Exp Ther 2005;312:726–32.

Pain Management: The Veterinary Technician's Perspective

Nancy Shaffran, CVT, VTS (ECC)

KEYWORDS

- Analgesia • Pain assessment
- Visual analogue scale • Dysphoria

As the practice of pain management becomes mainstream in veterinary medicine, experts continually offer up, and debate, the efficacy of analgesic drugs, combinations, methods of administration, and alternative therapies. The search also continues for the most objective scientific methods of measuring and assessing pain in our patients. A survey (Shaffran and colleagues, unpublished data, 1993) of veterinarians and technicians at four teaching hospitals revealed consistency in terms of answering the simple question: "How do you know when your patient is in pain?" The responses were quite similar among the different groups (ie, veterinarians, veterinary students, veterinary technicians) and across geographic areas. The only striking difference between veterinarians and the other groups was that nearly all the veterinarians responded "because my technician tells me," which was within the top 10 reasons on their lists. This is not surprising, given the huge role that human nurses have played in pain management for their nonverbal patients.[1] Human neonatal and pediatric nurses and veterinary technicians share the position of patient advocate, giving their patients voice and attending to their perceived needs. Unlike human medicine, however, veterinary technicians typically do this without the help of parents, who play a large role in advocating for their hospitalized children.

The quality of pain management in practices seems to be directly related to veterinary technicians. A study done in Canada in 1999 showed that pain management practice increased proportionately with the number of licensed veterinary technicians on staff and relative to the amount of continuing education the technicians received.[2]

The role of advocate for a nonverbal patient can be daunting. Veterinary technicians are in the unique position of being responsible for most of and the quality of patient care without the freedom to prescribe or initiate therapy. This often results in the recurring, and sometimes frustrating, pursuit of a positive response from veterinarians

88 Geigel Hill Road, Erwinna, PA 18920, USA
E-mail address: nancy.shaffran@pfizer.com

Vet Clin Small Anim 38 (2008) 1415–1428
doi:10.1016/j.cvsm.2008.07.002
vetsmall.theclinics.com

toward administration of analgesics. Knowledge of the physiology of pain and pharmacology of analgesics is essential for good communication between veterinarians and veterinary technicians. Optimally, the veterinarian regards the technician as an integral member of the pain management team. The skilled technician is a source of vital information required to choose and administer appropriate analgesics. He or she is a trusted caretaker for hospitalized patients. The success of this relationship is terribly important for all patients and applies to elective, routine, and extraordinary cases. The critical care setting may best demonstrate the crucial role that veterinary technicians play in providing optimum patient care, wherein the concentrated interactive nature of the nurse-patient relationship is coupled with severely diminished communication skills of the critically ill patient. Nowhere more than in the intensive care unit (ICU) is this relationship more apparent. Technicians in the ICU observe patients closely for extended periods and are usually the first to notice changes in status. Familiarity with patient personalities and reactions to stimuli give additional insight into how particular patients may react to painful stimuli. This includes the differences in expression between dogs and cats, the young and old, and variations among certain breeds. For example, Siberian huskies and Doberman pinschers, who vocalize regularly even in nonpainful situations, can be more difficult to assess with respect to pain. They are often thought to be more "sensitive" to pain, or to possess a lower pain threshold than other breeds, when, in fact, they are likely using a communication style typical of the breed to convey similar pain or stress to other patients. On the other hand, pit bulls and Labrador retrievers seem to remain stoical in the face of pain, also making pain assessment difficult. The skilled technician factors this into his or her pain assessments.

Many technicians perform daily responsibilities without adequate knowledge about the pharmacology of analgesics or the physiology of the pain process. This knowledge is essential, however, if the technician is to contribute maximally to the pain management strategies of his or her practice. Familiarity with the current principles of pain management, including preemptive and multimodal therapies, and prevention of the wind-up phenomenon are vital and must be put into practice. When technicians are appropriately trained in all these aspects of pain management, they become a vital force in the perpetuation of optimum care for surgical, medical, and chronically painful patients.

- Patient assessment
- Providing nonpharmacologic comfort and care
- Differentiating pain from other stress
- Requesting appropriate analgesia and sedation
- Administering medications and performing analgesic techniques
- Monitoring and treating drug effects
- Assessing patients after surgery
- Communicating with clients about hospital and at-home care
- Logging controlled substances

TREATMENT GOALS AND COMMUNICATION

The goal of providing the best pain management protocols for small animal patients is achieved when working together as a team. Communication among all members of the entire health care team, including veterinarians, veterinary technicians and nurses, assistants, and pet owners, is essential for consistent pain management. The veterinary nurse and veterinarian perpetuate optimum care through written and verbal communication. The veterinarian should write clear orders, including specific drug(s) and initial dosages. Veterinarians should not fall into trap of "ticking the box" when it comes to pain management, however. In that case, once a particular analgesic is ordered, the subject is closed. Veterinary technicians have the responsibility of continually monitoring their patients and often develop a sense of which analgesics seem to work best under various circumstances.

TECHNICIAN AND CLINICIAN

Discussion about each case directly with the clinician should address particular concerns or expectations, potential for adjustments in analgesic regimens (eg, as needed injections to a constant rate infusion [CRI]), changes or additions to drug protocols (eg, adding a nonsteroidal anti-inflammatory drug [NSAID] or an adjunctive analgesic), or the possible addition of sedatives if needed. Once these guidelines have been established, allowing the nursing staff to decide when the drug is needed creates the most appropriate approach to pain management. This also empowers the nursing team to use their critical thinking, observation, and interpretation skills.

As previously mentioned, veterinary technicians often complain that their requests for patient analgesia go unheeded. The actual method of communication plays a large part in achieving a positive outcome. For example: "Can I give Charlie something for pain?" is inadequate to convey the situation and often results in a negative response. To be effective, technicians must present two sets of information: (1) what the patient is doing that indicates painfulness and (2) that which already has been done and considered inadequate. For example: "My patient Charlie, the black lab, which had a cruciate repair yesterday, is not doing as well as I would like. Despite the fact that his bladder is empty and I have offered him food and water, he seems restless and has difficulty in getting comfortable. He is panting excessively, although his temperature is normal. I checked the bandage, and it does not seem too tight. The record says he got morphine last night at midnight, which allowed him to sleep for 4 hours, but he has not had any since. Could we try a repeat dose to see if it makes him more comfortable? Or, because his biochemical profile is normal, would you consider administering a nonsteroidal analgesic?"

This approach delivers the necessary information to gain the veterinarian's confidence in the technician's assessment skills and knowledge of the case. He or she is much more likely to agree to administer pain medication under these circumstances.

Technicians can also play a vital role in the administration of preemptive medication, which is often overlooked in a busy hospital setting. For example: "I have really noticed a difference in the recovery of the animals who receive a dose of NSAID or hydromorphone before surgery. We have the preoperative blood work and the renal values are normal. Would you like me to give an NSAID to this patient now?" This approach should also be used when suggesting the placement of transdermal analgesic patches, starting CRIs, and performing local or regional nerve blocks.

TECHNICIAN TO TECHNICIAN

Overlap in schedules provides the team members time to discuss the animal's case in detail before the shift change occurs. This exchange of information during rounds is vital in that it provides specific information, such as history, complications, current concerns, and treatment goals. Pain management issues, such as the appearance and behavior of the patient that prompted the administration of analgesics; the type, dose, and timing of previous analgesic administration; and the response and any adverse reactions after administration, should be described. This information can be used to guide treatment during the next shift and to improve the continuity of care. Treatment objectives should also be clearly expressed at this time. For example, is a plane of steady analgesia with regular dosing optimal, or is weaning off the goal? It can be quite frustrating for the day shift to work to achieve a steady state of pain management only to have the night shift omit scheduled dosages because of misunderstood objectives. Conversely, a shift change allows for a fresh perspective. It is not uncommon, after a long shift, for staff to become accustomed and nonreactive to behaviors that may indicate discomfort to the incoming team. Completing a patient summary at the end of every night shift, including comments on the patient's comfort level, provides a valuable source of information for incoming personnel who were not present for rounds and for retrospective pain management studies.

As Needed Orders

Giving technicians greater choice and control over pain management involves trusting their judgment and experience. After standing orders are established, the success of pain management relies on giving skilled technicians the freedom to give analgesics as needed, to adjust dosages when required, to administer adjunctive medications, and to potentially reverse drugs when severe adverse reactions occur. Most opioid orders should be on a set schedule; however, there must be the option to provide additional doses on an as needed basis. This gives the technician the ability to respond to patients quickly, without looking for authorization after the patient becomes painful. Conversely, as perioperative pain subsides, the requirement for every 4 hours dosing of an opioid may be reduced to every 5 or 6 hours, avoiding the unwanted adverse effects of too frequent dosing when not required. CRIs should be ordered with a dose range allowing the technician to titrate up or down easily depending on individual patient response. When appropriate, orders for additional sedation, if needed, can significantly improve pain management by removing the fear and anxiety that can exacerbate pain. When anxiety is assumed to be a component of abnormal behavior, bolus dosing or CRI using a low dose of an α_2-agonist can be quite effective; however, patients must be healthy otherwise. Alternatively, especially when the patient may be older or there are cardiovascular concerns, acepromazine administered intravenously at a dose of 0.01 mg/kg (Karol Mathews, DVM, DVSc, personal communication, 2008) is an excellent sedative or anxiolytic. This dosing has no effect on blood pressure, as noted on direct blood pressure monitoring. The reader is referred to specific articles elsewhere in this issue for suggested pain management regimens.

Working with painful patients for long hours often creates a stressful environment for veterinary technicians. Technicians should be entrusted with the responsibility and freedom to administer agreed-on analgesics. Giving technicians a voice in the pain management process creates a truly positive team environment in which their thoughts and skills are valued. Patients ultimately receive better care, and technicians are satisfied knowing that they are doing everything they can to ensure the well-being of patients in their charge.

PATIENT ASSESSMENT

In current human medicine, preventing and treating pain is recognized as an essential part of overall patient management. In fact, pain is considered to play such an important role in overall health and well-being that it is now considered to be a fifth vital sign, ranking it of equal importance with temperature, pulse, respiration, and blood pressure.[3] Not only do human health care providers view pain as a symptom of an underlying disease or condition, but they view pain as an important syndrome in its own right. This is attributable to the vast array of negative physiologic events attributable to pain, regardless of the patient's underlying disease or condition. There has been a lag in regulation of the approach to pain management in veterinary medicine; however, recent changes to the American Animal Hospital Association (AAHA) standards require that pain assessment be included in every veterinary patient assessment regardless of presenting complaint. Other requirements include making repeat regular assessments throughout hospitalization and recording of those assessments in the medical record. A full listing of the AAHA pain management standards can be found on the AAHA Web site.[4]

In people and animals, pain triggers a series of physiologic changes that increase stress. Although the nervous system is the main target of nociceptive (pain transmission) information and provides the means for the body to react to that information, the body's resulting response is not limited to the nervous system. Most, if not all, of the body's major systems are affected by inadequately controlled pain. For example, the increased cortisol levels that can accompany pain may interfere with wound healing and reduce the immune system's ability to work effectively. In addition to suppressing the immune system, increased sympathetic nervous system activity associated with unrelieved pain may result in increased catabolism and metabolic rate, anorexia, ileus, and atelectasis. The cardiovascular system is also adversely affected, resulting in increased heart rate and blood pressure, irregular heart rhythms, and coagulopathies. Reducing or suppressing the stress response by managing pain can minimize adverse effects on the cardiovascular system, including fewer cardiac arrhythmias. Given these potential consequences, it becomes obvious that, like human beings, animals in pain require more intensive medical care than those whose pain is adequately managed (see the article on The Stress and Distress Associated with Pain).

All patients should be evaluated for painfulness on admission and at regular intervals throughout the hospitalization period. Some pain signs may be obvious (eg, vocalization or agitation with increased heart rate, blood pressure, or respiratory rate). Subtle behavioral changes, such as restlessness, decreased appetite, insomnia, resistance to handling, and abnormal posture, are more common and often more significant signs.[5,6] The observer's subjective opinion and physiologic signs can be described using a pain scale, such as a visual analog scale (VAS).[7] A VAS designed for use in nonverbal human patients uses pictorial rather than numeric rating systems. The main difference between a human VAS and an animal VAS is that in human medicine, the patient is the reporter of his or her own pain level, whereas in veterinary medicine, VAS readings are most often provided by a veterinary technician who is describing pain for the patient. As an example of a veterinary pictorial rating scale, see **Fig. 1** for dogs and **Fig. 2** for cats, wherein any score greater than 0 indicates a need for varying degrees of analgesia. Patients scoring 1 may be manageable on NSAIDs alone, whereas patients with higher scores are likely to need additional therapy, such as opioids, CRI, epidural, and anti-windup drugs. Regardless of the specific tool used, pain assessments should be made at 4- to 6-hour intervals throughout hospitalization in the general patient population and much more frequently in the critical care setting, wherein patient status is more dynamic. During the immediate postoperative period, and throughout the critical phase, patients should be monitored as often as every 30 minutes. For consistency, assessments should be performed by the same person whenever possible. Repeated recorded assessments allow evaluation of the efficacy of analgesic protocols and make the response to specific drugs more obvious. A complete patient description, including physiologic signs (eg, temperature, pulse, respiration) and behavioral signs (eg, vocalization, posturing, eating and sleeping habits) should be documented in the medical record. A simple chart system allows evaluation of the efficacy of the analgesic protocol (**Fig. 3**). The way to move the

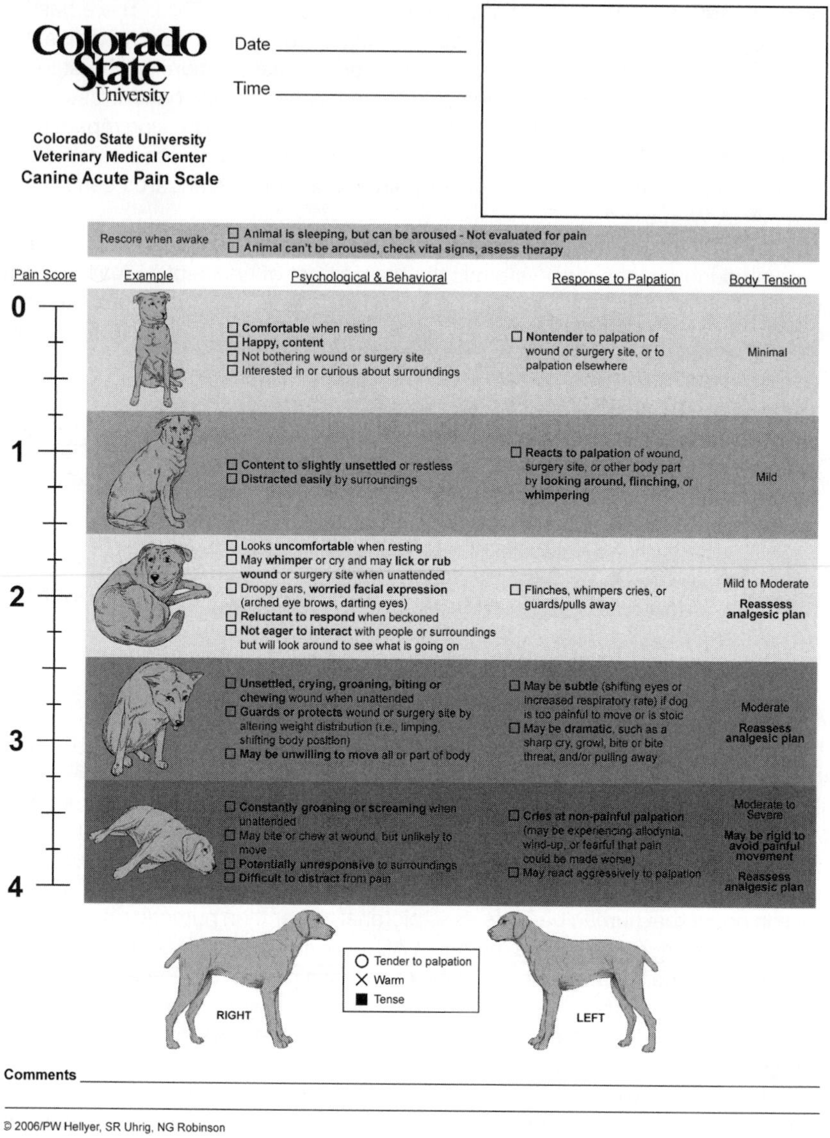

Fig. 1. Colorado State University Veterinary Medical Center Canine Acute Pain Scale. (*Courtesy of* P.W. Hellyer, DVM, MS, Fort Collins, CO.)

practice of pain management from a rote or happenstance event to a sound medical approach is by careful documentation of analgesic type, dose, frequency, and, most importantly, response throughout the treatment period. Documentation of the patient's response to the analgesic protocol also helps to determine when discontinuation of analgesics would be possible.

Experienced veterinary technicians rarely need to be trained to recognize an animal in distress. With experience, technicians become skillful observers of behavioral changes in their patients, noticing the subtlest expressions of potential pain. Most technicians also acquire a sense of how painful most procedures, conditions, and

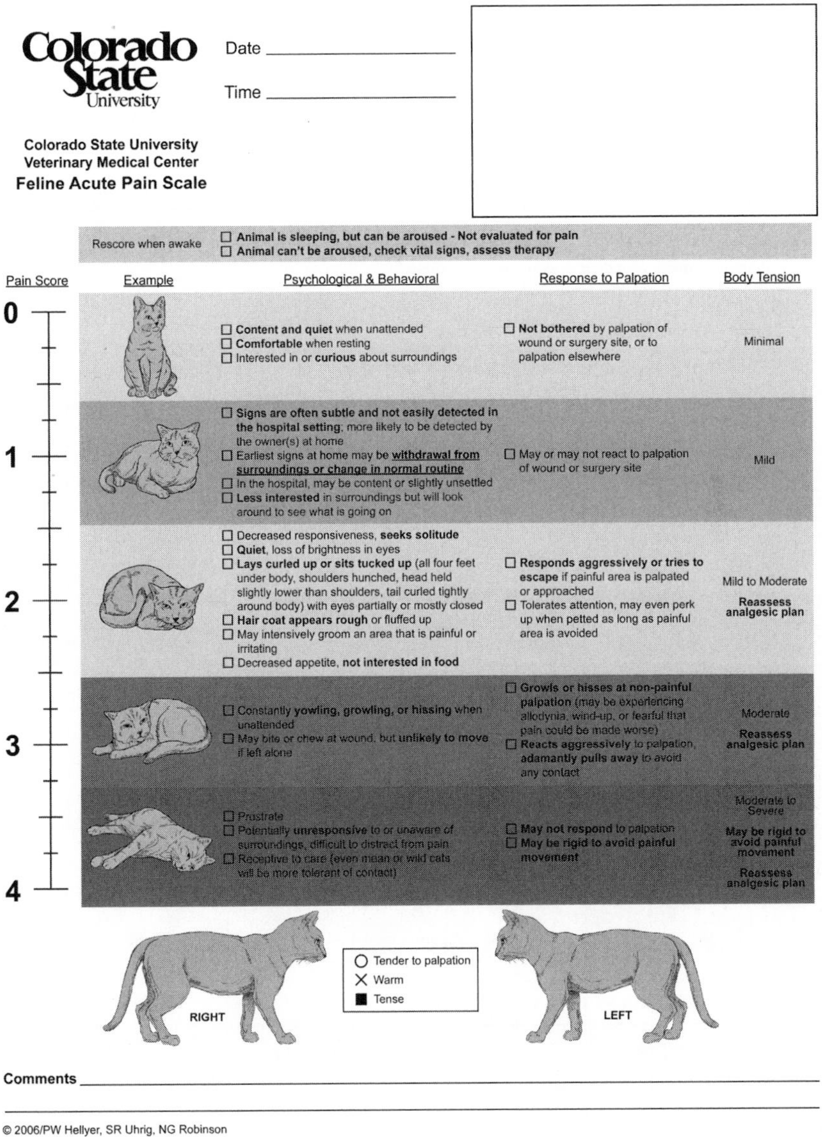

Fig. 2. Colorado State University Veterinary Medical Center Feline Acute Pain Scale. (*Courtesy of* P.W. Hellyer, DVM, MS, Fort Collins, CO.)

surgical procedures are likely to be, based on repeated prolonged exposure to animals in the recovery phase. Nevertheless, it is often difficult for even the most experienced technician to distinguish between pain and other stress (eg, fear, anxiety). Differentiating between pain and dysphoria after drug administration or anesthesia presents additional challenges.

Differentiating Pain from Other Stress or Dysphoria

Postoperative patients frequently display aberrant behavior for several minutes to hours after surgery. These behaviors may include vocalization, thrashing, rolling,

Analgesia/Response LOG

Date: ______ Start Time: _________

Patient Name: ________________________ Case #:___________

Procedure/Condition:____

OTHER PAIN MANAGEMENT THERAPIES INITIATED: ***(Include padding used, position, physical therapy-frequency/method, environmental changes)***

____

____

Drug Name	Dosage	Dose	Time Given	Route (CRI, IV, IM. SQ)	Time Effect Assessed	Observations	Interpretation	Scale Rating

Fig. 3. Analgesia/Response LOG. (*Courtesy of* Andrea Battaglia, Syracuse, NY.)

self-mutilation, and tachypnea. Often, it is difficult to discern between pain, other stress, and reaction to opioids or general anesthesia. Differentiation is critical for determining effective treatment (ie, additional analgesics, reversing the opioid, administering sedatives). Many veterinary professionals describe abnormal postoperative behaviors as "emergence delirium," attributing the events to residual inhalant anesthesia. Anesthesia-related behaviors should resolve within several minutes. Behaviors that persist beyond a few minutes require further investigation and attention. Most animals experiencing mild to moderate pain can be temporarily soothed by speaking in low tones during a petting interaction, although painful behaviors normally resume when the patient is left alone. These patients seem to recognize that someone is with them and usually make eye contact. A patient who stops the abnormal behaviors in the presence of a calming person is likely to be in pain rather than having a drug reaction; however, this may not typify the response of a patient who is consumed by severe pain or is extremely anxious and not painful. Claustrophobia, usually in medium- to large-sized dogs that occupy most of the cage, also contributes to anxiety and vocalization. Painful animals also respond when the area around the source of pain is gently palpated. This should confirm the suspicion of painfulness and prompt the administration of additional analgesics. Animals that are dysphoric or "delirious" because of opioid overdose rarely respond to soothing interaction or to light palpation of the painful area. These patients may benefit from sedation or partial opioid reversal using careful titration, which is usually reserved for patients who do not respond to distraction or sedation or have a physiologic condition that is of immediate medical concern. Recently, treating otherwise healthy patients with a combination sedative analgesia drug, such as a low-dose α_2–agonist, has become popular in the immediate postoperative period.

SOUND APPROACH TO ASSESSMENT

Historically, animal pain has been recognized and treated only in those patients that display overt behavioral signs, such as vocalization. By requiring animals to show dramatic signs, patients are forced to prove that they are in pain before they are given analgesics. In reality, many animals instinctively hide pain just as they would in the wild to avoid becoming prey. Some may be too ill or injured to have the resources available to commit to behavioral change.[8] By the time these animals do show obvious signs of pain, its intensity is likely to be severe. Patients should never be required to prove they are in pain. A sound approach to pain management favors anticipation of the severity and duration of pain that is likely to occur with any procedure, condition, or operation. A list of anticipated levels of pain associated with surgical procedures, illness, or injuries is available.[5]

Categorization of the expected severity (mild, moderate, or severe) of pain is used to establish the initial type of analgesia and the duration of treatment. Dosages can be adjusted later according to individual patient needs. Baseline treatment is chosen based on knowledge of the mechanisms of pain; drug dosages and expected duration; pain assessment; and the knowledge of the expected levels of pain for injury, surgery, or diseases. The initial approach should be based on the following questions:

- How painful is the condition, procedure, or surgery expected to be?
- Are there any underlying factors, such as stress, anxiety, fear, or preexisting chronic pain conditions, that could intensify acute symptoms?
- What is the normal behavior or disposition of the particular breed and for this animal in particular?
- Are there any contraindications to particular drugs or drug classes for this patient's condition?
- Does this animal have a history of drug sensitivities?

Nonpharmacologic Interventions

Pain likely has physical and psychologic components. Fear and anxiety can exacerbate pain and vice versa. Attending to an animal's physical and perceived emotional needs can reduce stress, and consequently minimize pain levels. A blind or deaf patient has special needs, because the stress is compounded by these disabilities. Also, environmental factors seem to affect the perception of pain in pets. The hospitalized patient is in unfamiliar surroundings and may be comforted by a favorite blanket or toy.

Veterinary technicians must be adept at "reading" patients, because the emotional needs of individual dogs and cats vary greatly. A comforting hand or a soothing voice can ease stress and make pain assessment easier. Skilled technicians know when a visit by the owner would be therapeutic and when it would more likely create anxiety in the patient. Astute technicians can also sense which animals are likely to recuperate better in a quiet environment and which patients are best distracted by exposure to a more active area of the hospital.

Patient comfort can be improved by minimizing painful procedures. Many nursing interventions, such as venipuncture and injections, cause pain. This can be reduced by coordination of required laboratory tests and treatments to minimize the total number of painful events. Increased technical skill also reduces the intensity of related pain. Patient protective policies such as a "two-stick rule" (any individual should attempt venipuncture or intravenous catheter placement no more than two times) should be instituted.

Animals have the potential to injure themselves in response to pain, such as an animal recovering from general anesthesia that may be weak and disoriented. Many problems can be avoided by providing a cage of appropriate size, with extra padding and careful positioning to reduce pressure on painful areas, also keeping in mind patients that have preexisting painful conditions, such as arthritis. Cages must be kept clean and dry, and patients should be groomed regularly. Fresh food and water should be available, and opportunities should be created for animals to receive sunshine and fresh air. Physical therapy and warm compresses help to relieve pain after orthopedic procedures.

Wherever the patient is housed in the hospital, environmental stressors caused by continual activity and disruption can be reduced by playing low soothing music or a white noise machine and by installing a dimming switch for the lights. The patient's cage should be designated as a safe zone, and all procedures considered noxious should be performed elsewhere whenever possible. This allows for the animal to feel comfortable and safe when in the cage.

Given the potential for a varying number of treatments required for the individual patient, care must be taken to allow for periods of undisturbed rest. Grouping treatments to reduce the number of disruptions is optimal. Also, so that animals do not associate contact with an unpleasant experience, initiate a "three-one rule". For every time the animal is exposed to an uncomfortable situation or invasive procedure, follow with three positive experiences, such as a petting, grooming, or feeding.

Providing these adjunctive nonpharmacologic actions can reduce pain and reduce the analgesic drug requirement by removing other stressors. Tending to patient's comfort needs should not be seen as a substitute for analgesia, however.

PRINCIPLES OF ADMINISTRATION OF ANALGESIA

Our improved understanding of the impact of pain on the body is shaping new philosophies in managing patient pain. Several basic principles are used in the approach to designing analgesic protocols and are particularly important in the perioperative period.

- Administering preemptive analgesics whenever possible seems to be much more effective than using the same agent to treat pain once it occurs. Analgesia given

before a noxious stimulus reduces postprocedure analgesia requirements, minimizes detrimental effects of pain, improves patient handling, lowers sedation or anesthetic requirements, and reduces hypersensitization.
- Use multimodal analgesia to take advantage of the synergistic effects obtained by combining two or more classes of analgesic drugs to alter more than one phase (transduction, transmission, modulation, and perception) of nociception. Drug combinations often produce better pain relief than single agents, thereby reducing the amount of each drug used and minimizing the risk for side effects.
- Match analgesics (based on dosage and duration of action) to the degree of expected surgical pain rather than to the patient's ability to express pain in a recognizable way.
- Maintain an analgesic plane once pain control is established. This may include scheduled intermittent dosing and additional administration (as needed) as indicated by patient response. For moderate to severely painful procedures or for more critical patients, the use of epidural analgesia and CRIs may be warranted.[9] Analgesics may be gradually tapered off as patients improve (see the articles by Dyson elsewhere in this issue).

Analgesics and Analgesic Techniques

There are a variety of techniques for administering analgesics. Trained technicians are able to deliver drugs by oral, transmucosal, subcutaneous, intramuscular, intravenous, transcutaneous, epidural, and CRI routes. Detailed descriptions of many analgesic techniques are available elswhere[10–12] and in various articles in this issue.

Given the fragile, transient, or unknown cardiovascular status of critically ill patients, opioids are often the analgesia of choice. The route of administration should be intravenous or intramuscular for maximal drug absorption. In conjunction with opioids, local and regional blocking techniques can be used safely in several patients. When specific nerves cannot be identified for blockade in dogs, lidocaine can be administered intravenously by CRI for systemic analgesia. Administering drugs by CRI provides excellent control and reduces the overall lower dose of individual agents.

When using an opiate alone, beginning in the middle of the recommended dose range is usually appropriate, with the option to increase the dose if pain behaviors persist or recur sooner than expected. Some animals may not exhibit typical signs of pain or may have a history of not reacting well to typical dosages of analgesics. In those situations, the dosage can be started at the low end and increased incrementally until effective pain control is achieved. With the titration approach, the technician monitors for subtle changes ensuring adequate analgesia and avoiding adverse drug reactions, such as nausea, panting, or an increase in anxiety. If an opioid is not effective, it may need to be given in conjunction with other analgesics. This may involve adding another analgesic class, such as an NSAID, CRI of lidocaine, ketamine, or α^2-agonist, or placing a fentanyl patch for long-term care. This approach may allow for a lower dose of opioids to be administered, avoiding the potential development of dysphoria seen with higher doses.

Monitoring Patients on Analgesics

One of the most common reasons given by veterinary professionals for withholding analgesics is fear of side effects. In reality, adverse side effects associated with appropriate doses of analgesic drugs are rare. Opioid-induced respiratory compromise is most often mentioned but is of much greater concern in human patients than in animals. In fact, pain can sometimes play a much greater role in limiting respiration than opioid effects.

Another concern often voiced is "the inability to monitor patients effectively" when analgesics are given. On the contrary, pain can cause several aberrant physiologic findings (eg, tachypnea, tachycardia, elevated body temperature, panting, increased blood pressure, restlessness) and severely limits the ability to assess other causes of this sympathetic response. Managing pain appropriately actually eliminates the pain-induced sympathetic response. Therefore, continuing tachycardia or tachypnea, for example, indicates a physiologic response to abnormal condition(s), allowing for more accurate monitoring of the true physiologic status in most cases. Veterinary technicians should also monitor for the possible adverse effects of analgesic agents during the perioperative period and throughout the course of treatment. Monitoring includes temperature, pulse, heart rate and rhythm, respiratory rate and ventilatory nature, and arterial blood pressure (**Table 1**). Activity level, behavior, and ability to move are also noted.

Weaning from Analgesic Therapy

As patients recover, the level or mode of pain management is decreased or altered to prepare for discharge from the hospital. CRIs are discontinued by slowly decreasing the dose (rate of administration) over a period of hours. Additional bolus injections may be necessary during the weaning phase if the animal begins to display an increased pain response. Fentanyl patches, oral opioids, or NSAIDs can be used in the transitional phase. A combination of analgesics is required until therapeutic levels of fentanyl are reached after the patch is applied. This time may range from 6 to 12 hours in the cat and from 12 to 24 hours in the dog. Do not supplement with butorphanol or buprenorphine. Keen observation is required during this phase so as not to allow managed pain to resume.

SPECIAL CONSIDERATIONS IN THE INTENSIVE CARE UNIT

Critically ill patients present unique challenges in terms of pain recognition and treatment options.[9] The analgesic needs for this patient population are likely to be increased over those of more stable patients. Choosing the correct analgesic therapy requires an understanding of the pharmacokinetics of a wide range of drugs and

Table 1
Recommended monitoring techniques for analgesic adverse events

Agent	Adverse Effect	Monitoring
Opioids	Sedation, dysphoria, low blood pressure, respiratory depression (rare), panting, hyperthermia	Mentation, blood pressure, respiratory rate, and nature of temperature
Local anesthetics	None unless given by CRI; then, nausea, vomiting, neurologic signs, and seizures	Observe regularly for muscle tremors and gastrointestinal upset
NSAIDs (ensure no contraindications before administration)	Gastrointestinal disturbances, gastrointestinal bleeding, renal disturbances	General observation, hydration status, stool quality, and urine production
α_2-Agonists	Bradycardia, cardiac arrhythmias, hypertension, and peripheral vasoconstriction	Palpate femoral pulse rate and quality, auscult heart and blood pressure

the levels or types of pain associated with various conditions. Failure to manage pain adequately in the critically ill impedes recovery and can contribute to patient morbidity and mortality. Although critically ill patients may be in the greatest need of pain relief, they are often the least likely to receive it because of persistent fears regarding drug side affects and overall ability to monitor progress. In fact, the physiologic signs accompanying pain, particularly tachypnea, tachycardia, and blood pressure changes, obscure the ability to provide true monitoring of patient condition. Until pain and its myriad of signs are removed from the equation, it is impossible to assess a critical patient's metabolic needs accurately.

Special considerations are raised for animals with specific critical disorders. For example, the selection of pharmaceutic pain management for an animal with head trauma must be approached with caution. Pharmacologic alteration of central nervous system activity can occur, making it difficult to assess changes in behavior and mentation. Similarly, analgesic selection for pregnant or lactating animals and for extremely young animals requires special consideration (see the articles by Mathews elsewhere in this issue).[13] Selection of analgesics may also need to be approached with caution in animals with other medical conditions, such as pancreatitis or other severe gastrointestinal disturbances, renal disease, or those receiving medication for unrelated problems.[14] Understanding the pharmacology of analgesic drugs and the associated side effects plays a key role in treatment for critical patients. Severe trauma or illness is never a reason to withhold using pharmaceutic pain management, however. It is a reason to be more creative with pain management protocols (see the article by Dyson elsewhere in this issue).

SUMMARY

Effective pain management is not an individual endeavor. It requires a team approach involving everyone who participates in patient care. Veterinary technicians constitute a vital force in this effort. A successful technician understands the goals of pain control and the analgesic options. Combining keen observation with good technical skills, the technician functions as a true patient advocate who appropriately assesses requests and administers analgesics to his or her patients. Veterinary technicians have played a vital role in bringing animal pain management to the forefront of veterinary practice. Through continued teaching and vigilant practice, technicians should be credited in large part for the continuing change in pain management standards.

REFERENCES

1. Coffman S, Alvarez Y, Pyngolil M, et al. Nursing assessment and management of pain in critically ill children. Heart Lung 1997;26(3):221–8.
2. Dohoo SE, Dohoo IR. Attitudes and concerns of Canadian animal health technologists toward postoperative pain management in dogs and cats. Can Vet J 1998; 39:491–6.
3. McCaffrey M. Pain ratings: the fifth vital sign. Am J Nurs 1997;97:15–6.
4. Available at: www.aaha.org.
5. Mathews KA. Pain assessment and general approach to management. Vet Clin North Am Small Anim Pract 2000;30(4):729–52.
6. Hansen B. Through a glass darkly: using behavior to assess pain. Semin Vet Med Surg (Small Anim) 1997;12(2):61–74.
7. Lascelles BD, Cripps PJ, Jones A, et al. Efficacy and kinetics of carprofen, administered preoperatively or postoperatively, for the prevention of pain in dogs undergoing ovariohysterectomy. Vet Surg 1998;27(6):568–82.

8. Robertson S. Assessment and management of acute pain in cats. J Vet Emerg Crit Care 2005;15(4):261–72.
9. Hansen BD. Analgesia and sedation in the critically ill. J Vet Emerg Crit Care 2005;15(4):285–94.
10. Tranquilli WJ, Grimm KA, Lamont LA. Pain management for the small animal practitioner. 2nd edition. Jackson (WY): Teton New Media; 2004.
11. Gaynor JS, Muir W. Handbook of veterinary pain management. St. Louis (MO): Mosby; 2002.
12. Mathews KA. PAIN—how to recognize treat stop (HURTS), version 1 [computer program]. Guelph, ON (Canada): Jonkar Veterinary Systems; 2003.
13. Mathews KA. Analgesia for the pregnant, lactating, neonatal, and pediatric cat and dog. J Vet Emerg Crit Care 2005;15(4):273–84.
14. Trepanier LA. Potential interactions between non-steroidal anti-inflammatory drugs and other drugs. J Vet Emerg Crit Care 2005;15(4):248–53.

Control of Cancer Pain in Veterinary Patients

James S. Gaynor, DVM, MS

KEYWORDS

• Dog • Cat • Cancer • Oncology • Pain

The treatment of cancer has become more commonplace in veterinary practice as knowledge, drugs, and therapeutic techniques evolve. Although some cancers still are not effectively treated, many owners attempt various measures at prolonging their pet's life. Regardless of the prognosis, it is vitally important to attempt to alleviate the pet's pain. It is estimated that cancer pain can be effectively managed in 90% of human beings with currently available drugs and techniques.[1] There is no reason to believe that the same success could not be achieved in small animals.

There are four main steps in ensuring that pain management is optimized in veterinary patients. The first step is to ensure that veterinarians have the appropriate education and training about the importance of alleviating pain, assessment of pain, available drugs and potential complications, and interventional techniques. The next step is educating the client about realistic expectations surrounding pain control and conveying the idea that most patients' pain can be managed. This involves letting the client know that owner involvement in evaluating the pet and providing feedback on therapy is crucial to success. The veterinarian and owner should all participate in developing effective strategies to alleviate pain. Client involvement also helps to decrease the potential feeling of helplessness. The third step is to assess the pet's pain thoroughly at the start and throughout the course of therapy, and not just when it gets severe. The fourth step is having good support from the veterinary practice or institution for the use of opioids and other controlled substances.

Effective alleviation of pain requires some basic understanding of pain itself. Pain is defined as "an unpleasant sensory and emotional experience associated with actual or potential tissue damage, or described in terms of such damage."[2–4] Although this definition was originally developed for use in human beings, it applies to animals as well. The emotional component is often overlooked and untreated. The physiology of pain has been described in great detail elsewhere.[5] It is important to realize that there are different types of pain that a patient can experience, necessitating different

Peak Performance Veterinary Group, 5520 North Nevada Avenue, Colorado Springs, CO 80918, USA
E-mail address: jgaynor@nopetpain.com

Vet Clin Small Anim 38 (2008) 1429–1448
doi:10.1016/j.cvsm.2008.06.009 vetsmall.theclinics.com
0195-5616/08/$ – see front matter

approaches to therapy (**Box 1**). Following are some basic definitions for terms used when discussing pain in general, and cancer pain in particular:

IMPORTANCE OF ALLEVIATING PAIN

The alleviation of pain is important for physiologic and ethical reasons.[6,7] Briefly, pain can induce a stress response in patients that is associated with elevations in corticotropin, cortisol, antidiuretic hormone (ADH), catecholamines, aldosterone, renin, angiotensin II, and glucose, along with decreases in insulin and testosterone. These changes can result in a general catabolic state with muscle protein catabolism and lipolysis, in addition to retention of water and sodium and excretion of potassium.[8] A prolonged stress response can decrease the rate of healing. In addition, the stress response can have adverse effects on the cardiovascular and pulmonary systems, fluid homeostasis, and gastrointestinal tract function.[7,9,10] It is important to minimize the stress response to have better overall health of the patient that has cancer.

Veterinarians have an ethical obligation to treat animal pain.[11,12] Most undertreatment of animal pain, however, is likely a result of lack of adequate knowledge and not a lack of concern. Outward show of concern for the pet and family is important for demonstrating a bond-centered approach to cancer therapy and pain management. Most owners who are willing to undergo the emotional stress and financial commitment to cancer therapy have already shown that they have a strong attachment to their pet. It is important for the veterinarian to foster good communication surrounding primary therapy and pain treatment and, at the same time, demonstrate empathy for

Box 1
Basic definitions for terms used when discussing pain in general, and cancer pain in particular

Acute pain follows some bodily injury, disappears with healing, and tends to be self-limiting.

Breakthrough pain is a transient flare-up of pain in the chronic pain setting and can occur even when chronic pain is under control.

Chronic pain lasts several weeks to months and persists beyond the expected healing time when nonmalignant in origin.

Cancer pain can be acute, chronic, or intermittent and is related to the disease itself or to the treatment.

Pre-emptive analgesia is the administration of an analgesic drug before stimulation to prevent sensitization of neurons, thus improving postoperative analgesia.

Local anesthesia is the temporary loss of sensation in a defined part of the body without loss of consciousness.

Neuropathic pain originates from injury or involvement of the peripheral or central nervous system and is described as burning or shooting, possibly associated with motor, sensory, or autonomic deficits.

Regional anesthesia is the loss of sensation in part of the body by interrupting the sensory nerves conducting impulses from that region of the body.

Somatic pain originates from damage to bones, joints, muscle, or skin and is described in human beings as localized, constant, sharp, aching, and throbbing.

Visceral pain arises from stretching, distention, or inflammation of the viscera and is described as deep, cramping, aching, or gnawing, without good localization

Wind-up is central sensitization attributable to an increase in the excitability of spinal neurons, contributing to the severity of postoperative pain.

the owner. This fosters the doctor-client-patient relationship and helps to build goodwill within and outside the practice.

ASSESSMENT OF PAIN

Assessment of pain in animals can be difficult and frustrating. Understanding types of pain and their causes can be helpful. Often, veterinarians need to rely on the experience in people to help define the pain in animals. Technicians and other staff members are usually the ones who experience the postoperative period more than the doctors. Pain assessment typically is delegated to these staff members. Recognition and assessment of pain is the first and probably the most difficult step in providing analgesia to dogs and cats. It is often easiest to assume that an animal is in pain if a person undergoing similar trauma or surgery would be in pain. A patient usually tolerates mild pain without a problem and does not exhibit any behavioral changes. Patients with mild pain often are not treated. Patients experiencing moderate pain usually exhibit changes in behavior, appetite, activity, positioning, or posture.[13,14] These patients also tend to respond significantly to palpation of the painful area. Severe pain can be thought of as intolerable, and is often manifested as unprovoked crying, whimpering, or howling associated with violent thrashing. Sometimes, the patient may not exhibit these behaviors, because the associated movements enhance the excruciating pain. Nonspecific physiologic responses to pain include elevated heart rate and blood pressure, abnormal cardiac rhythm, panting, salivation, dilated pupils, and behavior that presents as vicious and uncontrollable. It is important to remember that there are differences in variables among individuals, breeds, and species.

Cancer pain typically begins as acute mild pain and then potentially progresses to a chronic pain state that may be mild to severe in nature. Practitioners should attempt to intervene early to prevent wind-up and problem chronic pain.

Classification as to origin of pain is also important, because some drugs have greater efficacy for different types of pain. Somatic pain originates from damage to bones, joints, muscle, or skin and is described in human beings as localized, constant, sharp, aching, and throbbing. Osteosarcoma is an example of somatic pain. Visceral pain arises from stretching, distention, or inflammation of the viscera and is described as deep, cramping, aching, or gnawing, without good localization. An enlarging visceral tumor can elicit visceral pain. Neuropathic pain originates from injury or involvement of the peripheral or central nervous system and is described as burning or shooting, possibly associated with motor, sensory, or autonomic deficits. Many soft tissue tumors have neuropathic components because of compression or invasion of nervous components.

Assessment of pain can be accomplished systematically with a pain scoring scale.[14–16] The objective of a pain scoring system is to place a quantitative value on a specific variable, add up the variables, and compare the total with some predetermined assessment of pain. There are many different pain score scales, and no single scale is perfect. Some investigators have also used a visual analog scale (VAS). A VAS would need to be validated for several people at each practice to ensure consistent scoring. Every pain scale requires a subjective assessment of another individual's experience, however, and, by its nature, is inherently flawed. Response to analgesic therapy is important to note and guide the practitioner to the analgesic requirement for the degree of pain the patient is experiencing. When doubt exists as to whether the patient is in pain, or how painful, a trial of analgesic therapy must be instituted.

Failure to assess pain initially and throughout the course of cancer treatment is a leading factor in undertreatment. Pain should be assessed early, with the goal of characterizing the pain as to location, intensity, and probable cause. Client engagement in this process helps to determine aggravating and relieving factors. After a good assessment is performed, goals for pain control can be set with the client. In addition to examining patients frequently, clients should be consulted on a regular basis, at least by telephone, to ensure an accurate assessment of a pet's pain.

DRUGS AND TECHNIQUES FOR ALLEVIATION OF PAIN

Throughout this issue, doses are mentioned in the text. It can be assumed that the doses are appropriate to dogs and cats unless otherwise noted.

Drug treatment is the cornerstone of cancer pain management. It is effective and affordable for most patients and owners. The general approach to pain management should follow the World Health Organization ladder, which is a three-step hierarchy (**Fig. 1**).[3] Within the same category of drugs, there can be different side effects for individuals. Therefore, if possible, it may be best to substitute drugs within a category before switching therapies. It is always best to try to keep dosage scheduling as simple as possible. The more complicated the regimen, the more likely it is that noncompliance may occur. Mild to moderate pain should be treated with a nonopioid, such as a nonsteroidal anti-inflammatory drug (NSAID), ensuring that there are no systemic contraindications. As pain increases, some type of opioid should be added to the regimen. As pain becomes more severe, increase the dose of the opioid. It should be noted that tachyphylaxis is common with opioids when used chronically and increasing the dosage, potentially to higher than the "normal" range, does not necessarily mean increasing the likelihood of adverse affects. Drugs should be dosed on a regular basis and not just as needed as pain becomes moderate to severe.

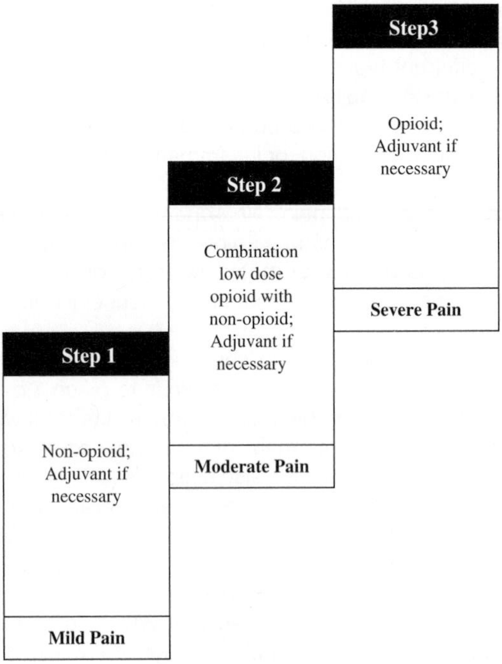

Fig. 1. World Health Organization cancer pain control ladder. (*Adapted from* http://www.who.int/cancer/palliative/painladder/en/. Accessed June 26, 2008; with permission.)

Continuous analgesia facilitates maintaining patient comfort. Additional doses of analgesics can then be administered as pain is intermittently more severe. Adjuvant drugs can be administered to help with specific types of pain and anxiety.

NONSTEROIDAL ANTI-INFLAMMATORY DRUGS

Nonopioid analgesics include such drugs as carprofen, etodolac, deracoxib, meloxicam, tepoxalin, firocoxib, aspirin, carprofen, ketoprofen, and acetaminophen (**Table 1**).[17] All except acetaminophen are considered NSAIDs. Despite the low anti-inflammatory activity of acetaminophen, it possesses beneficial effects of analgesia; minimal risk for bleeding in thrombocytopenic patients; decreased gastrointestinal effects; and synergism with opioid analgesics, such as codeine. Acetaminophen may also be helpful for breakthrough pain control in dogs already receiving NSAIDs. Acetaminophen should

Table 1
Non-opioid analgesic and adjunct drug doses in dogs and cats

Drug	Dog Dose	Cat Dose
Acetaminophen	10–15 mg/kg PO q 12 h for 5 days	Not recommended
Acetaminophen (300 mg) + codeine (30 or 60 mg)	Dose on acetaminophen, 10–15 mg/kg	Not recommended
Amantadine	3–5 mg/kg PO q 24 h	3–5 mg/kg PO q 24 h
Amitriptyline	0.5–2.0 mg/kg PO q 24 h	5–10 mg PO q 24 h
Carprofen	4.4 mg/kg SC single dose 4.4 mg/kg PO q 24 h	1–4 mg/kg SC single dose Not recommended for oral use
Deracoxib	1–2 mg/kg PO q 24 h 3–4 mg/kg PO q 24 h, 7-day limit	Not recommended
Firocoxib	10 mg/kg PO q 24 h	Not recommended
Gabapentin	2–40 mg/kg PO q 24 h	2–40 mg/kg PO q 24 h
Imipramine	0.5–1.0 mg/kg PO q 8 h	2.5–5.0 mg/kg PO q 12 h
Ketamine (as NMDA receptor antagonist rather than anesthetic)	0.5 mg/kg IV, followed by 10 μg/kg/min during surgery, followed by 2 μg/kg/min for next 24 h	0.5 mg/kg IV, followed by 10 μg/kg/min during surgery, followed by 2 μg/kg/min for next 24 h
Ketoprofen	1–2 mg/kg IV, IM, SC initial dose 1 mg/kg PO q 24 h up to 5 days	0.5–2 mg/kg IV, IM, SC initial dose 0.5–1 mg/kg PO q 24 h up to 5 days
Meloxicam	0.2 mg/kg IV, SC 0.2 mg/kg initial loading dose, then 0.1 mg/kg PO q 24 h	0.1 mg/kg SC 0.1 mg/kg PO on day 1, then 0.05 mg/kg PO q 24 h
Pamidronate	1–2 mg/kg diluted over 2–4 h IV, SC	1–1.5 mg/kg diluted over 2–4 h
Piroxicam	0.3 mg/kg PO q 24–48 h	0.3 mg/kg PO q 24–48 h 1 mg/cat PO q 24 h for a maximum of 7 days
Tramadol	2–4 mg/kg PO q 6–12 h	2–4 mg/kg PO q 6–12 h

Abbreviations: h, hours; IM, intramuscular; IV, intravenous; PO, per os; q, every; SC, subcutaneous.

be avoided in cats because of their inadequate cytochrome P-450–dependent hydroxylation.[18]

Mild to moderate pain, especially that arising from intrathoracic masses, intra-abdominal masses, and bone tumors and metastases, can be relieved with NSAIDs. When pain increases, NSAIDs have an opioid-sparing effect such that better analgesia can be achieved with lower doses of opioids. NSAIDs have central analgesic and peripheral anti-inflammatory effects mediated by means of inhibition of cyclooxygenase (COX). The choice of NSAID ultimately depends on available species information, clinical response, and tolerance of side effects. Most NSAIDs have been formally investigated only in dogs, leaving anecdotal information for use in cats, although good information does exist for meloxicam in cats.[19] The most common side effect of aspirin administration in dogs is gastric irritation and bleeding because of loss of gastric acid inhibition and cytoprotective mucous production normally promoted by prostaglandins. NSAIDs approved for use in dogs have a low incidence of side effects, most commonly, vomiting, diarrhea, and inappetence. Other less common side effects include renal failure and hepatic dysfunction that may lead to failure.[20]

NSAIDs that are more selective for inhibition of COX-2 seem to have fewer gastrointestinal effects and potentially fewer renal effects.[21,22] Therefore, more selective COX-2 inhibitors, such as carprofen, meloxicam, deracoxib, firocoxib, and the dual-inhibitor tepoxalin should be considered priority NSAIDs in patients that have cancer. A blood chemistry panel should be performed before initiating NSAID therapy. If there is evidence of liver or renal disease, dehydration, or hypotension, another approach to therapy should be considered. Therapy with older NSAIDs, such as aspirin and ketoprofen, may also inhibit platelet function, leading to bleeding and oozing. Therapy with NSAIDs should be stopped if this occurs. If clinical effectiveness is not achieved with one NSAID, it should be discontinued and another started 7 days later to avoid additive or synergistic COX inhibition effects. Aspirin should be avoided in dogs because of the increased possibility of gastrointestinal bleeding, even with buffered formulations.[2,23] Administering misoprostol as a synthetic prostaglandin can help to provide gastrointestinal protection during shorter switchover periods. All patients that have cancer should be closely monitored for gastrointestinal bleeding if receiving NSAID therapy during chemotherapy that may induce thrombocytopenia.

OPIOIDS

Opioids are the major class of analgesics used in the management of moderate to severe cancer pain. They are most effective and predictable and have low risk associated with them.[24] The most common parenteral opioids used in small animals are morphine, hydromorphone, oxymorphone, fentanyl, codeine, meperidine, buprenorphine, and butorphanol (**Table 2**). Parenteral opioids should be used in the perioperative period and should be discontinued when a patient can be switched to oral medication. Common oral opioids include morphine, oxycodone, buprenorphine, and codeine with or without acetaminophen (see **Table 2**).

As a patient's pain increases, the required dose of opioid also increases. Veterinarians may be reluctant to administer high doses of opioids for fear of adverse side effects. It is important to remember that veterinarians have an ethical obligation to benefit the patient by alleviating pain. Opioids can be administered while managing side effects to help the patient maximally. Side effects of opioid administration include diarrhea, vomiting, and dysphoria or sedation initially, with constipation with long-term use but, less commonly, sedation and dysphoria. The initial gastrointestinal effects occur most frequently with the first injection in the perioperative period and usually

Table 2
Injectable and oral opioid analgesic doses in dogs and cats

Drug	Dog Dose	Cat Dose
Buprenorphine	0.005–0.02 mg/kg SC, IM, IV q 4–8 h	0.005–0.02 mg/kg SC, IM, IV q 4–8 h 0.01–0.02 bucally q 6–12 h
Butorphanol	0.2–0.8 mg/kg SC, IM q 2–6 h 0.5–2 mg/kg PO q 6–8 h	0.1–0.4 mg/kg SC, IM q 2–6 h 0.1 mg/kg IV q 1–2 h 0.5–2 mg/kg PO q 6–8 h
Codeine	0.5–1 mg/kg PO q 4–6 h	0.5 mg/kg PO q 6 h
Fentanyl	0.01–0.04 mg/kg SC, IM 0.002–0.005 mg/kg IV 2–20 μg/kg/h IV	0.005–0.04 mg/kg SC, IM 0.002–0.005 mg/kg IV 2–20 μg/kg/h IV
Hydromorphone	0.05–0.2 mg/kg SC, IM 0.05–0.1 mg/kg IV q 2–6 h 0.05–0.1 mg/kg/h	0.05–0.1 mg/kg SC, IM q 2–6 h 0.03–0.05 mg/kg IV q 1 h 0.01–0.05 mg/kg/h
Morphine	0.25–1.0 mg/kg SQ, IM q 4–6 h 0.05–0.1 mg/kg IV q 1–2 h 0.05–0.1 mg/kg/h 0.1 mg/kg epidurally q 12–24 h	0.05–0.1 mg/kg IM, SC q 4–6 h
Morphine sulfate: sustained release	2–5 mg/kg q 12 h	Not recommended
Morphine sulfate tablets and oral liquid	1.0 mg/kg PO q 4–6 h	Not recommended
Oxymorphone	0.025–0.2 mg/kg IV, IM, SC	0.02–0.2 mg/kg IV, IM, SC
Oxycodone	0.1–0.3 mg/kg PO q 8–12 h	Not recommended

Abbreviations: h, hours; IM, intramuscular; IV, intravenous; PO, per os; q, every; SC, subcutaneous.

do not occur with subsequent dosing. Dosing to effect may reduce this occurrence. These effects usually do not occur with oral dosing. When sending a patient home with oral medications, it is important to discuss with the owner that dosing is individual. It is possible that a given dose is perfect, does not provide enough analgesia, induces sedation, or induces dysphoria or excitement. Adjusting of the dose requires excellent doctor-client interaction. Bradycardia is also possible after opioid administration but is most common if opioids are administered parenterally. If bradycardia occurs, an anticholinergic, such as atropine or glycopyrrolate, should be administered rather than discontinuing the opioid.

Opioids are classified as full μ-receptor agonists, partial agonists, and κ-agonist–μ-antagonists. Examples of the full μ-receptor agonists include morphine, oxymorphone, fentanyl, codeine, and meperidine. In normal healthy animals, opioids may produce sedation, which is usually acceptable, or dysphoria, an exaggerated unrest, which usually is undesirable. These adverse effects are noted when pain does not exist or is overestimated, and a relative overdose of the opioid was thus administered. Full μ-agonists induce the best analgesia in a dose-dependent manner and are not limited by a ceiling effect. As pain increases, larger doses may be administered, again stressing the importance of "dosing to effect." Morphine or hydromorphone should be the most commonly used injectable opioid for the acute treatment of cancer-related pain. Morphine is available in multiple injectable and oral formulations, including short-duration tablets and liquids and sustained-release tablets. Oral morphine may be the most effective method for providing longer term analgesia to dogs and cats with moderate to severe pain. Patients receiving nonopioid analgesics at set dosing intervals should also be provided with some short-duration opioid for breakthrough pain. Oxymorphone is only available as an injectable analgesic. Oxymorphone and most other opioids may induce panting by changing the temperature set point in the brain.[24] This usually is not an issue, except when attempting thoracic or abdominal radiography. This effect may be avoided by dosing to effect in many cases. Meperidine is short acting in animals, limiting its use as an analgesic in patients that have cancer. Codeine is available alone or with acetaminophen, allowing some flexibility in choice of oral medications. Fentanyl is an injectable drug that is potent and effective. All the previously mentioned parenteral opioids may be administered by an intermittent intravenous, intramuscular, or subcutaneous route. A problem with this type of intermittent dosing is that patients often become painful before their subsequent dose and then are extremely sedated after dosing. An alternate dosing regimen would use continuous infusion of an opioid. Fentanyl is an appropriate drug for continuous infusion because it is short acting. This enables the practitioner to alter the dose as necessary from minute to minute to achieve good analgesia and potentially minimal sedation if desired.

Oxycodone, an excellent oral analgesic in dogs, may be used for primary pain control or for the control of breakthrough pain. Oral oxycodone is currently being used more and more frequently for severe pain in dogs. It seems to induce less sedation and dysphoria than oral morphine and provides a greater degree of pain control than oral codeine. Buprenorphine is an example of a partial μ-agonist. It does not produce the same degree of analgesia as morphine and has a ceiling effect. The advantage of buprenorphine is that it has a long duration of action, 6 to 12 hours. It also has a long time to onset, approximately 40 minutes, even when given intravenously. Buprenorphine is a unique drug in that larger doses may actually produce less analgesia because of a bell-shaped dose-response curve. Tapering the dose to the individual may be difficult. If an animal does not have adequate analgesia after receiving buprenorphine, dosing with a morphine-like drug may not produce any results because of buprenorphine's strong affinity for μ-opioid receptors. Buprenorphine is not easily reversible. Experimentally, it takes 1000 times the normal dose of naloxone to reverse it in a normal dog.[25–27] Because of the inherent lack of maximal analgesia compared with morphine, buprenorphine should only be used for mild to moderate cancer pain in dogs. If any doubt exists as to severity of pain, one can start with a pure μ-opioid and adjust the dose to the desired effect. If a low dose produces analgesia, one can assume that buprenorphine is adequate for future management.

There are good data to suggest that cats get excellent analgesia when buprenorphine is administered intravenously or buccally. The buccal route seems to induce equivalent analgesia.[28,29] There is also some evidence that the buccal route may be effective in dogs.[30] It remains to be seen if this is beneficial in dogs based on actual pain relief and cost.

Another group of opioids available are the κ-agonist–μ-antagonists, of which butorphanol is an example. Butorphanol may reverse the effects of drugs like morphine, a pure μ-agonist, but provides analgesia and sedation of its own. Butorphanol is also reversible with naloxone and nalmefene. The analgesia is not as good as that produced by morphine. Even in large parenteral doses, butorphanol produces analgesia of short duration in dogs[31] and, as such, may not be useful for cancer pain.

An alternative to administering oral opioids to provide multiple-day analgesia is to apply a transdermal fentanyl patch. Fentanyl patches require 12 to 24 hours to take effect and last 2 to 4 days in dogs but require 12 hours to take effect in cats. Additional analgesia must be provided during the first 0.5 to 1 day after patch placement. If an opioid is selected, pure μ-agonists must be used. One problem with transdermal fentanyl is related to unreliable plasma levels in dogs,[32–34] probably because of failure of patch application or inappropriate dosing. Fentanyl patches may not provide enough analgesia for severe pain,[33] but they allow lower doses of additional drugs. Fentanyl patches are expensive and should not be the first approach to chronic therapy. Additionally, the usefulness of a fentanyl patch may be limited by sedation or dysphoria, necessitating removing the patch prematurely. Transdermal fentanyl is most appropriate in those patients that do not tolerate oral medication. Fentanyl patches should not be prescribed when young children are in the household, because potential removal with ingestion is a concern.

Epidural opioids, especially morphine, have been used as a method for perioperative analgesia. With placement of an epidural catheter, epidural opioids can be administered for days to weeks. This may be appropriate for long-term pain control in patients that have vertebral mass(es) or other forms of cancer that induce severe pain. The reader is referred to the discussion on epidural analgesia elsewhere in this issue.

Although not truly an opioid, tramadol, a serotonin reuptake inhibitor, can provide significant pain control in addition to an NSAID. Tramadol can bridge the gap between an NSAID alone and the addition of a potent oral opioid for extended periods. Although the pharmacokinetics of tramadol suggest high dose and frequent administration,[35] most canine and feline patients develop significant comfort at 2 to 3 mg/kg administered orally two to three times daily.

The appropriate dose of an opioid is the dose that produces analgesia with the fewest side effects. The need for increased doses often reflects progression of disease. Long-term use produces opioid tolerance, increasing doses or frequency to achieve equivalent results. As previously mentioned, veterinarians should not be afraid of increasing doses in patients and should remember the need for analgesia. A distinct advantage of using opioids for pain control is that they are reversible with naloxone or nalmefene if unacceptable side effects occur. Prolonged use may produce constipation. Oral laxatives can help to alleviate this problem.

α_2-AGONISTS

Xylazine, medetomidine, and dexmedetomidine are three α_2-agonists approved for use in small animals in the United States. They are noncontrolled parenteral agents and provide excellent visceral analgesia but only for 20 minutes to 2 hours.[36–39] Their effects can be virtually completely reversed with yohimbine or atipamezole, respectively. The α_2-agonists should not be the first or sole choice in providing analgesia around the time of surgery to patients that have cancer because they greatly reduce cardiac function and oxygenation.[36,40,41] α_2-Agonists have synergistic effects with opioids. When used in microdoses (0.5–1 μg/kg administered intravenously, 1–3 μg/kg/h), this effect can be useful after surgery for inducing additional analgesia and alleviating dysphoria and anxiety.

N-METHYL-D-ASPARTATE RECEPTOR ANTAGONISTS

Ketamine has been used for many years as an induction agent to general anesthesia in normal and compromised patients. It has been well established that ketamine provides reasonable somatic but poor visceral analgesia.[42] Ketamine has been identified as an *N*-methyl-D-aspartate (NMDA) receptor antagonist. NMDA receptors are believed to play a role in the processes leading up to central sensitization and wind-up. As an NMDA receptor antagonist, ketamine reduces postoperative pain and cumulative opioid requirements for a variety of procedures in human beings.[43] This is accomplished with doses that are much smaller than those for anesthesia. In fact, these doses of ketamine should not be considered as direct analgesic doses but as NMDA antagonist doses inducing an indirect analgesic effect, essentially allowing other analgesics to work more effectively. As such, it is uncommon for patients to develop behavioral or cardiovascular effects. In fact, microdose ketamine may actually decrease the incidence of opioid-induced dysphoria after surgery. Intraoperative microdose ketamine has been demonstrated to be effective for pain control long after discontinuing administration. Dogs recovering after this type of therapy for forelimb amputation are more comfortable in the perioperative period and after the dog has been sent home.[44] When used in this manner, ketamine should be administered as a bolus (0.5 mg/kg administered intravenously), followed by an infusion (10 μg/kg/min) before and during surgical stimulation. A lower infusion rate (2 μg/kg/min = 0.12 mg/kg/h) may be beneficial for the first 24 hours after surgery, with an even lower rate (1 μg/kg/min = 0.6 mg/kg/h) for the next 24 hours. In the absence of an infusion pump, ketamine can be mixed in a bag of crystalloid solutions for administration during anesthesia. Using anesthesia fluid administration rates of 10 mL/kg/h, ketamine at a dose of 60 mg (0.6 mL) should be added to a 1-L bag of crystalloid fluids to deliver ketamine at a rate of 0.6 mg/kg/h Higher doses of ketamine (1–2 mg/kg/h) may provide significant direct analgesia effects. It is unclear if an NMDA antagonist effect occurs at these higher doses.

Amantadine, an oral anti-influenza A medication that also has NMDA antagonist effects,[45] can be administered at 3 mg/kg orally once daily to prevent wind-up.[46] It should be part of the early intervention in patients that have osteosarcoma.[47] Although the specific pharmacokinetics have not been determined for amantadine, good information is available for rimantadine, a similar medication.[48]

TRANQUILIZERS

A concern that frequently arises with pain management is concurrent tranquilization and sedation. Most of the drugs used by veterinarians usually produce concurrent sedation. As mentioned previously, opioids have the greatest potential of producing dysphoria instead of sedation. Dysphoria becomes more likely when cats are administered canine doses of opioids and when a patient is already experiencing high anxiety in the hospital. Dysphoric patients can sometimes be treated simply by petting and soothing or by helping a patient to change position. Low-dose acepromazine (**Table 3**) administered intravenously or intramuscularly is reasonable drug therapy for dysphoria. Although acepromazine does not treat pain, it calms anxious patients well and also makes them care less about their pain. For patients in which acepromazine is contraindicated, such as those with bleeding disorders, the benzodiazepines (see **Table 2**) diazepam and midazolam often calm patients. Benzodiazepines should not be used by themselves in most alert patients because they frequently cause excitement. Combined with opioids, sedation usually results. In patients that are hemodynamically stable, a microdose of dexmedetomidine (0.0005–0.001 mg/kg administered intravenously) or medetomidine (0.001–0.002 mg/kg administered intravenously) administered intravenously or intramuscularly also can decrease dysphoria and increase analgesia.

Patients that develop dysphoria after oral analgesic medications often respond well to oral acepromazine or diazepam. It is important to discern whether the opioid dose is effective before changing the analgesia regimen, because dysphoria may occur with too high, too low, or an appropriate analgesic dose of the opioid.

Table 3
Tranquilizer and sedative doses in dogs and cats

Drug	Dog Dose	Cat Dose
Acepromazine	0.025–0.1 mg/kg; maximum of 4 mg IV, SC, IM 0.5–2 mg/kg PO	0.05–0.1 mg/kg; maximum of 1 mg IV 0.1–2.0 mg/kg PO
Alprazolam	0.025–0.1 mg/kg q 8 h	0.0125–0.025 mg/kg q 12 h
Dexmedetomidine	0.0005 mg/kg/h IV (preanesthetic) 0.0005–0.002 mg/kg IV bolus (short-term sedation/analgesia) 0.0005–0.001 mg/kg/h IV (extended sedation/ analgesia-CRI)	0.0010 mg/kg/h IV (preanesthetic) 0.0010–0.004 mg/kg IV bolus (short-term sedation/analgesia) 0.0010–0.002 mg/kg/h IV(extended sedation/analgesia-CRI)
Diazepam	0.1–0.5 mg/kg IV, IM 0.5–2.2 mg/kg PO	0.05–0.4 mg/kg IV, IM 0.5–2.2 mg/kg PO
Medetomidine	0.01–0.02 mg/kg IM 0.005–0.01 mg/kg IV (sedation/ analgesia) 0.005–0.01 mg/kg IM 0.003–0.005 mg/kg IV (preanesthetic) 0.01- 0.02 mg/kg/h IV (supplemental CRI during inhalant anesthesia) 0.001–0.003 mg/kg IV bolus (short-term sedation/analgesia) 0.001–0.002 mg/kg/h IV (extended sedation/analgesia CRI)	0.015–0.03 mg/kg IM 0.01–0.015 mg/kg IV (sedation/ analgesia) 0.01–0.01 IM 0.005–0.01 mg/kg IV (preanesthetic) 0.003–0.010 IV bolus (short-term sedation/analgesia)
Midazolam	0.1–0.25 mg/kg IV, IM	0.05–0.25 mg/kg IV, IM
Xylazine	1.1–2.2 mg/kg IM, SC 0.05–0.1 mg/kg IV prn 0.2 mg/kg SC, IM q 1–2 h	1.1 mg/kg IM, SC 0.05–0.1 mg/kg IV prn 0.2–0.4 mg/kg SC, IM q 1–2 h

Abbreviations: CRI, constant rate infusion; h, hours; IM, intramuscular; IV, intravenous; PO, per os; prn, as needed; q, every; SC, subcutaneous.

Alprazolam at a dosage of 0.1 to 0.5 mg/kg/d administered orally can be given as an anxiolytic. Diazepam and midazolam can be administered as alternative therapy for animals in which acepromazine is contraindicated.

ANTICONVULSANTS

Gabapentin is a structural analogue of γ-aminobutyric acid (GABA)[49] and was originally introduced as an antiepileptic drug. The mechanism of action of gabapentin is unclear and elusive. Although gabapentin is related to GABA, it does not seem to have any analgesic effect at GABA receptors.

Several rat studies have investigated the effects of gabapentin on signs of neuropathic pain, such as hyperalgesia and allodynia. Other studies indicate a role for gabapentin in decreasing incisional pain and arthritis. Although the exact indications and efficacy for gabapentin have not yet been determined, it seems to be useful for neuropathic cancer pain. When gabapentin is added to an opioid regimen for patients that are only partially opioid responsive, they experience significantly better analgesia.

These patients also experience less allodynia. Burning and lancinating pain is also more likely to respond to gabapentin compared with dull aching pain.

Although dosing has not been established in dogs or cats, the following recommendations are extrapolations from human beings. It is important to remember that there are no controlled or evidence-based studies in dogs and cats using gabapentin. Gabapentin has been investigated as an antiepileptic drug in dogs, with dosing between 800 and 1500 mg/d. Initial doses for pain range from 2.5 to 10 mg/kg administered orally two or three times daily but can be escalated up to 50 mg/kg administered orally two to three times daily depending on the analgesic effect achieved. Gabapentin may need to be compounded for smaller patients.

TRICYCLIC ANTIDEPRESSANTS

Tricyclic antidepressants, such as amitriptyline, clomipramine, and imipramine, block the reuptake of serotonin and norepinephrine in the central nervous system (see **Table 3**). They also have antihistaminic effects. These drugs have been used in human patients for the treatment of chronic and neuropathic pain at doses considerably lower than those used to treat depression.[50] Despite the lack of studies verifying the use of tricyclic antidepressants in this manner, clinical experience by many practitioners would substantiate this analgesic use in dogs and cats.

LOCAL ANESTHETICS

The use of local and regional anesthetic techniques in small animals was common in the early twentieth century. There has recently been increased interest in these techniques, probably because of their ability to provide pre-emptive analgesia and decrease wind-up.[51,52] Local anesthetic techniques can be used instead of general anesthesia in selected cases or, more commonly, in combination.

The most commonly used local anesthetics include lidocaine and bupivacaine. Lidocaine has a short onset (<1 minute) and lasts approximately 60 to 90 minutes. Doses of 1.5 to 2.0 mg/kg are safe in dogs and cats. Signs of toxicity are manifested as nausea and vomiting, followed by neurologic changes, including seizures. Bupivacaine takes approximately 20 minutes to take effect but may last for 5 to 8 hours. Although lidocaine has antidysrhythmic effects at low to moderate intravenous doses, bupivacaine has cardiotoxic effects when administered intravascularly. Inadvertent intravenous administration can result in death.[53,54] Epinephrine may be added to bupivacaine in a 1:200,000 dilution to cause local vasoconstriction and prolonged duration. Epinephrine should not be used for peripheral blocks, because there may not be collateral circulation to provide adequate perfusion to distal tissues. Combinations of lidocaine and bupivacaine are often used to achieve quick onset and long duration. This is especially necessary when using local anesthetics interpleurally. Because of its long onset, bupivacaine causes stinging discomfort. Lidocaine administered concurrently limits the discomfort to a period of seconds. When bupivacaine is used alone, a ratio of 1:10 sodium bicarbonate (1 mL) to bupivacaine 0.5% (10 mL) has been shown to reduce but not eliminate the discomfort of bupivacaine.

There are numerous uses for local anesthetics. They are often used epidurally to produce better analgesia in low doses or as anesthesia for caudal procedures in higher doses. They may be used interpleurally for thoracic and cranial abdominal pain. Intercostal nerve blocks are easily performed for lateral thoracotomy pain. Brachial plexus infiltration provides anesthesia for the proximal and distal forelimb. Maxillary, infraorbital, mandibular, and mental nerve blocks are commonly used for procedures involving the face and mouth. Local infiltration is common for procedures involving the ear. Ring blocks have also been used for distal limb and digit amputations. Many of these techniques have been well described.[55]

The 5% lidocaine patch produces local tissue concentrations far lower than those capable of producing toxicity but high enough to produce clinically effective local analgesia for periods of up to 24 hours without complete sensory block. The patches have been used to provide analgesia for skin abrasions, lacerations, and severe local skin irritation and itching (hot spots), and they are likely useful for localized pain related to cancer.

Epidural Drug Administration

Epidural administration of drugs requires additional skill and expertise that may not be available in all clinical settings. Details of the procedure are described in the companion article elsewhere in this issue. Epidural morphine is commonly administered in the perioperative period to provide analgesia but not anesthesia in the abdomen or more caudally. In some instances, analgesia may be effective for the thorax and forelimb. This analgesia may last up to 24 hours.[56] Local anesthetics may also be administered epidurally as a low dose to augment epidural morphine-induced analgesia or at a higher dose to produce anesthesia.

A catheter can also be placed in the epidural space for severe pain that may be intractable in the caudal portion of the body. Maintenance of this catheter requires veterinarian and client vigilance to ensure cleanliness and prevent infection migrating to the spinal cord. With proper care, an epidural catheter can remain in place for days to weeks.

OTHER PAIN-RELIEVING MODALITIES

Local or whole-body radiation can enhance analgesic drug effectiveness by reducing metastatic or primary tumor bulk.[57] The radiation dose should be balanced between the amount necessary to kill tumor cells and that which would affect normal cells. Mucositis of the oral cavity and pharynx can develop after radiation to the neck, head, or oral cavities, resulting in impaired ability to eat and drink. Mucositis therapies include analgesics, green tea rinses, sucralfate, 2% viscous lidocaine, and a 1:1 combination of 2% lidocaine viscous to aluminum hydroxide, 64 mg/mL (commonly referred to as "Pink Lady"). A mix of 50 mL of each for a total volume of 100 mL can be sent home with the patient. This mixture tends to assist adherence of the lidocaine to the lesions. When local anesthetics are used orally, the maximum dose of lidocaine should not be exceeded. Just enough should be given to coat the inside of the mouth to avoid swallowing and coating the pharynx, because this can desensitize the area, potentially predisposing to aspiration.

Osteosarcoma and bony metastases are common causes of pain in advanced cancer. Some tumors cause osteoblastic metastases, but most can cause osteolytic lesions. Administration of bisphosphonates, such as pamidronate, reduces pain and pathologic fractures in human beings.[58] Bisphosphonates accumulate on bone surfaces and inhibit osteoclast-induced resorption, favoring bone formation. This therapy is now reasonably priced and should be available to all veterinary clients. Pamidronate (1–2 mg/kg) is diluted in saline and administered intravenously over a 2- to 4-hour period at 3- to 5-week intervals. It decreases pain and potentially increases survival in dogs that have osteosarcoma.[59] A potential oral alternative to pamidronate is alendronate. Alendronate inhibits cell migration through mechanisms that depend on calcium.[60] It has been studied specifically in dogs and has been shown to have an antiosteosarcoma effect.[61] At reasonable doses, it has also been shown to have no significant adverse effects over a 3-year period.[62] Although alendronate therapy has not been clinically studied as a pain-relieving treatment for canine osteosarcoma, clinically, it seems to be effective.[63]

Acupuncture can be used as a pain-relieving modality, often in conjunction with other therapy or when conventional therapy does not work. In conjunction with other therapy, it can allow administration of lower doses of drugs that may have significant side effects. Although some practitioners have difficulty in accepting acupuncture because of traditional Chinese medical explanations, which may be scientifically untenable, it is important to remember that there exists well-documented physiologic theory and evidence for its clinical effects.[64–66] Electroacupuncture can be useful for cancer-related bone pain.[67] In general, acupuncture analgesia is extremely useful for pelvic, radius or ulna, and femoral bone pain in addition to cutaneous discomfort secondary to radiation therapy. Acupuncture also helps to increase appetite and alleviate nausea associated with chemotherapy and some analgesics in addition to promoting general well-being. For details, please refer to the article by Gaynor.[68]

SPECIFIC PAIN PROBLEMS

When developing a plan for alleviating pain in a patient that has cancer, it helps to have a paradigm to follow. A simple flow chart (**Fig. 2**) can help with the sequence of activities related to pain assessment and management.[69] This flow chart emphasizes the use of multiple modalities, beginning therapy with the least invasive methods and advancing treatment to meet the patient's needs. Although not all types of pain can be addressed here, pain relief should be considered achievable by following recommendations and paradigms in this article.

SURGICAL CASE EXAMPLES

The following generic examples, in conjunction with the flow chart, present useful approaches to specific types of pain encountered in oncology practice. The examples recommend specific techniques for the procedure rather than a complete analgesia program. Implicit in the recommendations is an appropriate opioid and an NSAID if not contraindicated.

- Lateral thoracotomy
  - Intercostal nerve block
  - Interpleural (intrapleural?) local anesthetic
  - Opioid epidural
- Sternotomy
  - Interpleural (intrapleural?) local anesthetic
  - Opioid epidural
- Forelimb amputation
  - Brachial plexus nerve block
  - Opioid epidural
- Rear limb amputation
  - Opioid epidural
- Cranial mandibular surgery
  - Mandibular nerve block
  - Mental nerve block
- Upper lip and nose (nasal?) procedure
  - Infraorbital nerve block
- Maxillary surgery
  - Maxillary nerve block

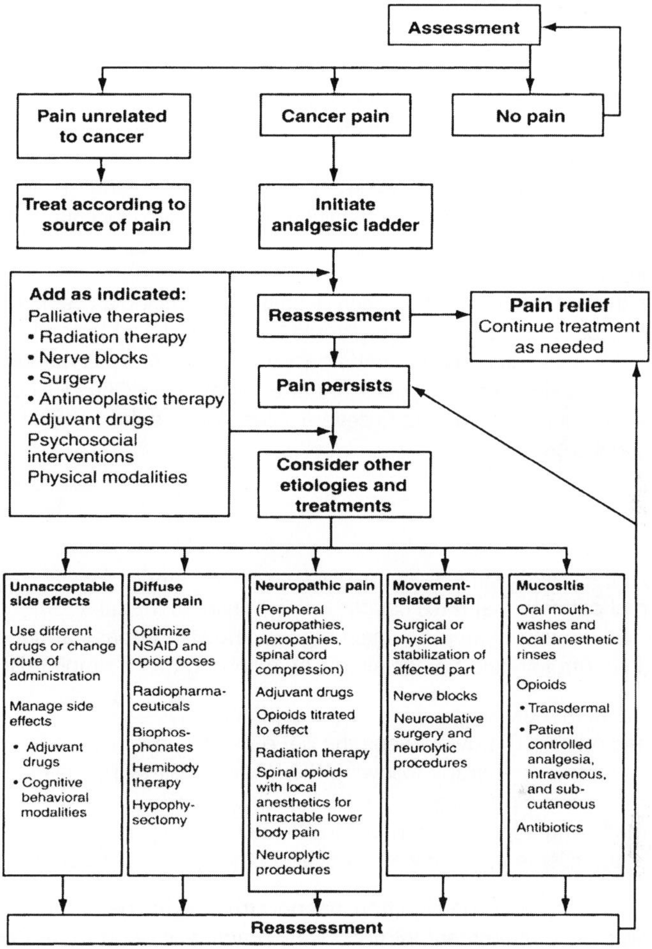

Fig. 2. Cancer pain flow chart. (*From* Jacox A, Carr DB, Payne R, et al. Management of cancer pain. Rockville (MD): Agency for Health Care Policy and Research; 1994. p. 13; with permission.)

For all these procedures, the addition of an NSAID administered intravenously, subcutaneously, or intramuscularly as is species and drug appropriate is an extremely valuable adjunct to the regimen.

- Midcaudal abdominal surgery
  - Opioid epidural (local anesthetic also if caudal abdomen)
- Cranial abdominal surgery
  - Interpleural local anesthetic
  - Opioid epidural

Although not all types of pain can be addressed, pain relief should be considered achievable by following recommendations and paradigms in this article.

Outpatient Case Examples

- Osteosarcoma (assuming the patient does not have an amputation)
  - Initial therapy with an approved NSAID for mild to moderate pain

Continuous therapy with amantadine to treat and prevent wind-up
Pamidronate, a bisphosphonate, every 3 to 4 weeks to decrease osteoclast function
Tramadol with the NSAID for moderate to severe pain
Oxycodone to replace tramadol as the pain gets worse

Chondrosarcoma
Initial therapy with an approved NSAID for mild to moderate pain
Gabapentin in progressively increasing doses for analgesia and to help prevent wind-up

Transitional cell carcinoma
This is the only tumor that has been definitively identified as being responsive to piroxicam. Hence, piroxicam should be administered for anticancer effects and for analgesia. The patient's packed cell volume (PCV) should be monitored closely, because piroxicam is a nonspecific COX-1/COX-2 inhibitor, predisposing to moderate to severe ulceration and the potential for gastrointestinal bleeding.

SUMMARY

Control of cancer pain is within the capabilities of most veterinarians and is achievable in most animal patients that have cancer with techniques that are currently available. Once veterinarians and technicians gain a good knowledge base about pain and its therapy, pain control should be achievable by following these simple ABCs:

A. Assess the pain. Ask for the owner's perceptions.
B. Believe the owner. The owner sees the pet each day in its own environment.
C. Choose appropriate therapy following the World Health Organization ladder and other more specific paradigms.
D. Deliver therapy in a logical coordinated manner.
E. Empower the clients to participate actively in their pet's well-being.

Great satisfaction can be derived from not only treating the pet's cancer but its pain. Incorporating pain management into oncology practice is good for the well-being of the pet, the owner, the staff, the veterinarians, and the practice.

REFERENCES

1. Goisis A, Gorini M, Ratti R, et al. Application of a WHO protocol on medical therapy for oncologic pain in an internal medicine hospital. Tumori 1989;75:470–2.
2. Bowersox TS, Lipowitz AJ, Hardy RM, et al. The use of a synthetic prostaglandin E1 analog as a gastric protectant against aspirin-induced hemorrhage in the dog. J Am Anim Hosp Assoc 1996;32:401–7.
3. World Health Organization. Cancer pain relief and palliative care. Report of a WHO expert committee. World Health Organ Tech Rep Ser 1990;804:1–75.
4. Mersky H. Clarification definition of neuropathic pain. Pain 2002;96:408–9.
5. Woolf CJ. Recent advances in the pathophysiology of acute pain. Br J Anaesth 1989;63:139–46.
6. Gaynor JS. Is postoperative pain management important in dogs and cats? Vet Med 1999;94:254–8.
7. Muir WW. Pain and stress. In: Gaynor J, Muir WW, editors. Handbook of veterinary pain management. 1st edition. St. Louis (MO): Mosby; 2002. p. 46–59.

8. Cousins MJ, Phillips GD. Acute pain management. New York: Churchill Livingstone; 1986; 19–48.
9. Hamill RJ. The physiologic and metabolic response to pain and stress. In: Hamill RJ, Rowlingson JC, editors. Handbook of critical care pain management. New York: McGraw-Hill; 1994. p. 39–52.
10. Cousins M. Acute and postoperative pain. In: Wall PD, Melzack R, editors. Textbook of pain. 3rd edition. Edinburgh (UK): Churchill Livingstone; 1994. p. 357–85.
11. McGuill MW. Our oath of kindness. J Am Vet Med Assoc 2002;221:1682–3.
12. Brown C, Thompson S, Vroegindewey G, et al. The global veterinarian: the why? The what? The how? J Vet Med Educ 2006;33:411–5.
13. Muir WW, Gaynor J. Pain behaviors. In: Gaynor J, Muir WW, editors. Handbook of veterinary pain management. 1st edition. St. Louis (MO): Mosby; 2002. p. 65–81.
14. Hellyer P. Objective, categoric methods for assessing pain and analgesia. In: Gaynor J, Muir WW, editors. Handbook of veterinary pain management. 1st edition. St. Louis (MO): Mosby; 2002. p. 82–110.
15. Holton LL, Scott EM, Nolan AM, et al. The development of a multidimensional scale to assess pain in dogs. Proceedings of the 6th International Congress on Veterinary Anesthesia 1997:106.
16. Holton LL, Scott EM, Nolan AM, et al. Comparison of three methods used for assessment of pain in dogs. J Am Vet Med Assoc 1998;212:61–6 [see comments].
17. Budsberg SC. Nonsteroidal antiinflammatory drugs. In: Gaynor J, Muir WW, editors. Handbook of veterinary pain management. St. Louis (MO): Mosby; 2002. p. 184–98.
18. Booth NH. Nonnarcotic analgesics. In: Booth NH, McDonald LE, editors. Veterinary pharmacology and therapeutics. 5th edition. Ames (IA): Iowa State University Press; 1982. p. 297–320.
19. Lascelles BD, Court MH, Hardie EM, et al. Nonsteroidal anti-inflammatory drugs in cats: a review. Vet Anaesth Analg 2007;34:228–50.
20. MacPhail CM, Lappin MR, Meyer DJ, et al. Hepatocellular toxicosis associated with administration of carprofen in 21 dogs. J Am Vet Med Assoc 1998; 212(12):1895–901.
21. Golden BD, Abramson SB. Selective cyclooxygenase-2 inhibitors. Rheum Dis Clin North Am 1999;25:359–78.
22. Rubin BR. Specific cyclooxygenase-2 (COX-2) inhibitors. J Am Osteopath Assoc 1999;99:300–1.
23. Shaw N, Burrows CF, King RR. Massive gastric hemorrhage induced by buffered aspirin in a greyhound. J Am Anim Hosp Assoc 1999;33:215–9.
24. Wagner A. Opioids. In: Gaynor J, Muir WW, editors. Handbook of veterinary pain management. St. Louis (MO): Mosby; 2002. p. 164–83.
25. Hoskin PJ, Hanks GW. Opioid agonist-antagonist drugs in acute and chronic pain states. Drugs 1991;41:326–44.
26. Rosland JH, Hole K. 1, 4-Benzodiazepines antagonize opiate-induced antinociception in mice. Anesth Analg 1990;71:242–8.
27. Heel RC, Brogden RN, Speight TM, et al. Buprenorphine: a review of its pharmacological properties and therapeutic efficacy. Drugs 1990;17:81–110.
28. Robertson SA, Taylor PM, Sear JW. Systemic uptake of buprenorphine by cats after oral mucosal administration. Vet Rec 2003;152:675–8.
29. Robertson SA, Taylor PM, Lascelles BD, et al. Changes in thermal threshold response in eight cats after administration of buprenorphine, butorphanol and morphine. Vet Rec 2003;153:462–5.

30. Mama K, Mich, P, Raske, T, et al. Buccal absorption of 3 formulations of buprenorphine in the dog. Annual Scientific Meeting of the American College of Veterinary Anesthesiologists, New Orleans, September 26–30, 2007.
31. Sawyer DC, Rech RH, Durham RA, et al. Dose response to butorphanol administered subcutaneously to increase visceral nociceptive threshold in dogs. Am J Vet Res 1991;52:1826–30.
32. Scherk-Nixon M. A study of the use of a transdermal fentanyl patch in cats. J Am Anim Hosp Assoc 1996;32:19–24.
33. Schultheiss PJ, Morse BC, Baker WH. Evaluation of a transdermal fentanyl system in the dog. Contemp Top Lab Anim Sci 1995;34(5):75–81.
34. Egger CM, Duke T, Archer J, et al. Comparison of plasma fentanyl concentrations by using three transdermal fentanyl patch sizes in dogs. Vet Surg 1998;27: 159–66.
35. KuKanich B, Papich MG. Pharmacokinetics of tramadol and the metabolite O-desmethyltramadol in dogs. J Vet Pharmacol Ther 2004;27:239–46.
36. Kuo WC, Keegan RD. Comparative cardiovascular, analgesic, and sedative effects of medetomidine, medetomidine-hydromorphone, and medetomidine-butorphanol in dogs. Proceedings of the Annual Meeting of the American College of Veterinary Anesthesiologists, Orlando, FL, October 10-11, 2002:34.
37. Benson GJ, Grubb TL, Neff-Davis C, et al. Effect of medetomidine on surgically-induced endocrine responses. Proceedings of the 5th International Congress of Veterinary Anesthesia, September 17–18, 1994:165.
38. Granholm M, McKusick BC, Westerholm FC, et al. Evaluation of the clinical efficacy and safety of intramuscular and intravenous doses of dexmedetomidine and medetomidine in dogs and their reversal with atipamezole. Vet Rec 2007; 160:891–7.
39. Leppanen MK, McKusick BC, Granholm MM, et al. Clinical efficacy and safety of dexmedetomidine and buprenorphine, butorphanol or diazepam for canine hip radiography. J Small Anim Pract 2006;47:663–9.
40. Serteyn D, Coppens P, Jones R, et al. Circulatory and respiratory effects of the combination medetomidine-ketamine in beagles. J Vet Pharmacol Ther 1993; 16:199–206.
41. Savola JM. Cardiovascular actions of medetomidine and their reversal by atipamezole. Acta vet scand 1989;85:39–47.
42. Haskins SC, Peiffer RL, Stowe CM. A clinical comparison of CT-1341, ketamine, and xylazine in cats. Am J Vet Res 1975;36:1537–43.
43. Fu ES, Miguel R, Scharf JE. Preemptive ketamine decreases postoperative narcotic requirements in patients undergoing abdominal surgery. Anesth Analg 1997;84:1086–90.
44. Wagner AE, Walton JA, Hellyer PW, et al. Use of low doses of ketamine administered by constant rate infusion as an adjunct for postoperative analgesia in dogs. J Am Vet Med Assoc 2002;221:72–4.
45. Blanpied TA, Clarke RJ, Johnson JW. Amantadine inhibits NMDA receptors by accelerating channel closure during channel block. J Neurosci 2005;25:3312–22.
46. Lascelles BD, Gaynor JS, Smith ES, et al. Amantadine in a multimodal analgesic regimen for alleviation of refractory osteoarthritis pain in dogs. American College of Veterinary Internal Medicine Conference. Seattle, WA. J Vet Intern Med 2007; 21:606–7 [absract].
47. Pud D, Eisenberg E, Spitzer A, et al. The NMDA receptor antagonist amantadine reduces surgical neuropathic pain in cancer patients: a double blind, randomized, placebo controlled trial. Pain 1998;75:349–54.

48. Hoffman HE, Gaylord JC, Blasecki JW, et al. Pharmacokinetics and metabolism of rimantadine hydrochloride in mice and dogs. Antimicrobial Agents Chemother 1988;32:1699–704.
49. Radulovic LL, Turck D, von Hodenberg A, et al. Disposition of gabapentin (Neurontin) in mice, rats, dogs, and monkeys. Drug Metab Dispos 1995;23:441–8.
50. Merskey H. Pharmacologic approaches other than opioids in chronic non-cancer pain management. Acta Anaesthesiol Scand 1997;41:187–90.
51. Bader AM, Datta S, Flanagan H, et al. Comparison of bupivacaine- and ropivacaine-induced conduction blockade in the isolated rabbit vagus nerve. Anesth Analg 1989;68:724–7.
52. Moller R, Covino BG. Cardiac electrophysiologic properties of bupivacaine and lidocaine compared with those of ropivacaine, a new amide local anesthetic. Anesth 1990;72:322–9.
53. Badgwell JM, Heavner JE, Kytta J. Bupivacaine toxicity in young pigs is age-dependent and is affected by volatile anesthetics. Anesth 1990;73:297–303.
54. Lacombe P, Blaise G, Loulmet D, et al. Electrophysiologic effects of bupivacaine in the isolated rabbit heart. Anesth Analg 1991;72:62–9.
55. Gaynor JS, Mama KR. Local and regional anesthetic techniques for alleviation of perioperative pain. In: Gaynor J, Muir WW, editors. Handbook of veterinary pain management. 1st edition. St. Louis (MO): Mosby; 2002. p. 261–80.
56. Robinson TM, Kruse-Elliott KT, Markel MD, et al. A comparison of transdermal fentanyl versus epidural morphine for analgesia in dogs undergoing major orthopedic surgery. J Am Anim Hosp Assoc 1999;35:95–100.
57. Friedland J. Local and systemic radiation for palliation of metastatic disease. Urol Clin North Am 1999;26:391–402.
58. Veri A, D'Andrea MR, Bonginelli P, et al. Clinical usefulness of bisphosphonates in oncology: treatment of bone metastases, antitumoral activity and effect on bone resorption markers. Int J Biol Markers 2007;22:24–33.
59. Fan TM, de Lorimier LP, O'Dell-Anderson K, et al. Single-agent pamidronate for palliative therapy of canine appendicular osteosarcoma bone pain. J Vet Intern Med 2007;21:431–9.
60. Molinuevo MS, Bruzzone L, Cortizo AM. Alendronate induces anti-migratory effects and inhibition of neutral phosphatases in UMR106 osteosarcoma cells. Eur J Pharmacol 2007;562:28–33.
61. Farese JP, Ashton J, Milner R, et al. The effect of the bisphosphonate alendronate on viability of canine osteosarcoma cells in vitro. In Vitro Cell Dev Biol Anim 2004;40:113–7.
62. Balena R, Markatos A, Seedor JG, et al. Long-term safety of the aminobisphosphonate alendronate in adult dogs. II. Histomorphometric analysis of the L5 vertebrae. J Pharmacol Exp Ther 1996;276:277–83.
63. Tomlin JL, Sturgeon C, Pead MJ, et al. Use of the bisphosphonate drug alendronate for palliative management of osteosarcoma in two dogs. Vet Rec 2000;147:129–32.
64. Kavoussi B, Ross BE. The neuroimmune basis of anti-inflammatory acupuncture. Integr Cancer Ther 2007;6:251–7.
65. Janssens LAA, Rogers PAM, Schoen AM. Acupuncture analgesia: a review. Vet Rec 1988;122:355–8.
66. Wright M, McGrath CJ. Physiologic and analgesic effects of acupuncture in the dog. J Am Vet Med Assoc 1981;178:502–7.

67. Zhang RX, Li A, Liu B, et al. Electroacupuncture attenuates bone cancer pain and inhibits spinal interleukin-1 beta expression in a rat model. Anesth Analg 2007;105:1482–8, table of contents.
68. Gaynor JS. Acupuncture for management of pain. Vet Clin North Am 2000;30(4):875–84.
69. Jacox A, Carr DB, Payne R, et al. Management of cancer pain. Rockville (MD): Agency for Health Care Policy and Research; 1994.

Nonsurgical Management of Osteoarthritis in Dogs

Spencer A. Johnston, VMD[a,*], Ronald M. McLaughlin, DVM, DVSc[b], Steven C. Budsberg, DVM, MS[a]

KEYWORDS

- Osteoarthritis • Nonsteroidal anti-inflammatory drug
- Disease-modifying agent of osteoarthritis • Physiotherapy
- Medical management • Evidence-based

Occam's razor is a philosophical statement that is often used as a guideline in the practice of medicine. Originally referred to as the Law of Parsimony, it essentially states that the simplest explanation of a problem is frequently the best.[1] In medicine, it is often used to suggest that a patient's clinical signs can usually be explained by one disease process instead of a complex interaction of multiple disease processes. By extension, it is often suggested that the abnormality is treated in the least complex manner possible.

Although Occam's razor can be used to explain how a multitude of clinical signs can be attributed to a condition like osteoarthritis (OA), it does not necessarily extend to the treatment of this condition. OA, although superficially considered to be deterioration of the joint associated with pain and dysfunction, is actually quite a complex condition. When considering treatment of OA, a multitude of biochemical, physical, and pathologic alterations must be recognized.[2] Because our knowledge of OA and factors contributing to its development suggest that OA has existed for as long as the diarthrodial joint has existed, and because no known cure or even universally accepted treatment for OA exists, it is probably safe to assume that a single simple treatment does not exist. This does not seem to hinder the quest to find one, however. The search for the Holy Grail of OA treatment continues, and is likely to continue, well past the career longevity of the authors of this article.

Treatment for OA is effectively limited to the available products. The number of products proved to provide safe and effective treatment does not change rapidly. The approved pharmaceutic agents are the most extensively reviewed products. There is a constant search to find new and improved treatments, however, and

[a] Department of Small Animal Medicine and Surgery, College of Veterinary Medicine, University of Georgia, 501 D.W. Brooks Drive, Athens, GA 30602, USA
[b] Department of Clinical Sciences, Mississippi State University, College of Veterinary Medicine, PO Box 6100, Mississippi State, MS 39762, USA
* Corresponding author.
E-mail address: spencerj@uga.edu (S.A. Johnston).

Vet Clin Small Anim 38 (2008) 1449–1470
doi:10.1016/j.cvsm.2008.08.001 **vetsmall.theclinics.com**

nonpharmaceutic treatments are often suggested and embraced despite a lack of proved efficacy or safety. Journal articles, podium presentations at major and minor veterinary meetings, and popular press articles frequently address the treatment of OA. Seemingly, most of these presentations are based on the same data, or include that author's or speaker's opinion variably based on scientific data or anecdotal experience.

In practice, the decision of when and how to treat OA is often based on a combination of factors. These factors include the available data regarding efficacy but also incorporate the frequency of administration, product formulation, cost, promotions and advertisements by the manufacturer or distributor of the drug or supplement, personal experience, and success or failure of prior treatments used by the client and patient. Treatment is further influenced by the ability or willingness of the client to understand or implement weight control, exercise modification, and physical therapy as part of the management strategy. This article presents a review of the published material regarding various treatments for OA. When there are no data regarding a specific treatment or when a statement is the opinion of the authors, such a deficiency is identified.

TREATMENT OF OSTEOARTHRITIS

Treatment of OA has traditionally been directed toward palliation of the painful symptoms associated with the condition. It is generally recognized that a variable degree of pathologic change, including bone and soft tissue alterations, exists, and the degree of pathologic change and clinical signs associated with OA must be considered on a continuous scale. The severity of discomfort, often manifest as lameness, can be inconsistent with the degree of pathologic or radiographic change. Furthermore, the severity of the associated symptoms may be related to recent use, or stress, placed on the articular and periarticular tissues. The combination of these variables may lead to chronic pain, often characterized as a dull ache, or acute pain, more typically characterized as a sharp shooting pain. The wide range of factors affecting joint health and pain status makes it difficult to provide a specific recommendation for the treatment of OA that is applicable in all situations. Part of the challenge of OA treatment is that the goal is often variable between patients or within an individual patient. As a result, multimodal therapy is often necessary to address this complex problem.

NONSTEROIDAL ANTI-INFLAMMATORY DRUGS

Nonsteroidal anti-inflammatory drugs (NSAIDs) are the most frequently recommended treatment for OA. The popularity of this class of drugs is typically attributed to the effectiveness of NSAIDs for palliating the painful symptoms associated with OA and their relative ease of administration. An excellent thorough review of NSAIDs approved in the United States for use in small animals was recently published.[3] It is not the intention of this article to repeat such an extensive review but to focus on the use of these products for the treatment of OA.

Although acetaminophen, an analgesic, is often recommended for the treatment of OA in human beings because of a decreased side effect profile, NSAIDs remain popular despite well-known side effects that may occur with their use.[4–6] When used by people who have OA, NSAIDs are generally considered to provide a greater global relief score than does acetaminophen.[7] A greater global relief score is generally a result of treatment effect (including decreased pain, improved functioning, or both), decreased side effects, and patient (or client) expectation.[8] Although use of acetaminophen is considered to be an option for the treatment of OA in dogs, no controlled clinical trials have been performed to evaluate the safety and efficacy of this drug.[9]

The efficacy of NSAIDs, when compared with placebo administration, for the treatment of OA is unquestioned. Studies comparing one NSAID with another NSAID for the treatment of people with OA most frequently demonstrate that each NSAID is superior to placebo with respect to pain relief but that no significant difference exists among NSAIDs.[10] Although some studies using veterinary-approved NSAIDs suggest a difference with respect to analgesic quality,[11] it is generally accepted that, when comparing large groups of patients, there is little difference among the approved NSAIDs with respect to the level of symptom relief. Nevertheless, there is evidence, through n-of-1 studies published in the human literature, that one NSAID is often more beneficial than another for a specific individual.[12] It is reasonable to presume that dogs have a similar response to NSAIDs. Veterinary NSAIDs are often prescribed based on convenience of dosing, product formulation, risk or concern for the patient developing side effects, marketing issues (including manufacturer support and promotional efforts), cost, and demonstrated efficacy for an individual.

A recent review article by Aragon and colleagues[13] identified the evidence-based literature related to clinical trials evaluating the treatment of OA in dogs. This review included NSAIDs in addition to other treatments. Articles published since that review are included in the following discussion. The rating system used by Aragon and colleagues[13] is included in the Appendix.

Aspirin

There have been no clinical trials assessing aspirin for the relief of painful symptoms associated with OA in dogs. The recommended dosage of aspirin, based on pharmacologic studies and clinical experience, is 10 to 25 mg/kg administered orally two to three times daily. In the authors' clinical experience, vomiting is often associated with a dosage of 25 mg/kg administered orally three times daily, whereas 10 mg/kg administered orally one or two times daily is better tolerated.[9] Endoscopic studies have documented that aspirin is more likely to cause gastric bleeding and erosions than most other NSAIDs.[14–16]

Carprofen

Carprofen was the first of the newer NSAIDs to be approved for canine use. Aragon and colleagues[13] evaluated five clinical trials designed to assess the use of carprofen to alleviate the clinical symptoms associated with OA. They concluded there was a moderate level of comfort that the substance and disease relation is scientifically valid. Since that evaluation, three more clinical trials have been published evaluating carprofen for the treatment of OA.[17–19] These three trials support the efficacy of carprofen for the treatment of OA. The strength of evidence ranking is likely to increase from moderate to high as the number of clinical trials supporting carprofen use for the treatment of OA increases.

The recommended dosage of carprofen is 2.2 mg/kg administered orally twice daily or 4.4 mg/kg administered orally once daily. Adverse effects reported with carprofen include gastrointestinal toxicity and idiopathic hepatocellular toxicosis. Because of different methods of reporting, it is difficult to assess the incidence of adverse effects related to the hepatic and gastrointestinal systems. Clinical trials evaluating the administration of carprofen for 60 days or longer suggest a combined incidence of approximately 6% or less.[17,20,21] A study directly comparing firocoxib and carprofen reported the incidence of health problems (including adipsia, anorexia, anxiety, constipation, diarrhea, emesis, and polydipsia) associated with firocoxib and carprofen use as 20% and 34%, respectively, but there was no statistical difference between the two treatment groups.[19] The study did not include an untreated group for comparison with the overall incidence of health problems in the study population.

One experimental study[22] suggested the possibility of decreased cartilage damage and subchondral bone remodeling in dogs with cranial cruciate ligament transection. This finding has not been evaluated in a clinical trial.

Etodolac

Etodolac was the second veterinary NSAID to obtain the approval of the US Food and Drug Administration (FDA). It was demonstrated to be effective for alleviating the painful symptoms associated with coxofemoral OA in one randomized placebo-controlled study.[23] Based on this study, Aragon and colleagues[13] concluded there was a moderate level of comfort that the substance and disease relation is scientifically valid. Etodolac was used as a noninferiority comparator in a clinical study of dogs with OA.[24] Although evaluation of the efficacy of etodolac was not the primary emphasis of that study, etodolac seemed to be effective for the treatment of OA. The recommended dose of etodolac is 10 to 15 mg/kg orally once daily.

Keratoconjunctivitis sicca (KCS) has been reported with etodolac administration.[25] The mean duration of etodolac administration before the development of KCS was approximately 8 to 9 months. Most dogs that developed KCS did not respond to treatment. The incidence of KCS development is unknown.

The product prescribing information states that oral administration of etodolac at a daily dosage of 10 mg/kg (4.5 mg/lb) for 12 months, or at 15 mg/kg (6.8 mg/lb) for 6 months, resulted in some dogs showing a mild weight loss, fecal abnormalities (loose, mucoid, mucosanguineous feces or diarrhea), and hypoproteinemia. Diarrhea was reported to occur in 2.6% of dogs receiving etodolac in the clinical trial reported by Budsberg and colleagues[23] and in 8.3% of dogs evaluated by Hanson and colleagues.[24]

Deracoxib

In one scientific abstract, deracoxib was reported to be effective for alleviating lameness associated with OA in dogs.[26] The recommended dosage is 1 to 2 mg/kg administered orally once daily for chronic pain. Deracoxib has been reported to cause gastrointestinal ulceration, although most cases reported were associated with concurrent administration of prednisone, another NSAID, or administration of deracoxib exceeding the recommended dose.[27] Because no clinical trials have been published regarding deracoxib use, Aragon and colleagues[13] were not able to evaluate the clinical evidence regarding deracoxib for the treatment of OA.

Meloxicam

Meloxicam has been evaluated in four clinical trials targeting dogs affected with OA.[20,28–30] All four of these studies are classified as type I.[13] In all studies, meloxicam was demonstrated to be effective for alleviating clinical symptoms. Aragon and colleagues[13] evaluated these four clinical trials and concluded there was a high level of comfort that the substance and disease relation is scientifically valid.

The recommended dosage of meloxicam is 0.1 mg/kg administered orally once daily. Administration of a single loading dose of 0.2 mg/kg administered orally can be given to hasten establishment of steady-state blood levels. The product insert for meloxicam indicates an incidence of diarrhea of approximately 12%. Two clinical trials[29,30] suggest an approximately 12% incidence of mild gastrointestinal side effects, although two other clinical studies[20,28] suggest that adverse gastrointestinal events occur less frequently. Meloxicam has been demonstrated not to affect gastrointestinal motility or gastrointestinal mucosa permeability when administered for 6 or 8 days, respectively.[31,32]

Tepoxalin

Tepoxalin is a unique member of the stable of drugs available to the small animal practitioner. It is classified as a dual inhibitor of cyclooxygenase (COX) and lipoxygenase (LOX). Tepoxalin inhibits the LOX pathway of arachidonic acid (AA) metabolism, and therefore decreases the production of leukotrienes, specifically LTB_4, which is a potent chemoattractant for neutrophils and other inflammatory cells.[33] Leukotrienes are known to increase the production of proinflammatory cytokines, such as interleukin-1β.[34] It is speculated that inhibition of the COX and LOX pathways provides greater analgesia than inhibition of COX inhibition alone. Despite the attractiveness of this theory, there are no published clinical studies demonstrating efficacy of tepoxalin for the treatment of OA in dogs. The recommended dosage is 10 mg/kg administered orally once daily. A loading dose of 20 mg/kg may be given to hasten increasing plasma levels to a minimum effective concentration. Commercially, tepoxalin is available as a rapidly dissolving tablet.

Firocoxib

Firocoxib is the most recently approved NSAID for the canine market. Three clinical trials have demonstrated that firocoxib is effective when administered to dogs with OA.[19,24,35] These trials were not evaluated by Aragon and colleagues.[13] Two of these trials[19,24] were study design type I, and one[35] was study design type III. Using the criteria employed by Aragon and colleagues,[13] the authors conclude there is a moderate level of comfort that the substance and disease relation is scientifically valid for firocoxib. The recommended dose is 5 mg/kg orally once daily.

The incidence of vomiting, diarrhea, or both was reported as 4.7% or less in one study evaluating firocoxib use.[24] The incidence of an adverse health event, not necessarily related to the gastrointestinal tract, was 20% by Pollmeier and colleagues[19] and could not be determined from the information presented in the study by Ryan and colleagues.[35]

ANALGESICS USED AS PART OF MULTIMODAL THERAPY

Because of the complex neurobiology of pain,[36] it is reasonable to believe that multimodal pharmacologic and nonpharmacologic therapy is advantageous for the treatment of OA.[4,37] Similarly, it is often suggested that the dosage of any drug be decreased to the lowest effective dose, particularly when used as part of multimodal therapy, to avoid potential side effects. However, since demonstrating efficacy of a single drug or modality for the treatment of OA is challenging, demonstrating the efficacy of an altered dosage, or the addition of a subsequent treatment or a combination of treatments for a condition with such variable pathologic and clinical signs as OA is more challenging and requires a considerable investment of time and resources.[37] Therefore, there are few clinical studies documenting the efficacy of an altered dosage of a single drug or the use of a combination of drugs. The following analgesics have been suggested based on a sound understanding of the neurobiology of chronic pain. Although these drugs may be used clinically in human beings and dogs, further studies are required to confirm efficacy.

Tramadol

Tramadol is considered to be an opioid analgesic that is unlike typical opioid analgesics. The mechanism of action is through weak inhibition of opioid receptors, along with interference of the release and reuptake of noradrenaline and serotonin in the descending inhibitory pathways.[38] Central inhibition of proinflammatory cytokines and nuclear factor (NF)-κB may also occur with tramadol use,[39] and tramadol may also work by influencing various neuronal cation channels and other receptors.[40] A once-daily formulation of tramadol has been demonstrated to be effective for treatment of OA in people.[41,42] The use of the combination of tramadol and an NSAID or paracetamol has been demonstrated to be effective for the treatment of OA in people.[43–46]

Although the combination of an NSAID and tramadol is commonly used clinically in veterinary medicine, no published clinical trials have demonstrated clinical efficacy of this combination for the treatment of OA in dogs. One study of the combination of ketoprofen and tramadol has been reported in abstract form.[47] Although no clinical trials have confirmed a safe dosage range, clinical use at a dosage of 2 to 5 mg/kg administered orally every 8 to 12 hours has been effective in the authors' experience.

Side effects reported with the use of tramadol in human beings include nausea, vomiting, constipation, dizziness, drowsiness, and seizures.[48] Infrequently, tramadol has been associated with serotonin syndrome, a condition of excessive serotonergic activity producing cognitive behavioral changes, neuromuscular hyperactivity, and autonomic activation.[49] Serotonin syndrome has been reported in human beings with tramadol alone, or when coadministered with other drugs that may inhibit reuptake of serotonin, such as tricyclic antidepressants.[49] Because of the possibility of this interaction, coadministration of tramadol and a tricyclic antidepressant, such as amitriptyline, should probably be avoided.

Amantadine

Amantadine inhibits the *N*-methyl-D-aspartate (NMDA) receptor. NMDA receptors are found in the dorsal spinal horn. Activation of these receptors is associated with chronic pain. When aδ and c fibers are chronically stimulated, glutamate is released from the afferent terminal. Glutamate then activates the NMDA receptor in the dorsal spinal horn, resulting in transmission of an ascending impulse along the second-order neuron.[36,50] Despite sound theory suggesting that NMDA receptor blockade results in decreased pain, a truly effective NMDA inhibitor has not been identified for treatment of neuropathic pain in human beings.[51] Although an NMDA inhibitor may not be an effective primary analgesic, it may provide benefit if coadministered with an opioid or other analgesic.

An interesting study by Lascelles and colleagues[52] demonstrated that administration of meloxicam to dogs with OA resulted in significant improvement in client-specific outcome measures. Additionally, it was demonstrated that the combination of amantadine (3–5 mg/kg administered once daily) and an NSAID (meloxicam), given for 21 days, provided greater treatment effect than meloxicam alone. This is the first clinical trial in human beings or dogs to demonstrate an effective analgesic effect of an NMDA inhibitor for the treatment of OA.

Gabapentin

It has been speculated that other drugs, such as gabapentin, may also be beneficial adjunctive treatment for OA. Gabapentin is structurally similar to γ-aminobutyric acid (GABA). Although the mechanism of action was initially thought to be through

GABAergic transmission, it is now believed to be through the blockade of voltage-gated calcium channels.[53] Gabapentin is thought to work primarily by influence within the central nervous system and is recognized as being beneficial for the treatment of neurogenic pain. To the authors' knowledge, no studies have been published evaluating the use of gabapentin for the treatment of OA in dogs.

Amitriptyline

Amitriptyline is a tricyclic antidepressant that has been used to treat chronic and neuropathic pain in human beings. Amitriptyline is thought to act centrally by inhibiting neuronal reuptake of norepinephrine and serotonin.[54] The result of this action is an increase in the activity of the descending inhibitory pathways that modulate afferent nociceptive input.[55,56] Amitriptyline may also act peripherally by inhibiting sodium channels.[54,57] There are no published clinic trials evaluating the use of amitriptyline for the treatment of OA in dogs.

ADDITIONAL THERAPEUTIC AGENTS

Polysulfated Glycosaminoglycan

Polysulfated glycosaminoglycan (PSGAG) is approved for use in dogs as a disease-modifying agent of osteoarthritis (DMOAD). Two studies are published providing information on the treatment of OA in dogs using PSGAG.[58,59] One study[58] was a type I study. The study subjectively suggested a potential positive effect without statistical significance. Aragon and colleagues[13] gave the study a quality rating that suggests some uncertainties exist relating to the scientific quality. The study does provide information to conclude there was some suggestion that the effect is physiologically meaningful and achievable. A more recent study[59] was a type II study and was not evaluated by Aragon and colleagues.[13] Using the criteria as applied by Aragon and colleagues,[13] this study receives a good quality rating. The overall rating of the strength of the evidence concludes that one can have a moderate level of comfort with the results of these two studies.

Although numerous dose recommendations have been reported for the use of Adequan Canine (Novartis Animal Health US, Inc., Greensboro, North Carolina) in dogs, a dosage of 5 mg/kg administered intramuscularly twice weekly for 4 weeks is the current labeled dosage in dogs. No data are available in regard to dosing beyond 4 weeks. PSGAG is a heparin analogue, and its use in animals with bleeding disorders should be avoided. Concurrent use with NSAIDs that exhibit strong antithromboxane (COX-1) activity should be avoided in all patients.

Pentosan Polysulfate

Pentosan polysulfate (PPS) is approved in human medicine to treat interstitial cystitis. It is also an antithrombotic/lipidemic agent and has had recurring popularity as a potential DMOAD. Two trials in dogs with OA have been published.[60,61] Both studies were prospective in design, were randomized, and are classified with a type I rating.[13] One study subjectively showed a positive effect,[61] and the other subjectively showed no positive effect.[60] Aragon and colleagues[13] gave the studies a quality rating that suggests some uncertainties exist relating to the scientific quality and a low consistency rating, meaning the results were inconsistent. The studies do provide information to conclude there was some suggestion that the effect is physiologically meaningful and achievable. An overall rating of the strength of the evidence concludes that one can have a moderate level of comfort with the results of the aforementioned studies.

Hyaluronan

Hyaluronan (HA) is a nonsulfated glycosaminoglycan that is a major component of synovial fluid. It is administered primarily by intra-articular injection, although a form of HA for intravenous administration is available for use in horses (Legend, Bayer HealthCare, LLC, Shawnee Mission, Kansas). One experimental study evaluated OA progression 32 weeks after intra-articular administration of HA.[62] This prospective nonrandomized study is rated as a type III study. No clinical improvement or preventative effects were identified. The study received a negative quality factor rating, which means it did not adequately address issues of scientific quality.[13] The influence of intravenous HA on synovial fluid quality was evaluated in one clinical trial.[63] Although this study was not a clinical trial assessing functional outcome, it did demonstrate that HA had no influence on the synovial fluid parameters assessed. Another study evaluated intra-articular sodium hyaluronate in dogs with naturally occurring OA.[64] Although not evaluated by Aragon and colleagues,[13] this study is considered to be a type III study with a negative quality factor rating. Based on the available evidence evaluating the use of HA in dogs, the overall rating of strength of the evidence concludes that one can have a low comfort level with the results of these studies.

NUTRITIONAL SUPPLEMENTS

Chondroitin Sulfate and Glucosamine Hydrochloride Preparations

Two trials were identified describing the use of compounds, with chondroitin sulfate and glucosamine hydrochloride as major components, for improving clinical signs associated with OA in dogs.[18,20] Both study designs were prospective, were randomized, and received a type I classification.[13] One study[18] subjectively showed a positive effect, whereas the other[20] showed no positive effect. Examination of the quality of the studies showed that they had adequately addressed issues of scientific quality relating to data collection, analysis, bias, and generalizability. There is a low consistency rating, meaning that the results were inconsistent between the studies. The studies do provide information to conclude there was some suggestion that the effect is physiologically meaningful and achievable. An overall rating of the strength of the evidence concludes that one can have a moderate level of comfort with the results of the aforementioned studies.

Green-Lipped Mussel Preparation

Two trials were identified by Aragon and colleagues[13] as evaluating use of a compound in which the main ingredient was green-lipped mussel (*Perna canaliculus*) for the treatment of OA in dogs.[65,66] Both studies were prospective and randomized in design and received a type I rating. Although both studies subjectively showed a positive effect, these studies were assigned a quality rating that suggests some uncertainties exist relating to the scientific quality. Two other studies[67,68] were not evaluated by Aragon and colleagues.[13] Using the criteria of Aragon and colleagues,[13] these studies were classified as type I studies but had questionable quality ratings. Of the four studies addressing use of green-lipped mussel, three studies suggested mild to moderate improvement, whereas one suggested no difference between placebo and treated groups. Therefore, there is a moderate level of consistency between the studies. The studies do provide information to conclude there was some suggestion that the effect is physiologically meaningful and achievable. An overall rating of the strength of the evidence concludes that one can have a low level of comfort with the results of the aforementioned studies.

P54FP

P54FP is an extract of the Indian and Javanese turmerics *Curcuma domestica* and *Curcuma xanthorrhiza*. A randomized, blind, placebo-controlled, parallel-group clinical trial of P54FP as a treatment for OA of the canine elbow or hip was performed.[60] This study is classified as type I study.[13] The study subjectively suggested a potential positive effect. Examination of the quality of the study showed that the issues of scientific quality relating to data collection, analysis, bias, and generalizability had been adequately addressed. The study does provide information to conclude there was some suggestion that the effect is physiologically meaningful and achievable. An overall rating of the strength of the evidence concludes that one can have a moderate level of comfort with the results of the aforementioned study.

Resin Extract of Boswellia Serrata

One trial with a herbal dietary supplement consisting of a natural resin extract of *Boswellia serrata*, a tree that grows in the hills of India,[69] was conducted to evaluate the effect on OA in dogs.[70] The study is classified with a type III rating. Subjective clinical improvements were identified. As for a quality rating, the study did not adequately address important issues of scientific quality as defined by Aragon and colleagues.[13] Using the criteria of Aragon and colleagues,[13] a low overall rating of the strength of the evidence is given for *B serrata*, indicating that one can have a low level of comfort with the results of the aforementioned study.

Omega-3 (n-3)–Based Diets

Increased omega-3 (n-3) fatty acid dietary supplementation has been advocated as an adjunctive therapy to degenerative and inflammatory arthritic conditions. The theory behind this idea is based on the fact that polyunsaturated fatty acids (PUFAs) are incorporated into cell membrane phospholipids. The amounts of PUFAs in cell membranes depend on dietary fatty acid content. AA is the predominant PUFA in cell membranes; however, supplementation with increased levels of n-3 fatty acids results in increased eicosapentaenoic acid (EPA) content in membrane phospholipids.[71] When eicosanoid metabolism is induced, the EPA competes with available AA as a substrate for the COX enzymes, altering the levels and even the particular inflammatory mediator produced.[71–73] The metabolism of EPA produces relatively less inflammatory prostaglandins (eg, PGE_3). Classic Western diets (human and canine) contain an abundance of n-6 PUFAs and a rather low proportion of n-3 PUFAs. Several canine food products that have a high n-3–to–n-6 fatty acid ratio, and are touted to be of therapeutic benefit in dogs with OA, have recently entered the market. Although most of the data supporting these diets is anecdotal, one abstract presented recently found significant increases in ground reaction forces in dogs with OA after 90 days of the feeding trial.[74]

Weight Control and Weight Loss

Weight reduction has been shown to ameliorate the clinical signs associated with OA in dogs.[75–79] In a nonblind prospective study of 9 overweight dogs with hip OA, Impellizeri and colleagues[75] found that an 11% to 18% reduction in body weight significantly decreased the severity of hind limb lameness. Mlacnik and colleagues[78] reported the results of a prospective randomized clinical trial in which 29 overweight dogs were treated with a combination of caloric restriction and physiotherapy. This treatment was shown to improve patient mobility and facilitate weight loss. Kealy and colleagues[76] reported that the prevalence and severity of OA were less in dogs with long-term reduced food intake (25% less food than control dogs). In another study, Kealy and colleagues[77] reported that long-term 25% restriction in food intake delayed the onset of signs of chronic disease, including OA, and also increased the mean lifespan in these dogs. In a longitudinal cohort study, Smith and colleagues[79] found that a restricted diet delayed or prevented development of radiographic signs of hip joint OA in a population of Labrador retrievers. These studies indicate that weight control is an important aspect of managing osteoarthritic dogs and that weight loss alone may substantially improve clinical signs in overweight dogs with OA.

PHYSICAL REHABILITATION FOR PATIENTS THAT HAVE OSTEOARTHRITIS

Physical rehabilitation is the treatment of diseases and injuries with physical agents, such as heat, cold, water, sound, electricity, massage, and exercise.[80] Its benefits may result from increasing blood and lymph flow through the affected area, resolving inflammation, preventing or minimizing muscle atrophy, preventing periarticular contraction, and providing positive psychologic effects for the patient and owner.[80] There is a paucity of scientific literature documenting effectiveness of physical rehabilitation techniques in small animals. Much of the available information is extrapolated from human physiotherapy, knowledge, and experience and is based on an understanding of basic physiology and pathophysiology. In recent years, however, interest in veterinary physical therapy has grown substantially. On the coattails of this increasing interest, more and more objective research is underway to develop physical therapy techniques specifically for animals (and for specific medical conditions) and to better understand the mechanisms by which rehabilitative techniques may benefit veterinary patients. Until this body of scientific literature increases, currently established physiotherapy techniques are used to manage canine patients that have OA and may reduce pain, control inflammation, improve strength and balance, increase range of motion, prevent muscle spasms, and help to restore more normal joint function.[81–87] In many cases, physiotherapy also helps to reduce the dose of analgesics necessary to maintain patient comfort.[87] Rehabilitation for patients that have OA generally consists of a combination of modalities.[81,82,86,87]

Cryotherapy

Cryotherapy, or local hypothermia, is used in acute inflammation. It promotes vasoconstriction and skeletal muscle relaxation and decreases nerve conduction.[88–93] Vasoconstriction limits blood flow into the area, thereby reducing edema. Muscle relaxation can decrease edema formation by improving venous return and by preventing endothelial damage caused by local acidosis. Decreased nerve conduction produces mild analgesia.

Cryotherapy is applied to osteoarthritic joints using ice packs, ice wraps, and cold compression wraps (**Fig. 1**). A "ziplock bag" containing a solution of two parts water and one part alcohol works well as a reusable cold pack.[82] Multiple-use ice packs and cold water circulating systems are also available. A light bandage can be applied to the limb after treatment.[89] Use of a compression bandage, such as an elastic wrap, can further lower the temperature of the deeper tissues.[89,91]

Superficial cryotherapy can penetrate to a tissue depth of 1 to 4 cm, with the greatest temperature change occurring to a depth of 1 cm.[82] Treatments usually last no more than 30 minutes and should be performed two to four times daily. Longer treatment times may lead to lower temperatures, resulting in protective vasodilation and local edema.[90]

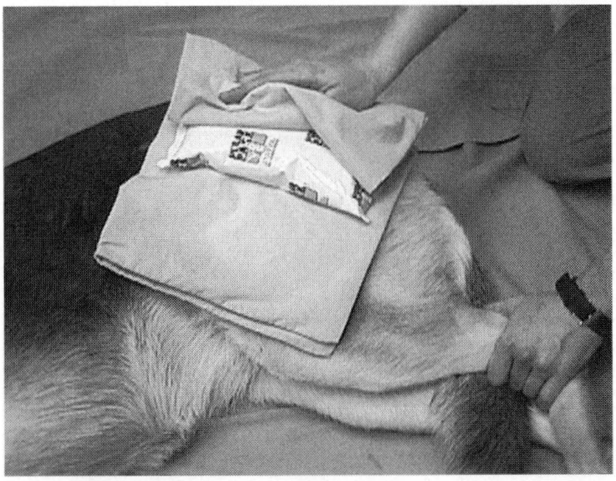

Fig. 1. Cold compress is applied to a dog's limb.

Moist Heat

Moist heat is typically used in chronic cases of OA after acute inflammation has resolved and is often applied before stretching, massage therapy, passive range-of-motion (PROM) exercises, or active excercise.[81,82,87] It has been shown to reduce muscle spasms and increase blood flow to the region.[89,93–95] Superficial hyperthermia reaches a tissue depth of 1 to 2 cm, causing vasodilation, mild sedation, relief of muscular pain, resorption of extravasated fluids, and increased local circulation.[94] Increased circulation enhances local metabolism and improves the delivery of nutrients. Heat also increases the compliance of joint capsules, tendons, and scar tissue and reduces joint stiffness, thereby countering much of the stimulus for pain.[92]

Moist heat is typically applied using moist hot packs, warm baths, warm towels, or hydrocollators.[96] It is applied directly over the affected joints for 15 to 20 minutes two to three times daily. The temperature of the heat source should be between 104°F and 109°F (40°C–45°C).[89] Electric heating pads can burn the patient's skin and are not recommended. The skin should be monitored every 2 to 3 minutes; if hot to the touch, more insulating towels should be applied. Heat is often combined with other forms of physiotherapy; specifically, massage and passive exercise if reduced swelling is the goal. Mild exercise in ambulatory patients within 1 hour of the hyperthermia leads to prolonged and increased effects from the treatment.[93] Superficial hyperthermia is contraindicated in the absence of skin sensation, because the patient can neither sense nor respond to the heat. Premature application of heat (during acute inflammation) may lead to increased edema and pain in the injured area.

Passive Range-of-Motion Exercises

PROM exercises are effective when performed appropriately and help to restore more normal joint motion in patients that have OA. The objective is to advance the joint through a comfortable range of motion. At no time should the patient experience discomfort from strenuous manipulation of the limb, because this can lead to reflex inhibition, limited use of the limb, fibrosis, and, ultimately, delayed return to function.[84] In many cases, analgesics are administered before PROM therapy to improve patient comfort. The patient should be muzzled before any manipulations.[80]

During PROM therapy, the therapist moves the joints without effort on the part of the patient (**Fig. 2**). It is intended to maintain normal range of motion in joints, prevent contracture, improve blood and lymphatic circulation, and stimulate sensory

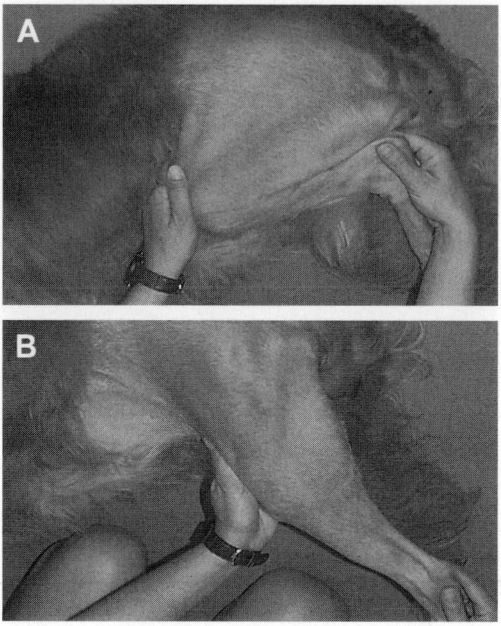

Fig. 2. PROM of the left stifle. The limb is placed in flexion (*A*) and extension (*B*).

awareness. Passive motion has been shown to reduce the catabolic effects of immobility on articular cartilage.[95,97] PROM therapy is commonly used whenever a patient has a lack of motor control or is unwilling to use the limb because of pain. The therapist moves a joint through an unrestricted pain-free motion for 10 to 15 repetitions two to three times a day.[98] It is important that passive motion be performed slowly with the muscles relaxed. The joint is grasped on either side and gently manipulated until the desired flexion or extension angle is reached.[85] After treatment of the individual joints, the entire limb is moved through a range of motion similar to that of ambulation for a minimum of 10 times.[95] A recent study by Crook and colleagues[83] evaluated the effect of passive stretching on the range of motion in osteoarthritic joints of 10 Labrador retrievers. After 21 days of passive stretching (10 repetitions performed twice daily), the range of motion in the affected joints was significantly increased.

Stretching Exercises

Stretching exercises are used to increase tissue extensibility and are performed several times daily after the application of moist heat or therapeutic ultrasound therapy. The muscles are stretched and held for 10 to 30 seconds. This procedure is repeated 10 times during each session.[95,96]

Balance and Proprioception Exercises

Balance exercises focus on weight shifting and are performed several times daily when possible.[95] This can be achieved by moving the standing patient, such that weight is shifted from limb to limb. Alternatively, the therapist can encourage weight shifting by exercising the patient on an uneven surface. Commonly, rocker boards are used to improve balance and proprioception.[81,87]

Massage Therapy

Massage therapy is often combined with other therapeutic techniques. Massage is used to increase arterial, venous, and lymphatic flow; to stretch and breakdown adhesions; to provide muscle relaxation; and to produce analgesia. Massage has no effect on muscle mass, strength, or rate of atrophy.[99] The five components of massage are rhythm, rate, pressure, direction, and frequency. The rhythm should be even. If the intent is to improve circulation, reduce edema, and provide relaxation, the rate should be slow.[100] The rate is increased when friction massage is used to loosen adhesions and break down fibrin clots in deeper structures. The appropriate pressure applied during massage also varies. Light to moderate pressure is used to achieve relaxation or reduce edema. Firmer pressures are used in frictional massage. Pressure also varies over the course of a massage, beginning with light pressure and proceeding to moderate pressure at the end of the session.[101]

There are many types of massage. Two commonly performed techniques in dogs are effleurage and pétrissage.[82,89] Effleurage is performed by running the hands gently over the surface of the skin beginning distally and moving toward the heart. The therapist maintains light contact with the skin, allowing the skin to glide gently over the underlying fascia, which reduces adhesions.[100] Pétrissage is performed by lifting and kneading the soft tissues and rhythmically squeezing the deeper muscles. Intermittently, small circles are made with the heel of the hands at a moderate rate with increasing pressure.[101] A massage session may last 10 to 20 minutes, beginning with effleurage and proceeding to pétrissage. After pétrissage, effleurage is again used to aid in blood and lymph flow from the treated area. Therapy may be performed every 24 to 48 hours.

Therapeutic Ultrasound

Therapeutic ultrasound can be used if heating of deeper tissues is required to help control pain and improve tissue extensibility. The sounds waves are converted to heat as they are absorbed in the muscles.[101] A depth of 5 cm can be reached, causing an elevation in temperature to 40°C to 45°C. Ultrasound is also thought to promote healing by stimulating fibroblastic activity, increasing cellular metabolism, improving circulation, and increasing the strength and pliability of tendons.[95] Nonthermal effects include increased cell membrane permeability, calcium transport, removal of blood cells from the interstitial space, and increased phagocytic activity of macrophages.[102,103] Ultrasound is frequently used to treat muscle injuries and OA and can be delivered at 1 MHz or 3 MHz.[81] The 1-MHz probe penetrates 3 to 5 cm and is used for deep tissues, primarily muscle. The 3-MHz probe achieves only superficial penetration and is used over bony areas. The units have a continuous mode and a pulsed mode.[93]

Ultrasound therapy begins by clipping the area and applying gel to promote ultrasound transmission. Various protocols may be used, depending on the condition being treated. Typically, pulsed ultrasound is applied (0.5–1.5 W/cm^2) to painful areas and continuous ultrasound is applied to stiff joints and muscles two to three times per week.[81]

Laser

Application of laser (light amplification of stimulated emission of radiation) energy in the red and near-infrared light regions may help to reduce pain and inflammation.[96] It has been shown to be effective in controlling OA pain without side effects.[104] The laser probe is held directly over the painful region. The number of joules applied depends on the size of the area and the condition being treated.

Electrical Stimulation

Electrical stimulators are used to increase muscle strength, improve joint range of motion, re-educate muscles, and decrease edema and pain.[105] The stimulator can be pulsed alternating current (biphasic) or pulsed direct current (monophasic). Transcutaneous electrical nerve stimulation (TENS) is used to treat the area of pain and to combat muscle atrophy.[96] One electrode is placed over the motor point of the muscle, and the other is placed along the muscle belly, after shaving the appropriate sites (**Fig. 3**). Typically, treatments last 20 to 30 minutes.[82]

The neuromuscular stimulator can be set with a specific frequency (hertz, pulses per second), amplitude, and pulse duration. The amplitude and the duration of the pulse should be adjusted to make the workout more comfortable for the patient. The location of the electrodes on the skin is marked so that they can be placed in the same location for each treatment. Research has shown that at a frequency of 50 pulses per second at a duration of 175 microseconds, a muscle may contract up to 50% of the normal isometric contraction.[106] Often, the stimulator is set so that the muscle contracts for 10 seconds and relaxes for 50 seconds (duty cycle), for a total of 10 cycles.[95] The optimal duty cycle depends on the condition being treated, however. One study found that neuromuscular stimulation effectively promoted an early return to function and reduced the amount of OA in dogs undergoing cranial cruciate repair.[107,108] This study used 35 pulses per second at 250 microseconds with a duty cycle of 12 seconds on and 25 seconds off for 30 minutes, 3 seconds ramp up, and 2 seconds ramp down.

Active Exercise

Active exercise improves muscular strength, endurance, cardiovascular function, and coordination while reducing joint stiffness and muscle atrophy.[81,82,87,109] It also helps to control body weight. Exercise also provides periodic cartilage loading, which may increase cartilage metabolism and synthesis of proteoglycans.[85,109] Low-impact exercises are preferred, such as leash walking, treadmill walking, jogging, swimming, or climbing stairs or ramps.[81,87] Initially, several shorter sessions (three 20-minute periods) are preferred over a single long session.[87] At first, exercise may be accomplished using active assisted exercise, in which the therapist assists the patient to overcome the force of gravity. Slings, harnesses, "towel walking," or aquatic therapy is commonly used.

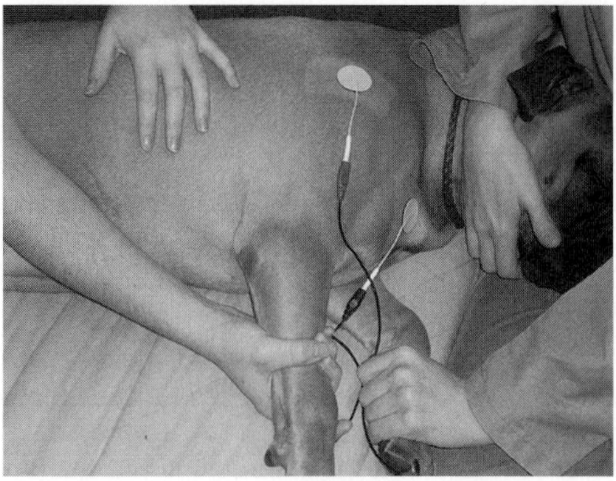

Fig. 3. Electrical stimulator is applied to a dog's right front limb to treat the shoulder.

Aquatic therapy is a special form of active exercise and was developed to help reduce the amount of weight that the patient supports during activity. The amount of weight bearing can be adjusted by varying the depth of the water in which the animal is placed. A water depth to the patient's midthorax promotes walking, whereas deeper water encourages swimming.[89] Swimming promotes the use of all limbs, whereas buoyancy permits mass muscle movement patterns that have instinctively low synaptic resistance pathways in the central nervous system.[110] Underwater treadmills are an increasingly common form of aquatic therapy and can be used for walking and swimming exercises.[87] If the water depth reaches the level of the greater trochanter, the weight borne by the dog is reduced by more than 50%.[96] The speed of the treadmill is typically set at 0.5 to 5 mph. Aquatic therapy using an underwater treadmill enhances cardiovascular endurance, improves muscle strength, reduces pain, and improves balance and range of motion.[87] The patient must be monitored closely during aquatic therapy to prevent exhaustion and hyperthermia.[82]

Active resistive exercises, in which the patient is required to perform specific tasks, are used to restore the animal's strength, stamina, and coordination. Examples include sit-stand exercises, wheelbarrowing, dancing, and approximation.[82,85,87] Approximation involves applying downward pressure over the limbs as the animal is standing, approximating the forces generated while walking. Figure-of-eight exercises may be used to develop medial leg muscles. Other resistive exercises include the use of a physioball to strengthen the forelimbs or hind limbs, and cavaletti rails to improve range of motion and proprioception (**Fig. 4**).[96] Stair climbing and leash walks are also useful resistive exercises and can be gradually increased in duration as the patient improves.

Therapy Monitoring

Rehabilitation programs are customized for individual patients and should be designed to encourage increased weight bearing, to enlarge muscle mass, and to reduce body fat, thereby breaking the cycle of disuse often seen in patients that

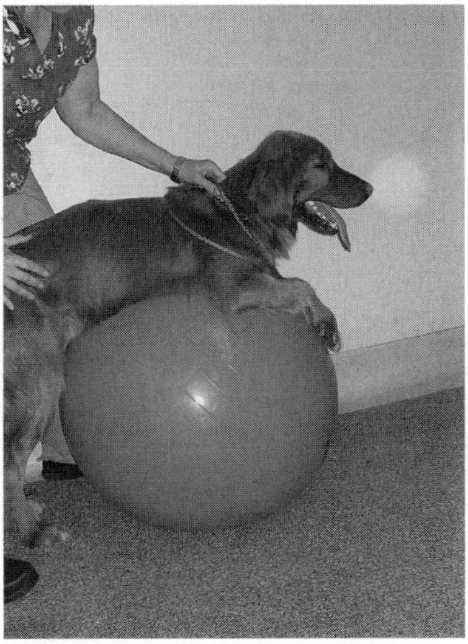

Fig. 4. Patient uses a physioball for active resistance therapy.

have OA.[82,85,87] It is important to maintain a consistent level of activity on a daily basis and to avoid intermittent bursts of activity surrounded by long periods of rest.[80,87] The program should be monitored regularly to determine the efficacy of treatment. Monitoring may include subjective and objective observations, such as goniometric assessment of range of motion, measurement of limb circumference (girth) to assess muscle mass, lameness scoring, documenting changes in muscle mass using CT, dual-energy x-ray absorptiometry (DEXA) analysis, and force plate gait analysis.[82]

APPENDIX

Evidence-Based Classification from Aragon and Colleagues[13]

Study design rating

Type I: randomized controlled interventional trials

Type II: prospective observational cohort studies

Type III: nonrandomized intervention trials with concurrent or historical controls, or case-control studies

Type IV: cross-sectional studies or analyses of secondary disease end points in intervention trials or case series

Quality factor rating

+ study has adequately addressed the issues of scientific quality relating to data collection, analysis, inclusion and exclusion, bias, and generalizability

ø some uncertainties exist relating to the scientific quality

− study has not adequately addressed issues of scientific quality

The total body of evidence rating[13] is a rating given on a combined evaluation of quantity, consistency, and relevance to disease risk reduction (RDRR), with each ranked according to the following criteria:

Quantity

*** numbers of studies (type I, type II, and + only) and individuals tested are sufficiently large enough to generalize comfortably to the target population

** sufficient numbers of studies and individuals, but uncertainties remain regarding generalizing

* numbers of studies and individuals are insufficient for generalization

Consistency

*** sufficient numbers of studies of high quality (+) that are type I or II studies and have consistent results

** moderate consistency across all study types

* results are inconsistent

RDRR

*** magnitude of the effect observed in the studies (type I, type II, and + only) is physiologically meaningful and achievable

** some suggestion that the effect is physiologically meaningful and achievable

* magnitude of the effect in the studies is not likely to be physiologically meaningful or achievable

Strength of evidence ranking

High level of comfort: indicates that qualified scientists agree that a specific claim is scientifically valid. This highest level of ranking indicates an extremely low level of probability of new scientific data overturning the conclusion that the relation in question is valid or significant. This rank is based on relevant high-quality studies of study design types I and II with sufficient numbers of individuals, resulting in a high degree of confidence that the results are relevant to the target population.

Moderate level of comfort: indicates that a relation is promising but not definitive. The claim is based on relevant high- to moderate-quality studies of study design type III and higher and sufficient numbers, resulting in a moderate degree of confidence that the results could be extrapolated to the target population.

Low level of comfort: ranking indicates a low consistency. The relation is based on moderate- to low-quality studies of study design type III and insufficient numbers of individuals tested, resulting in a low degree of confidence that the results could be extrapolated. Uncertainties exist as to whether the proposed benefits would be physiologically meaningful and achievable.

Extremely low level of comfort: ranking indicates extremely low consistency. The relation is based on moderate- to low-quality studies of design type III and insufficient numbers, resulting in an extremely low degree of confidence that the results could be extrapolated.

REFERENCES

1. Lo Re V 3rd, Bellini LM. William of Occam and Occam's razor. Ann Intern Med 2002;136:634–5.
2. Todhunter RJ, Johnston SA. Osteoarthritis. In: Slatter D, editor. Textbook of small animal surgery, vol. 2. 3rd edition. Philadelphia: W.B. Saunders Co.; 2003. p. 2208–46.
3. Clark TP. The clinical pharmacology of cyclooxygenase-2–selective and dual inhibitors. Vet Clin North Am Small Anim Pract 2006;36:1061–85.
4. Zhang W, Moskowitz RW, Nuki G, et al. OARSI recommendations for the management of hip and knee osteoarthritis, part II: OARSI evidence-based, expert consensus guidelines. Osteoarthritis Cartilage 2008;16:137–62.
5. Nikles CJ, Yelland M, Glasziou PP, et al. Do individualized medication effectiveness tests (n-of-1 trials) change clinical decisions about which drugs to use for osteoarthritis and chronic pain? Am J Ther 2005;12:92–7.
6. Nikles CJ, Yelland M, Del Mar C, et al. The role of paracetamol in chronic pain: an evidence-based approach. Am J Ther 2005;12:80–91.
7. Towheed TE, Maxwell L, Judd MG, et al. Acetaminophen for osteoarthritis. Cochrane Database Syst Rev 2006;1:CD004257.
8. Farrar JT, Young JP Jr, LaMoreaux L, et al. Clinical importance of changes in chronic pain intensity measured on an 11-point numerical pain rating scale. Pain 2001;94:149–58.
9. Johnston SA, Budsberg SC. Nonsteroidal anti-inflammatory drugs and corticosteroids for the management of canine osteoarthritis. Vet Clin North Am Small Anim Pract 1997;27:841–62.
10. Chen YF, Jobanputra P, Barton P, et al. Cyclooxygenase-2 selective nonsteroidal anti-inflammatory drugs (etodolac, meloxicam, celecoxib, rofecoxib, etoricoxib, valdecoxib and lumiracoxib) for osteoarthritis and rheumatoid arthritis: a systematic review and economic evaluation. Health Technol Assess 2008;12:1–178.
11. Hazewinkel HA, van den Brom WE, Theyse LF, et al. Comparison of the effects of firocoxib, carprofen and vedaprofen in a sodium urate crystal induced synovitis model of arthritis in dogs. Res Vet Sci 2008;84:74–9.

12. Wegman AC, van der Windt DA, de Haan M, et al. Switching from NSAIDs to paracetamol: a series of n of 1 trials for individual patients with osteoarthritis. Ann Rheum Dis 2003;62:1156–61.
13. Aragon CL, Hofmeister EH, Budsberg SC. Systematic review of clinical trials of treatments for osteoarthritis in dogs. J Am Vet Med Assoc 2007;230:514–21.
14. Ward DM, Leib MS, Johnston SA, et al. The effect of dosing interval on the efficacy of misoprostol in the prevention of aspirin-induced gastric injury. J Vet Intern Med 2003;17:282–90.
15. Sennello KA, Leib MS. Effects of deracoxib or buffered aspirin on the gastric mucosa of healthy dogs. J Vet Intern Med 2006;20:1291–6.
16. Reimer ME, Johnston SA, Leib MS, et al. The gastroduodenal effects of buffered aspirin, carprofen, and etodolac in healthy dogs. J Vet Intern Med 1999;13:472–7.
17. Mansa S, Palmer E, Grondahl C, et al. Long-term treatment with carprofen of 805 dogs with osteoarthritis. Vet Rec 2007;160:427–30.
18. McCarthy G, O'Donovan J, Jones B, et al. Randomised double-blind, positive-controlled trial to assess the efficacy of glucosamine/chondroitin sulfate for the treatment of dogs with osteoarthritis. Vet J 2007;174:54–61.
19. Pollmeier M, Toulemonde C, Fleishman C, et al. Clinical evaluation of firocoxib and carprofen for the treatment of dogs with osteoarthritis. Vet Rec 2006;159: 547–51.
20. Moreau M, Dupuis J, Bonneau NH, et al. Clinical evaluation of a nutraceutical, carprofen and meloxicam for the treatment of dogs with osteoarthritis. Vet Rec 2003;152:323–9.
21. Raekallio MR, Hielm-Bjorkman AK, Kejonen J, et al. Evaluation of adverse effects of long-term orally administered carprofen in dogs. J Am Vet Med Assoc 2006; 228:876–80.
22. Pelletier JP, Lajeunesse D, Jovanovic DV, et al. Carprofen simultaneously reduces progression of morphological changes in cartilage and subchondral bone in experimental dog osteoarthritis. J Rheumatol 2000;27:2893–902.
23. Budsberg SC, Johnston SA, Schwarz PD, et al. Efficacy of etodolac for the treatment of osteoarthritis of the hip joints in dogs. J Am Vet Med Assoc 1999;214: 206–10.
24. Hanson PD, Brooks KC, Case J, et al. Efficacy and safety of firocoxib in the management of canine osteoarthritis under field conditions. Vet Ther 2006;7:127–40.
25. Klauss G, Giuliano EA, Moore CP, et al. Keratoconjunctivitis sicca associated with administration of etodolac in dogs: 211 cases (1992–2002). J Am Vet Med Assoc 2007;230:541–7.
26. Johnston SA, Conzemius MG, Cross AR, et al. A multi-center clinical study of the effect of deracoxib, a COX-2 selective drug, on chronic pain in dogs with osteoarthritis. [abstract]. Vet Surg 2001;30:497.
27. Lascelles BD, Blikslager AT, Fox SM, et al. Gastrointestinal tract perforation in dogs treated with a selective cyclooxygenase-2 inhibitor: 29 cases (2002–2003). J Am Vet Med Assoc 2005;227:1112–7.
28. Peterson KD, Keefe TJ. Effects of meloxicam on severity of lameness and other clinical signs of osteoarthritis in dogs. J Am Vet Med Assoc 2004;225: 1056–60.
29. Nell T, Bergman J, Hoeijmakers M, et al. Comparison of vedaprofen and meloxicam in dogs with musculoskeletal pain and inflammation. J Small Anim Pract 2002;43:208–12.
30. Doig PA, Purbrick KA, Hare JE, et al. Clinical efficacy and tolerance of meloxicam in dogs with chronic osteoarthritis. Can Vet J 2000;41:296–300.

31. Narita T, Okabe N, Hane M, et al. Nonsteroidal anti-inflammatory drugs induce hypermotilinemia and disturbance of interdigestive migrating contractions in instrumented dogs. J Vet Pharmacol Ther 2006;29:569–77.
32. Craven M, Chandler ML, Steiner JM, et al. Acute effects of carprofen and meloxicam on canine gastrointestinal permeability and mucosal absorptive capacity. J Vet Intern Med 2007;21:917–23.
33. Agnello KA, Reynolds LR, Budsberg SC. In vivo effects of tepoxalin, an inhibitor of cyclooxygenase and lipoxygenase, on prostanoid and leukotriene production in dogs with chronic osteoarthritis. Am J Vet Res 2005;66:966–72.
34. Jovanovic DV, Fernandes JC, Martel-Pelletier J, et al. In vivo dual inhibition of cyclooxygenase and lipoxygenase by ML-3000 reduces the progression of experimental osteoarthritis: suppression of collagenase 1 and interleukin-1beta synthesis. Arthritis Rheum 2001;44:2320–30.
35. Ryan WG, Moldave K, Carithers D. Clinical effectiveness and safety of a new NSAID, firocoxib: a 1,000 dog study. Vet Ther 2006;7:119–26.
36. Schaible HG, Schmelz M, Tegeder I. Pathophysiology and treatment of pain in joint disease. Adv Drug Deliv Rev 2006;58:323–42.
37. Kidd BL, Langford RM, Wodehouse T. Arthritis and pain. Current approaches in the treatment of arthritic pain. Arthritis Res Ther 2007;9:214.
38. Raffa RB, Friderichs E, Reimann W, et al. Opioid and nonopioid components independently contribute to the mechanism of action of tramadol, an 'atypical' opioid analgesic. J Pharmacol Exp Ther 1992;260:275–85.
39. Hassanzadeh P. Tramadol attenuates hyperalgesia, activation of NF-κB, and production of proinflammatory cytokines in rate model of neuropathic pain. [abstract]. Eur J Pain 2007;11:S65.
40. Marincsak R, Toth BI, Czifra G, et al. The analgesic drug, tramadol, acts as an agonist of the transient receptor potential vanilloid-1. Anesth Analg 2008;106: 1890–6.
41. Babul N, Noveck R, Chipman H, et al. Efficacy and safety of extended-release, once-daily tramadol in chronic pain: a randomized 12-week clinical trial in osteoarthritis of the knee. J Pain 2004;28:59–71.
42. Malonne H, Coffiner M, Sonet B, et al. Efficacy and tolerability of sustained-release tramadol in the treatment of symptomatic osteoarthritis of the hip or knee: a multicenter, randomized, double-blind, placebo-controlled study. Clin Ther 2004;26:1774–82.
43. Schnitzer TJ, Kamin M, Olson WH. Tramadol allows reduction of naproxen dose among patients with naproxen-responsive osteoarthritis pain: a randomized, double-blind, placebo-controlled study. Arthritis Rheum 1999;42:1370–7.
44. Wilder-Smith CH, Hill L, Spargo K, et al. Treatment of severe pain from osteoarthritis with slow-release tramadol or dihydrocodeine in combination with NSAIDs: a randomised study comparing analgesia, antinociception and gastrointestinal effects. Pain 2001;91:23–31.
45. Schug SA. Combination analgesia in 2005—a rational approach: focus on paracetamol-tramadol. Clin Rheumatol 2006;25(Suppl 1):S16–21.
46. Schug SA. The role of tramadol in current treatment strategies for musculoskeletal pain. Ther Clin Risk Manag 2007;3:717–23.
47. Lambert C, Bianchi E, Keroack S, et al. Reduced dosage of ketoprofen alone or with tramadol for long-term treatment of osteoarthritis in dogs [abstract]. Vet Anaesth Analg 2004;31:23.
48. Dworkin RH, O'Connor AB, Backonja M, et al. Pharmacologic management of neuropathic pain: evidence-based recommendations. Pain 2007;132:237–51.

49. Kitson R, Carr B. Tramadol and severe serotonin syndrome. Anaesthesia 2005;60:934–5.
50. Riedel W, Neeck G. Nociception, pain, and antinociception: current concepts. Z Rheumatol 2001;60:404–15.
51. Childers WE Jr, Baudy RB. N-methyl-D-aspartate antagonists and neuropathic pain: the search for relief. J Med Chem 2007;50:2557–62.
52. Lascelles BD, Gaynor JS, Smith ES, et al. Amantadine in a multimodal analgesic regimen for alleviation of refractory osteoarthritis pain in dogs. J Vet Intern Med 2008;22:53–9.
53. Curros-Criado MM, Herrero JF. The antinociceptive effect of systemic gabapentin is related to the type of sensitization-induced hyperalgesia. J Neuroinflammation 2007;4:15.
54. Vadalouca A, Siafaka I, Argyra E, et al. Therapeutic management of chronic neuropathic pain: an examination of pharmacologic treatment. Ann N Y Acad Sci 2006;1088:164–86.
55. Ho KY, Huh BK, White WD, et al. Topical amitriptyline versus lidocaine in the treatment of neuropathic pain. Clin J Pain 2008;24:51–5.
56. Mico JA, Ardid D, Berrocoso E, et al. Antidepressants and pain. Trends Pharmacol Sci 2006;27:348–54.
57. Dick IE, Brochu RM, Purohit Y, et al. Sodium channel blockade may contribute to the analgesic efficacy of antidepressants. J Pain 2007;8:315–24.
58. de Haan JJ, Goring RL, Beale BS. Evaluation of polysulfated glycosaminoglycan for the treatment of hip dysplasia in dogs. Vet Surg 1994;23:177–81.
59. Fujiki M, Shineha J, Yamanokuchi K, et al. Effects of treatment with polysulfated glycosaminoglycan on serum cartilage oligomeric matrix protein and C-reactive protein concentrations, serum matrix metalloproteinase-2 and -9 activities, and lameness in dogs with osteoarthritis. Am J Vet Res 2007;68:827–33.
60. Innes JF, Fuller CJ, Grover ER, et al. Randomised, double-blind, placebo-controlled parallel group study of P54FP for the treatment of dogs with osteoarthritis. Vet Rec 2003;152:457–60.
61. Read RA, Cullis-Hill D, Jones MP. Systemic use of pentosan polysulphate in the treatment of osteoarthritis. J Small Anim Pract 1996;37:108–14.
62. Brandt KD, Smith GN, Myers SL. Hyaluronan injection affects neither osteoarthritis progression nor loading of the OA knee in dogs. Biorheology 2004;41:493–502.
63. Canapp SO, Cross AR, Brown MP, et al. Examination of synovial fluid and serum following intravenous injections of hyaluronan for the treatment of osteoarthritis in dogs. Vet Comp Orthop Traumatol 2005;18:169–74.
64. Hellstrom LE, Carlsson C, Boucher JF, et al. Intra-articular injections with high molecular weight sodium hyaluronate as a therapy for canine arthritis. Vet Rec 2003;153:89–90.
65. Bierer TL, Bui LM. Improvement of arthritic signs in dogs fed green-lipped mussel (Perna canaliculus). J Nutr 2002;132:1634S–6S.
66. Bui LM, Bierer TL. Influence of green lipped mussels (Perna canaliculus) in alleviating signs of arthritis in dogs. Vet Ther 2003;4:397–407.
67. Dobenecker B, Beetz Y, Kienzle E. A placebo-controlled double-blind study on the effect of nutraceuticals (chondroitin sulfate and mussel extract) in dogs with joint diseases as perceived by their owners. J Nutr 2002;132:1690S–1S.
68. Pollard B, Guilford WG, Ankenbauer-Perkins KL, et al. Clinical efficacy and tolerance of an extract of green-lipped mussel (Perna canaliculus) in dogs presumptively diagnosed with degenerative joint disease. N Z Vet J 2006;54:114–8.

69. Kimmatkar N, Thawani V, Hingorani L, et al. Efficacy and tolerability of Boswellia serrata extract in treatment of osteoarthritis of knee—a randomized double blind placebo controlled trial. Phytomedicine 2003;10:3–7.
70. Reichling J, Schmokel H, Fitzi J, et al. Dietary support with Boswellia resin in canine inflammatory joint and spinal disease. Schweiz Arch Tierheilkd 2004; 146:71–9.
71. Goodnight SH Jr, Harris WS, Connor WE, et al. Polyunsaturated fatty acids, hyperlipidemia, and thrombosis. Arteriosclerosis 1982;2:87–113.
72. Siess W, Roth P, Scherer B, et al. Platelet-membrane fatty acids, platelet aggregation, and thromboxane formation during a mackerel diet. Lancet 1980;1: 441–4.
73. Smith WL. Cyclooxygenases, peroxide tone and the allure of fish oil. Curr Opin Cell Biol 2005;17:174–82.
74. Roush JK, Cross AR, Renberg WC, et al. Effects of feeding a high omega-3 fatty acid diet on serum fatty acid profiles and force plate analysis in dogs with osteoarthritis [abstract]. Vet Surg 2005;34:E21.
75. Impellizeri JA, Tetrick MA, Muir P. Effect of weight reduction on clinical signs of lameness in dogs with hip osteoarthritis. J Am Vet Med Assoc 2000;216:1089–91.
76. Kealy RD, Lawler DF, Ballam JM, et al. Evaluation of the effect of limited food consumption on radiographic evidence of osteoarthritis in dogs. J Am Vet Med Assoc 2000;217:1678–80.
77. Kealy RD, Lawler DF, Ballam JM, et al. Effects of diet restriction on life span and age-related changes in dogs. J Am Vet Med Assoc 2002;220:1315–20.
78. Mlacnik E, Bockstahler BA, Muller M, et al. Effects of caloric restriction and a moderate or intense physiotherapy program for treatment of lameness in overweight dogs with osteoarthritis. J Am Vet Med Assoc 2006;229:1756–60.
79. Smith GK, Paster ER, Powers MY, et al. Lifelong diet restriction and radiographic evidence of osteoarthritis of the hip joint in dogs. J Am Vet Med Assoc 2006;229:690–3.
80. Tanger GH. Physical therapy in small animal patients: basic principles. Compend Cont Educ Pract Vet 1984;6:933–8.
81. Bockstahler B, Levine D, Millis DL. Arthritis. In: Bockstahler B, Levine D, Millis DL, editors. Essential facts of physiotherapy in dogs and cats—rehabilitation and pain management. Germany: BE VetVerlag; 2004. p. 6–33.
82. Clark B, McLaughlin RM. Physical rehabilitation for the small animal orthopedic patient. Vet Med 2001;96:234–46.
83. Crook T, McGowan C, Pead M. Effect of passive stretching on the range of motion of osteoarthritic joints in 10 Labrador retrievers. Vet Rec 2007;160:545–7.
84. Millis DL. Postoperative rehabilitation. North American Veterinary Conference. Orlando, FL, January 2000.
85. Millis DL, Levine D. The role of exercise and physical modalities in the treatment of osteoarthritis. Vet Clin North Am Small Anim Pract 1997;27:913–30.
86. Saunders DG, Walker JR, Levine D. Joint mobilization. Vet Clin North Am Small Anim Pract 2005;35:1287–316.
87. Taylor RA, Millis DL, Levine D, et al. Physical rehabilitation for geriatric and arthritic patients. In: Millis DL, Levine D, Taylor RA, editors. Canine rehabilitation and physical therapy. St. Louis: W.B. Saunders Co.; 2004.
88. Gucker T. The use of heat and cold in orthopedics. In: Light SJ, editor. Therapeutic heat and cold. Baltimore (MD): Waverly Press; 1965. p. 398–407.
89. Hodges CO, Palmer RH. Postoperative physical therapy. Surgical complication and wound healing in small animal practice. Philadelphia: W.B. Saunders; 1993. p. 389–405.

90. Marone PJ. Orthopedic rehabilitation. In: Gartland JJ, editor. Fundamentals of orthopedics. 4th edition. Philadelphia: W.B. Saunders; 1987. p. 409–24.
91. Merrick MA, Knight KL, Ingersoll CD, et al. The effects of ice and compression wraps on intramuscular temperatures at various depths. J Athl Train 1993;28: 236–45.
92. Michlovitz SL. Thermal agents in rehabilitation. Philadelphia: F.A. Davis Co.; 1990.
93. Whitney SL. Physcial agents: heat and cold modalities. In: Scully RM, Barnes MR, editors. Physical therapy. Philadelphia: J.B. Lippincott; 1989. p. 489.
94. Hayes KW. Conductive heat. In: Hayes KW, editor. Manual for physical agents. East Norwalk (CT): Appleton & Lang; 1993. p. 9–15.
95. Taylor RA. Postsurgical physical therapy: the missing link. Compend Contin Educ Pract Vet 1992;14(12):1583–93.
96. Saunders DG. Rehabilitation of the osteoarthritic patient. NAVC Clinician's Brief 2008;6(2):27–30.
97. Salter RB, Simmonds DF, Malcolm BW, et al. The biological effect of continuous passive motion on the healing of full-thickness defects in articular cartilage. An experimental investigation in the rabbit. J Bone Joint Surg Am 1980;62: 1232–51.
98. Downer AH. Physical therapy for animals—selected techniques. Springfield (IL): Thomas Books; 1978.
99. Geiringer SR. Traction, manipulation and massage. In: DeLisa JA, editor. Rehabilitation medicine: principles and practice. Philadelphia: J.B. Lippincott Co.; 1988. p. 276–94.
100. Blaser HW. Massage: current concepts. In: Peat M, editor. Current physical therapy. Toronto (Ontario): B.C. Decker Co.; 1988. p. 65–8.
101. Manning AM. Physical therapy for critically ill veterinary patients. Part II: the musculoskeletal system. Compend Contin Educ Pract Vet 1997;803–9.
102. Dyson M. Stimulation of tissue repair by therapeutic ultrasound. Infect Surg 1982;37–44.
103. Enwemeka CS, Rodriguez O, Mendosa S. The biomechanical effects of low-intensity ultrasound on healing tendons. Ultrasound Med Biol 1990;16:801–7.
104. Di Domenica F, Sarzi-Puttini P, Cazzola M, et al. Physical and rehabilitative approaches in osteoarthritis. Semin Arthritis Rheum 2005;34:62–9.
105. Greathouse DG. Effects of neuromuscular stimulation on skeletal muscle ultrastructure. In: Nelson RM, editor. Clinical electrotherapy. Philadelphia: F.A. Davis Co.; 1992.
106. Currier DP, Ray JM, Nyland J, et al. Effects of electrical and electromagnetic stimulation after anterior cruciate ligament reconstruction. J Orthop Sports Phys Ther 1993;17:177–84.
107. Johnson JM. Rehabilitation with electrical muscle stimulation for dogs with treated cranial cruciate ligament deficient stifles. Vet Surg 1994;23:405.
108. Johnson JM, Johnson AL, Pijanowski GJ, et al. Rehabilitation of dogs with surgically treated cranial cruciate ligament-deficient stifles by use of electrical stimulation of muscles. Am J Vet Res 1997;58:1473–8.
109. Palmoski MJ. Effects of altered load on articular cartilage in vivo and in vitro. Int J Sports Med 1984;5:79.
110. Downer AH. Whirlpool therapy for animals. Mod Vet Pract 1977;58:39–42.

Index

Note: Page numbers of article titles are in **boldface** type.

A

Acepromazine
  dosage of, 1314
  for trauma patients, 1333
  in pain management
    cancer-related, 1439
    for ongoing pain, 1343
    in pediatric cats and dogs, 1303
Acetaminophen
  codeine and, in cancer pain management, 1433
  in cancer pain management, 1433
  in small animals, 1250–1252
Active exercise, for osteoarthritis in dogs, 1462
Acupuncture
  for chronic neuropathic pain in cats and dogs, 1402–1403
  for neuropathic pain in hospitalized cats and dogs, 1399
  in cancer pain management, 1442
Acute pain, defined, 1430
Adjunctive analgesic therapy, **1187–1203.** See also *Analgesia/analgesics, adjunctive.*
α_2-Adrenergic agonists, intravenous administration of, continuous rate infusion
  in, for critically ill cats and dogs, 1358–1359
α_2-Adrenoreceptor agonists, for pain management in cats, 1281
Aggression, analgesia and chemical restraint for, 1330–1335
α_2-Agonists, 1188, 1189–1191
  in cancer pain management, 1437
  in dogs and cats, 1220–1221
Airway obstruction, upper, analgesia and chemical restraint for, 1336
Allodynia, defined, 1174
Alprazolam, in cancer pain management, 1439
Amantadine
  for chronic neuropathic pain in cats and dogs, 1401
  for osteoarthritis in dogs, 1454
  in cancer pain management, 1433
Amitriptyline
  for osteoarthritis in dogs, 1455
  in cancer pain management, 1433
Amputation, in cats and dogs, 1384
Analgesia/analgesics
  acting at descending antinociceptive pathways, 1180
  acting at dorsal horn, 1178–1179
  acting at nociceptors, 1176
  acting at primary afferent fibers, 1177–1178

Vet Clin Small Anim 38 (2008) 1471–1490
doi:10.1016/S0195-5616(08)00180-0
vetsmall.theclinics.com
0195-5616/08/$ – see front matter

Analgesia/analgesics (*continued*)
acting at thalamocortical structures, 1179
adjunctive, **1187–1203**
α_2-agonists, 1188, 1189–1191
anticonvulsants, 1188, 1194–1195
bisphosphonates, 1188, 1196
dexmedetomidine, 1188, 1189–1191
gabapentin, 1188, 1194–1195
intravenous lidocaine, 1188, 1195–1196
medetomidine, 1188, 1189–1191
NMDAs, 1188, 1192–1194
nonpharmacologic, 1196
pamidronate, 1188, 1196
pharmacologic, 1187–1196
prescribing of, guidelines for, 1197
systemic local anesthetics, 1188, 1195–1196
tramadol, 1188, 1191–1192
types of, 1187
chemical restraint and, for emergent veterinary patient, **1329–1352**
adjuvant agents, 1349–1350
described, 1329–1330
for aggression, 1330–1335
for arrhythmias, 1345–1346
for cardiovascular compromise, 1340, 1344, 1345
for chest trauma, 1337–1340
for dehydration, 1345
for diaphragmatic hernia, 1337
for gastric or dilation volvulus, 1346–1347
for gastrointestinal or visceral pain, 1346–1348
for intra-arterial or intravenous catheter placement, 1348
for lower respiratory system injury, 1336–1337
for neurologic compromise, 1335–1336
for pancreatitis, 1347–1348
for peritonitis, 1347–1348
for respiratory compromise, 1336
for shock, 1345
for upper airway obstruction, 1336
in urinary catheter placement, 1348
nursing care with, 1350
defined, 1174
development of, targets for, 1175
epidural, in dogs and cats, **1205–1230.** See also *Epidural analgesia, in dogs and cats.*
for critically ill cats and dogs
intravenous administration of, continuous rate infusion in, 1357–1359
update on, **1353–1363**
approach to, 1359–1361
intravenous administration of, continuous rate infusion in, 1357–1359
for osteoarthritis in dogs, 1453–1455
for pain management
in cats, 1270, 1282–1283
in dogs and cats, 1341–1344

in pediatric cats and dogs, **1299–1304.** See also *Pain management, in pediatric cats and dogs.*
in pregnant cats and dogs, 1291–1297
veterinary technician's perspective on, principles of administration of, 1424–1426
in central sensitization management, 1183
in pain management
in nursing cats and dogs, **1297–1299**
in perioperative pain management, advance application of, 1310–1311
in peripheral sensitization management, 1181–1182
multimodal, defined, 1173
postoperative, 1321
pre-emptive, defined, 1430
regional, for neuropathic pain in hospitalized cats and dogs, 1397
Anesthesia/anesthetics
epidural, in dogs and cats. See also *Epidural anesthesia, in dogs and cats.*
in dogs and cats, **1205–1230**
local
defined, 1430
for critically ill cats and dogs, 1354–1357
for pain management
in cats, 1280–1281
in pediatric cats and dogs, 1304–1305
in cancer pain management, 1440–1441
systemic, 1188, 1195–1196
regional, defined, 1430
systemic local, 1188, 1195–1196
Anticonvulsant(s), 1188, 1194–1195
in cancer pain management, 1439–1440
Antidepressant(s), tricyclic
for chronic neuropathic pain in cats and dogs, 1401–1402
in cancer pain management, 1440
Anti-inflammatory drugs, nonsteroidal
for neuropathic pain in hospitalized cats and dogs, 1397–1398
for osteoarthritis in dogs, 1450–1453
for pain management
in cats, 1278–1279
long-term use of, 1279–1280
vs. opioids, 1279
in nursing cats and dogs, **1297–1299**
in pediatric cats and dogs, 1304
in pregnant cats and dogs, 1294–1296
in cancer pain management, 1433–1434
in small animals, **1242–1266**
acetaminophen, 1250–1252
adverse effects of, 1255–1260
gastrointestinal toxicity, 1255–1256
hepatic injury, 1259–1260
renal injury, 1256–1258
sensitivity-related, 1258–1259
aspirin-triggered lipoxin, 1253–1254
assays for, 1246–1247

Anti-inflammatory (*continued*)
clinical drug selection, 1260–1261
COX-2 inhibitors, 1248–1249
COX-3 inhibitors, 1245
dual inhibitors, 1250
in vitro tests in predicting in vivo performance, 1247–1248
inconsistencies among studies, 1245–1246
mechanism of action of, 1243–1245
pharmacokinetic features, 1252
pharmacokinetic-pharmacodynamic modeling, 1246–1247
prostaglandin inhibition, 1248
update on, **1243–1266**
washout period, 1252–1255
indications, dosage, and duration of, 1313
Antinociceptive pathways, descending, 1179–1180
analgesics acting at, 1180
Aquatic therapy, for osteoarthritis in dogs, 1463
Arrhythmia(s), analgesia and chemical restraint for, 1345–1346
Ascending spinal tracts, dorsal horn neurons and, 1178
Aspirin, for osteoarthritis in dogs, 1451
Aspirin-triggered lipoxin, in small animals, 1253–1254

B

Back pain, in cats and dogs, 1386
Balance exercises, for osteoarthritis in dogs, 1460
Bisphosphonate(s), 1188, 1196
Boswellia serrata, resin extract of, for osteoarthritis in dogs, 1457
Brachial plexus
in dogs, clinical anatomy of, 1232–1235
paravertebral blockade of, in dogs, **1231–1241**
complications of, 1236
electrical nerve locators in, 1238–1240
indications for, 1235
modified technique for, 1236–1237
complications of, 1237
indications for, 1236–1237
radial, ulnar, median, and musculocutaneous nerves techniques for, 1237–1238
technique for, 1235–1236
Breakthrough pain
defined, 1430
in cats and dogs, 1377
treatment of, 1392
Bupivacaine
for ongoing pain, 1343
for upper airway obstruction or trauma, 1339
Buprenorphine
for ongoing pain, 1343
for pain management
in cats, 1273–1274
in pediatric cats and dogs, 1302

in cancer pain management, 1435
indications, dosage, and duration of, 1312
Butorphanol
continuous rate infusion of, 1319
for ongoing pain, 1343
for pain management
in cats, 1273
in pediatric cats and dogs, 1302
for trauma patients, 1332
for upper airway obstruction or trauma, 1338, 1339
in cancer pain management, 1435
indications, dosage, and duration of, 1312

C

Cancer pain
assessment of, 1431–1432
control of, **1429–1448**
α_2-agonists in, 1437
anticonvulsants in, 1439–1440
described, 1429–1430
drugs in, epidural administration of, 1441
importance of, 1430–1431
local anesthetics in, 1440–1441
local or whole-body irradiation in, 1441–1442
NMDAs receptor antagonists in, 1437–1438
NSAIDs in, 1433–1434
opioids in, 1434–1437
problems associated with, 1442
surgery in, case examples, 1442–1444
TCAs in, 1440
tranquilizers in, 1438–1439
defined, 1430
Cardiorespiratory system, epidural analgesic and anesthetic effects on, in dogs and cats, 1217–1218
Cardiovascular compromise, analgesia and chemical restraint for, 1340, 1344, 1345
Carprofen
for ongoing pain, 1343
for osteoarthritis in dogs, 1451–1452
for pain management in cats, 1278–1279
in cancer pain management, 1433
Cat(s)
as pets, prevalence of, 1267
critically ill, analgesia for, update on, **1353–1363.** See also *Analgesia/analgesics, for critically ill cats and dogs, update on.*
epidural analgesia and anesthesia in, **1205–1230.** See also *Epidural analgesia, in dogs and cats.*
epidural anesthesia in, **1205–1230.** See also *Epidural anesthesia, in dogs and cats.*
neuropathic pain in, **1365–1414.** See also *Neuropathic pain, in cats and dogs.*
nursing, pain management in, **1297–1299**
pain in

Cat(s) (*continued*)
analgesics for, 1341–1344
assessment of, 1268–1269
pain management in, **1267–1290**
α_2-adrenoreceptor agonists in, 1281
analgesics in, 1270, 1282–1283
drug metabolism effects on, 1269
ketamine in, 1281–1282
local anesthetic drugs in, 1280–1281
multimodal approach to, 1282
NSAIDs in
long-term use of, 1279–1280
vs. opioids, 1279–1280
opioids in, 1270–1278. See also *Opioid(s), for pain management in cats.*
surgery-related pain, opioids vs. NSAIDS in, 1279
tramadol in, 1277–1278
pediatric, pain management in, **1299–1304.** See also *Pain management, in pediatric cats and dogs.*
pregnant, pain management for, **1291–1297.** See also *Pain management, for cats and dogs, during pregnancy.*
Catheter(s), placement of, analgesia and chemical restraint for, 1348
Central nervous system (CNS), of cats and dogs, 1368–1370
tumors in, 1388–1389
Central pain syndrome, in cats and dogs, 1388–1389
Central sensitization, multimodal pain management in, 1182–1183
Cesarean section, perioperative pain management during, 1323
Chemical restraint, analgesia and, for emergent veterinary patient, **1329–1352.** See also *Analgesia/analgesics, chemical restraint and, for emergent veterinary patient.*
Chest trauma, analgesia and chemical restraint for, 1337–1340
Chondroitin sulfate, for osteoarthritis in dogs, 1456–1458
Chronic pain, defined, 1430
CNS. See *Central nervous system (CNS).*
Codeine
acetaminophen and, in cancer pain management, 1433
for ongoing pain, 1343
for pain management
in pediatric cats and dogs, 1300
in pregnant cats and dogs, 1295
in cancer pain management, 1435
Communication, in pain management, veterinary technician's perspective on, 1416–1417
Congenital/developmental lesions, neuropathic pain due to, in cats and dogs, 1388–1389
Continous rate infusions, of opioids, for pain management in cats, 1276–1277
Continuous rate infusions
in perioperative pain management, 1316–1320
of intravenous analgesics, for critically ill cats and dogs, 1357–1359
of ketamine, 1320
of lidocaine, 1319
of morphine/lidocaine/ketamine, 1320
of opioids, 1318–1319
COX-2 inhibitors, in small animals, 1248–1249
COX-3 inhibitors, in small animals, 1245

Critically ill cats and dogs, analgesia for, update on, **1353–1363.** See also *Analgesia/analgesics, for critically ill cats and dogs, update on.*
Cryotherapy, for osteoarthritis in dogs, 1458
Cystitis, feline interstitial, neuropathic pain due to, 1389

D

Dehydration, analgesia and chemical restraint for, 1345
Deracoxib
for osteoarthritis in dogs, 1452
in cancer pain management, 1433
Descending antinociceptive pathways, 1179–1180
analgesics acting at, 1180
Descending inhibitory pathway, in neuropathic pain in cats and dogs, 1376
Descending inhibitory system, of cats and dogs, 1371
Dexamethazone, for upper airway obstruction or trauma, 1338
Dexmedetomidine, 1188, 1189–1191
in cancer pain management, 1439
Dextromethorphan, for chronic neuropathic pain in cats and dogs, 1401
Diabetic neuropathy, neuropathic pain due to, in cats and dogs, 1387–1388
Diaphragmatic hernia, analgesia and chemical restraint for, 1337
Diazepam
dosage of, 1314
for ongoing pain, 1343
for pain management, in pediatric cats and dogs, 1303
for trauma patients, 1333
for upper airway obstruction or trauma, 1338, 1339
in cancer pain management, 1439
ketamine and, for upper airway obstruction or trauma, 1338
propofol and, for upper airway obstruction or trauma, 1338, 1339
Diet(s), omega-3–based, for osteoarthritis in dogs, 1457
Dilation volvulus, analgesia and chemical restraint for, 1346–1347
Discospondylitis, in cats and dogs, 1386
Dog(s)
brachial plexus in
clinical anatomy of, 1232–1235
paravertebral blockade of, **1231–1241.** See also *Brachial plexus, paravertebral blockade of, in dogs.*
critically ill, analgesia for, update on, **1353–1363.** See also *Analgesia/analgesics, for critically ill cats and dogs, update on.*
epidural analgesia and anesthesia in, **1205–1230.** See also *Epidural analgesia, in dogs and cats.*
epidural anesthesia in, **1205–1230.** See also *Epidural anesthesia, in dogs and cats.*
neuropathic pain in, **1365–1414.** See also *Neuropathic pain, in cats and dogs.*
NSAIDS for, currently available, 1244
nursing, pain management in, **1297–1299**
osteoarthritis in, nonsurgical management of, **1449–1470.** See also *Osteoarthritis, in dogs, nonsurgical management of.*
pain in, analgesics for, 1341–1344
pediatric, pain management in, **1299–1304.** See also *Pain management, in pediatric cats and dogs.*

Dog(s) (*continued*)
pregnant, pain management for, **1291–1297.** See also *Pain management, for cats and dogs, during pregnancy.*
Dorsal horn, analgesic drugs acting at, 1178–1179
Dorsal horn neurons, ascending spinal tracts and, 1178
Drug(s). See also specific types, e.g., *Opioid(s).*
Drug metabolism, in cats, pain management effects of, 1269
Dual inhibitors, in small animals, 1250
Dysphoria, differentiating pain from, veterinary technician's perspective on, 1421–1423

E

Elderly, perioperative pain management in, 1323
Electrical nerve locators, in paravertebral blockade of brachial plexus in dogs, 1238–1240
Electrical stimulation, for osteoarthritis in dogs, 1462
Emergency cases, perioperative pain management for, 1323
Endogenous facilitatory systems, of cats and dogs, 1370
Epidural administration, 1441
of opioids, for pain management in cats, 1273, 1278
Epidural analgesia, in dogs and cats, **1205–1230**
absorption from epidural space, 1214–1215
adverse side effects of, 1218–1219
anatomic considerations in, 1205–1208
cardiorespiratory effects of, 1217–1218
opioids, 1215–1217
pharmacologic considerations in, 1213–1223
position and volume in, 1208–1210
preservatives, 1222–1223
technique for, 1210–1213
Epidural anesthesia, in dogs and cats, **1205–1230**
absorption from epidural space, 1214–1215
adverse side effects of, 1218–1219
α_2-agonists, 1220–1221
anatomic considerations in, 1205–1208
cardiorespiratory effects of, 1217–1218
ketamine, 1221
local agents, 1219–1220
opioids, 1215–1217
pharmacologic considerations in, 1213–1223
position and volume in, 1208–1210
preservatives, 1222–1223
technique for, 1210–1213
Etodolac, for osteoarthritis in dogs, 1452
Exercise(s)
active, for osteoarthritis in dogs, 1462
balance, for osteoarthritis in dogs, 1460
PROM, for osteoarthritis in dogs, 1459–1460
proprioception, for osteoarthritis in dogs, 1460
stretching, for osteoarthritis in dogs, 1460

F

Fecainide, for neuropathic pain in hospitalized cats and dogs, 1396
Feline interstitial cystitis, neuropathic pain due to, 1389
Fentanyl
continuous rate infusion of, 1318–1319
for gastrointestinal compromise, 1347
for ongoing pain, 1342
for pain management
in cats, 1274–1275
in pediatric cats and dogs, 1300, 1302, 1303
for trauma patients, 1332
in cancer pain management, 1435
indications, dosage, and duration of, 1312
Fentanyl transdermal patch
for ongoing pain, 1342
in pain management, in pediatric cats and dogs, 1300
indications, dosage, and duration of, 1312
Fibrocartilaginous embolic myelopathy, in cats and dogs, 1386
Firocoxib
for osteoarthritis in dogs, 1453
in cancer pain management, 1433
Fracture(s), pelvic, in cats and dogs, 1382–1383

G

Gabapentin, 1188, 1194–1195
dosage of, 1344
for chronic neuropathic pain in cats and dogs, 1401
for critically ill cats and dogs, 1361
for emergent veterinary patient, 1349–1350
for neuropathic pain in hospitalized cats and dogs, 1398–1399
for osteoarthritis in dogs, 1454–1455
in cancer pain management, 1433
Gastric volvulus, analgesia and chemical restraint for, 1346–1347
Gastrointestinal pain, analgesia and chemical restraint for, 1346–1348
Gastrointestinal system, neuropathic pain associated with, in cats and dogs, 1390
Gastrointestinal toxicity, NSAIDs and, in small animals, 1255–1256
Glucosamine hydrochloride preparations, for osteoarthritis in dogs, 1456–1458
Green-lipped mussel preparation, for osteoarthritis in dogs, 1456

H

Heat, moist, for osteoarthritis in dogs, 1459
Hepatic injury, NSAIDs and, in small animals, 1259–1260
Hernia(s)
diaphragmatic, analgesia and chemical restraint for, 1337
inguinal, repair of, in cats and dogs, 1382
Hyaluronan, for osteoarthritis in dogs, 1456
Hydromorphone
for gastrointestinal compromise, 1347
for ongoing pain, 1342

Hydromorphone (*continued*)
for pain management
in cats, 1275
in pediatric cats and dogs, 1300, 1303
in pregnant cats and dogs, 1295
for trauma patients, 1332
in cancer pain management, 1435
indications, dosage, and duration of, 1312
Hyperalgesia, defined, 1174

I

IASP. See *International Association for the Study of Pain (IASP).*
Imipramine, in cancer pain management, 1433
Immune response mechanisms, in neuropathic pain in cats and dogs, 1375–1376
Inflammatory bowel disease, neuropathic pain due to, in cats and dogs, 1390
Inguinal hernia, repair of, in cats and dogs, 1382
Intensive care unit, pain management in, veterinary technician's perspective on, 1426–1427
International Association for the Study of Pain (IASP), 1366
Intervertebral disc herniation, in cats and dogs, 1385–1386
Intra-arterial catheter placement, analgesia and chemical restraint for, 1348
Intravenous catheter placement, analgesia and chemical restraint for, 1348
Irradiation, local or whole-body, in cancer pain management, 1441–1442

K

Ketamine
continuous rate infusion of, 1320
diazepam and
for upper airway obstruction or trauma, 1338
indications, dosage, and duration of, 1312
dosage for, 1344
for critically ill cats and dogs, intravenous administration of, continuous rate infusion in, 1359
for emergent veterinary patient, 1349
for neuropathic pain in hospitalized cats and dogs, 1394–1395
for ongoing pain, 1342
for pain management
in cats, 1281–1282
in dogs and cats, 1221
in nursing cats and dogs, 1299
in perioperative pain management, 1315
in pregnant cats and dogs, 1296–1297
indications, dosage, and duration of, 1312
for trauma patients, 1333
for upper airway obstruction or trauma, 1339
in cancer pain management, 1433
Ketoprofen
for ongoing pain, 1342
for pain management in cats, 1279
in cancer pain management, 1433

L

Lamotrigine, for chronic neuropathic pain in cats and dogs, 1402
Laser, for osteoarthritis in dogs, 1461
Lesion(s)
  congenital/developmental, neuropathic pain due to, in cats and dogs, 1388–1389
  lumbosacral, in cats and dogs, 1384–1385
Lidocaine
  continuous rate infusion of, 1319
  dosage for, 1344
  for criticaaly ill cats and dogs, intravenous administration of, continuous rate infusion in, 1359
  for emergent veterinary patient, 1349
  for neuropathic pain in hospitalized cats and dogs, 1396
  in perioperative pain management, 1315
  indications, dosage, and duration of, 1313
  intravenous, 1188, 1195–1196
Lidocaine dermal patches, for chronic neuropathic pain in cats and dogs, 1402
Limb nerve entrapment, in cats and dogs, 1383–1384
Lipoxin, aspirin-triggered, in small animals, 1253–1254
Local anesthesia
  defined, 1430
  for critically ill cats and dogs, 1354–1357
  for pain management
    in cats, 1280–1281
    in pediatric cats and dogs, 1304–1305
  in cancer pain management, 1440–1441
  systemic, 1188, 1195–1196
Lower respiratory system, injury to, analgesia and chemical restraint for, 1336–1337
Lumbosacral lesions, in cats and dogs, 1384–1385

M

Massage therapy, for osteoarthritis in dogs, 1461
Medetomidine, 1188, 1189–1191
  for ongoing pain, 1343
  for trauma patients, 1333
  in cancer pain management, 1439
  in pain management, for ongoing pain, 1343
  indications, dosage, and duration of, 1313
Meloxicam
  for ongoing pain, 1342
  for osteoarthritis in dogs, 1452–1453
  for pain management in cats, 1279
  in cancer pain management, 1433
Meperidine
  for ongoing pain, 1343
  for pain management
    in cats, 1275
    in pediatric cats and dogs, 1302, 1303
  for trauma patients, 1332

Meperidine (*continued*)
for upper airway obstruction or trauma, 1338
indications, dosage, and duration of, 1313
Methadone
for gastrointestinal compromise, 1347
for ongoing pain, 1342
for pain management
in cats, 1275
in pediatric cats and dogs, 1300, 1302, 1303
in pregnant cats and dogs, 1295
N-Methyl-D-aspartate (NMDA) receptor antagonists, 1188, 1192–1194
for neuropathic pain in hospitalized cats and dogs, 1394
in cancer pain management, 1437–1438
Mexiletine, for neuropathic pain in hospitalized cats and dogs, 1396
Midazolam
dosage of, 1314
for ongoing pain, 1343
for pain management, in pediatric cats and dogs, 1303
for trauma patients, 1333
in cancer pain management, 1439
Moist heat, for osteoarthritis in dogs, 1459
Morphine
continuous rate infusion of, 1318
for gastrointestinal compromise, 1347
for ongoing pain, 1342
for pain management
in cats, 1276
in pediatric cats and dogs, 1300, 1302, 1303
in pregnant cats and dogs, 1295
for trauma patients, 1332
in cancer pain management, 1435
in perioperative pain management, 1316
indications, dosage, and duration of, 1313
Morphine syrup, for ongoing pain, 1343
Morphine/lidocaine/ketamine, continuous rate infusion of, 1320
Multimodal analgesia, defined, 1173
Multimodal pain management, **1173–1186.** See also *Pain management, multimodal.*
Myelopathy, fibrocartilaginous embolic, in cats and dogs, 1386

N

Nalbuphine, for pain management in cats, 1276
Neck pain, in cats and dogs, 1386
Nervous system sensitization, 1180–1183
multimodal pain management in
central sensitization, 1182–1183
peripheral sensitization, 1180–1182
Neurologic compromise, analgesia and chemical restraint for, 1335–1336
Neuron(s), dorsal horn, ascending spinal tracts and, 1178
Neuropathic pain
defined, 1430

in cats and dogs, **1365–1414**
back pain, 1386
breakthrough pain, 1377
central pain syndrome, 1388–1389
CNS tumors, 1388–1389
CNS–related, 1368–1370
conditions associated with, 1381–1387
congenital/developmental lesions, 1388–1389
descending inhibitory pathway in, 1376
descending inhibitory system in, 1371
described, 1365–1366, 1372
diabetic neuropathy–related, 1387–1388
diagnosis of, 1377–1381
discospondylitis, 1386
endogenous facilitatory systems in, 1370
feline interstitial cystitis–related, 1389
fibrocartilaginous embolic myelopathy, 1386
gastrointestinal system–related, 1390
immune response mechanisms in, 1375–1376
inflammatory bowel disease–related, 1390
neck pain, 1386
of visceral origin, 1389–1391
pancreatic pain–related, 1390–1391
pancreatitis-related, 1390–1391
pathophysiology of, 1367–1371
peripheral nervous system lesions, 1387
peripheral nervous system–related, 1367–1368
physiology of, 1367–1371
polyradiculoneuritis, 1386–1387
prevention of, intraoperative considerations in, 1379–1380
sensory-sympathetic coupling, 1372–1375
spinal cord injury–related, 1390
spinal pain, vascular innervation–related, 1387
trauma-related, 1381–1386
amputation, 1384
inguinal hernia repair, 1382
intervertebral disc herniation, 1385–1386
limb nerve entrapment, 1383–1384
lumbosacral lesions, 1384–1385
pelvic fractures, 1382–1383
pudendal nerve entrapment, 1383
spinal cord injury, 1385
treatment of, 1391–1404
acupuncture in, 1399, 1402–1403
amantadine in, 1401
dextromethorphan in, 1401
flecainide in, 1396
for breakthrough pain, 1392
for chronic pain, 1399–1403
for stimulus-evoked pain, 1391–1392
future modalities, 1403–1404

Nalbuphine (*continued*)
gabapentin in, 1398–1399, 1401
in hospitalized patients, 1392–1399
ketamine in, 1394–1395
lamotrigine in, 1402
lidocaine dermal patches in, 1402
lidocaine in, 1396
mexiletine in, 1396
NMDA receptor antagonists in, 1394
norepinephrine reuptake inhibitors in, 1403–1404
NSAIDs in, 1397–1398
opioids in, 1392–1393, 1399
pregabalin in, 1401
α_2-receptor agonists in, 1396–1397
regional analgesia in, 1397
serotonin reuptake inhibitors in, 1403–1404
sodium channel blockers in, 1395–1396
TCAs in, 1401–1402
tocainide in, 1396
tramadol in, 1400–1401
vanilloid receptor-1 antagonists in, 1403
vasculitis-related, 1389
vertebral osteomyelitis, 1386
stimulus-evoked, in cats and dogs, treatment of, 1391–1392
Neuropathy(ies), diabetic, neuropathic pain due to, in cats and dogs, 1387–1388
NMDAs. See *N-Methyl-D-aspartate receptor antagonists (NMDAs).*
Nociception, 1174–1179
defined, 1174
described, 1175
peripheral nociceptors in, 1175–1176
primary afferent fibers in, 1176–1177
Nociceptor(s)
analgesic drugs acting at, 1176
peripheral, 1175–1176
Norepinephrine reuptake inhibitors, for chronic neuropathic pain in cats and dogs, 1403–1404
Noxious, defined, 1174
NSAIDs. See *Anti-inflammatory drugs, nonsteroidal.*
Nursing cats and dogs, pain management in, **1297–1299**
Nutritional supplements, for osteoarthritis in dogs, 1456–1458

O

Omega-3–based diets, for osteoarthritis in dogs, 1457
Opioid(s)
continuous rate infusion of, 1318–1319
for chronic neuropathic pain in cats and dogs, 1399
for critically ill cats and dogs, intravenous administration of, continuous rate infusion in, 1358
for neuropathic pain in hospitalized cats and dogs, 1392–1393
for ongoing pain, 1343

for pain management
in cats, 1270–1278
buprenorphine, 1273–1274
butorphanol, 1273
combinations of, 1276
constant rate infusion of, 1276–1277
described, 1270
dose-related effects of, 1272
epidural administration of, 1273, 1278
evaluation of, 1270
fentanyl, 1274–1275
hydromorphone, 1275
individual variability with, 1271–1272
long-term use of, 1277
meperidine, 1275
methadone, 1275
morphine, 1276
nalbuphine, 1276
NSAIDs in, 1278–1279
oral administration of, 1272
oxymorphone, 1276
routes of administration of, 1272–1273
side effects of, 1270–1271
transdermal delivery systems for, 1273–1274
transmucosal uptake of, 1273
vs. NSAIDs, 1279
in dogs and cats, 1215–1217
in nursing cats and dogs, 1298–1299
in pediatric cats and dogs, 1301–1304
in perioperative pain management, 1315
in pregnant cats and dogs, 1293–1294
for trauma patients, 1332
in cancer pain management, 1434–1437
Opioid antagonists, for pain management, in pregnant cats and dogs, 1294
Osteoarthritis, in dogs
evidence-based classification of, 1464–1465
nonsurgical management of, **1449–1470**
active exercise, 1462
amantadine, 1454
amitriptyline, 1455
analgesics, 1453–1455
aquatic therapy, 1463
aspirin, 1451
balance exercises, 1460
carprofen, 1451–1452
chondroitin sulfate, 1456–1458
cryotherapy, 1458
deracoxib, 1452
described, 1449–1450
electrical stimulation, 1462
etodolac, 1452

Osteoarthritis (*continued*)
firocoxib, 1453
gabapentin, 1454–1455
glucosamine hydrochloride preparations, 1456–1458
green-lipped mussel preparation, 1456
hyaluronan, 1456
laser, 1461
massage therapy, 1461
meloxicam, 1452–1453
moist heat, 1459
monitoring of, 1463–1464
NSAIDs, 1450–1453
nutritional supplements, 1456–1458
omega-3–based diets, 1457
P54FP, 1457
pentosan polysulfate, 1455
physical rehabilitation, 1458–1464
PROM exercises, 1459–1460
proprioception exercises, 1460
PSGAG, 1455
resin extract of *Boswellia serrata,* 1457
stretching exercises, 1460
tepoxalin, 1453
therapeutic ultrasound, 1461
tramadol, 1454
weight control and loss, 1457–1458
Osteomyelitis, vertebral, in cats and dogs, 1386
Oxycodone
for pain management
in pediatric cats and dogs, 1300
in pregnant cats and dogs, 1295
in cancer pain management, 1435, 1436
Oxymorphone
for pain management
in cats, 1276
in pregnant cats and dogs, 1295
in cancer pain management, 1435, 1436

P

P54FP, for osteoarthritis in dogs, 1457
Pain
acute, defined, 1430
alleviation of
drugs for, 1432–1441
importance of, 1430–1431
techniques for, 1432–1433
assessment of, 1431–1432
veterinary technician's perspective on, 1418–1423
approach to, 1423–1424
back, in cats and dogs, 1386

biochemical basis of, understanding of, new directions in, 1183
breakthrough
defined, 1430
in cats and dogs, 1377
treatment of, 1392
cancer. See also *Cancer pain.*
control of, **1429–1448.** See also *Cancer pain, control of.*
chronic, defined, 1430
defined, 1173
differentiating from other stress or dysphoria, veterinary technician's perspective on, 1421–1423
emergent conditions–related, 1330–1331
gastrointestinal, analgesia and chemical restraint for, 1346–1348
in cats, assessment of, 1268–1269
in cats and dogs, analgesics for, 1341–1344
neck, in cats and dogs, 1386
neuropathic
defined, 1430
in cats and dogs, **1365–1414.** See also *Neuropathic pain, in cats and dogs.*
ongoing, management of, 1342–1343
pancreatic, neuropathic pain due to, in cats and dogs, 1390–1391
perioperative, management of, **1309–1327.** See also *Perioperative pain, management of.*
somatic, defined, 1430
spinal, vascular innervation–related, in cats and dogs, 1387
visceral
analgesia and chemical restraint for, 1346–1348
defined, 1430
Pain management
for cats, **1267–1290.** See also *Cat(s), pain management in.*
for cats and dogs, during pregnancy, **1291–1297**
analgesia for, 1291–1297
ketamine in, 1296–1297
NSAIDs in, 1294–1296
opioid antagonists in, 1294
opioid(s) in, 1293–1294
for nursing cats and dogs, **1297–1299**
for pediatric cats and dogs, **1299–1304**
NSAIDs in, 1304
opioids in, 1301–1304
sedatives in, 1304
in perioperative cats and dogs, 1321–1322
multimodal, **1173–1186**
for nociception, 1175–1180. See also *Nociception.*
nervous system sensitization–related, 1180–1183
nociception-related, 1175–1180
zoledronate, 1188, 1196
perioperative, **1309–1327.** See also *Perioperative pain, management of.*
veterinary technician's perspective on, **1415–1428**
analgesics in, principles of administration of, 1424–1426
clinician in, 1417

Pain (*continued*)
communication in, 1416–1417
described, 1415–1416
differentiating pain from other stress or dysphoria, 1421–1423
in intensive care unit, 1426–1427
nonpharmacologic interventions in, 1423–1424
technician to technician in, 1417–1418
treatment goals in, 1416–1417
Pamidronate, 1188, 1196
in cancer pain management, 1433
Pancreatic pain, neuropathic pain due to, in cats and dogs, 1390–1391
Pancreatitis
analgesia and chemical restraint for, 1347–1348
neuropathic pain due to, in cats and dogs, 1390–1391
Paravertebral blockade, of brachial plexus, in dogs, **1231–1241.** See also *Brachial plexus, paravertebral blockade of, in dogs.*
Passive range-of-motion (PROM) exercises, for osteoarthritis in dogs, 1459–1460
Pelvic fractures, in cats and dogs, 1382–1383
Pentosan polysulfate, for osteoarthritis in dogs, 1455
Perioperative pain, management of, **1309–1327**
adjuncts to, 1309–1310
advance application of, 1310–1311
agents in
induction of, 1315
maintenance of, 1316
preparation for recovery, 1320–1321
continuous rate infusions in, 1316–1320
for cesarean section, 1323
for common elective surgical procedures, 1322–1323
in children, 1321–1322
in emergency cases, 1323
in the elderly, 1323
premedication, 1311–1315
Peripheral nervous system, of cats and dogs, 1367–1368
lesions of, neuropathic pain due to, 1387
Peripheral nociceptors, 1175–1176
Peripheral sensitization, multimodal pain management in, 1180–1182
Peritonitis, analgesia and chemical restraint for, 1347–1348
Physical rehabilitation, for osteoarthritis in dogs, 1458–1464
Piroxicam, in cancer pain management, 1433
Polysulfated glycosaminoglycan (PSGAG), for osteoarthritis in dogs, 1455
Postoperative analgesia, in pain management, 1321
Pre-emptive analgesia, defined, 1430
Pregabalin, for chronic neuropathic pain in cats and dogs, 1401
Pregnant cats and dogs, pain management for, **1291–1297.** See also *Pain management, for cats and dogs, during pregnancy.*
Premedication, in pain management, 1311–1315
Preservative(s), in dogs and cats, 1222–1223
Primary afferent fibers
analgesics acting at, 1177–1178
in nociception, 1176–1177

PROM exercises. See *Passive range-of-motion (PROM) exercises.*
Propofol
diazepam and, for upper airway obstruction or trauma, 1338, 1339
dosage of, 1314
Proprioception exercises, for osteoarthritis in dogs, 1460
Prostaglandin inhibition, in small animals, 1248
PSGAG. See *Polysulfated glycosaminoglycan (PSGAG).*
Pudendal nerve entrapment, in cats and dogs, 1383

R

α_2-Receptor agonists, for neuropathic pain in hospitalized cats and dogs, 1396–1397
Regional analgesia, for neuropathic pain in hospitalized cats and dogs, 1397
Regional anesthesia, defined, 1430
Rehabilitation, physical, for osteoarthritis in dogs, 1458–1464
Renal injury, NSAIDs and, in small animals, 1256–1258
Resin extract of *Boswellia serrata,* for osteoarthritis in dogs, 1457
Respiratory compromise, analgesia and chemical restraint for, 1336
Restraint(s), chemical, analgesia and, for emergent veterinary patient, **1329–1352.** See also *Analgesia/analgesics, chemical restraint and, for emergent veterinary patient.*

S

Sedative(s), in pediatric cats and dogs, 1304
Sensitivity, NSAIDs-related, in small animals, 1258–1259
Sensitization
central, multimodal pain management in, 1182–1183
nervous system, multimodal pain management in, 1180–1183. See also *Nervous system sensitization, multimodal pain management in.*
peripheral, multimodal pain management in, 1180–1182
Sensory-sympathetic coupling, in neuropathic pain, in cats and dogs, 1372–1375
Serotonin reuptake inhibitors, for neuropathic pain in cats and dogs, 1403–1404
Shock, analgesia and chemical restraint for, 1345
Small animals, NSAIDs in, update on, **1243–1266.** See also *Anti-inflammatory drugs, nonsteroidal, in small animals.*
Sodium channel blockers, for neuropathic pain in hospitalized cats and dogs, 1395–1396
Somatic pain, defined, 1430
Spinal cord injury, in cats and dogs, 1385
neuropathic pain due to, 1390
Spinal pain, vascular innervation–related, in cats and dogs, 1387
Spinal tracts, ascending, dorsal horn neurons and, 1178
Stimulation, electrical, for osteoarthritis in dogs, 1462
Stimulus-evoked neuropathic pain, in cats and dogs, treatment of, 1391–1392
Stress, pain vs., veterinary technician's perspective on, 1421–1423
Stretching exercises, for osteoarthritis in dogs, 1460
Systemic local anesthetics, 1188, 1195–1196

T

TCAs. See *Tricyclic antidepressants (TCAs).*
Tepoxalin, for osteoarthritis in dogs, 1453

Thalamocortical structures, analgesics acting at, 1179
Thalamocortical system, 1179
Therapeutic ultrasound, for osteoarthritis in dogs, 1461
Tocainide, for neuropathic pain in hospitalized cats and dogs, 1396
Toxicity, gastrointestinal, NSAIDs and, in small animals, 1255–1256
Tramadol, 1188, 1191–1192
  for chronic neuropathic pain in cats and dogs, 1400–1401
  for osteoarthritis in dogs, 1454
  for pain management in cats, 1277–1278
  in cancer pain management, 1433
Tranquilizers, in cancer pain management, 1438–1439
Transdermal delivery systems, for opioid administration, in cats, 1273–1274
Transmucosal uptake, in opioid administration, in cats, 1273
Trauma
  chest, analgesia and chemical restraint for, 1337–1340
  neuropathic pain associated with, in cats and dogs, 1381–1386
Tricyclic antidepressants (TCAs)
  for chronic neuropathic pain in cats and dogs, 1401–1402
  in cancer pain management, 1440
Tumor(s), CNS, in cats and dogs, 1388–1389

U

Ultrasound, therapeutic, for osteoarthritis in dogs, 1461
Upper airway obstruction, analgesia and chemical restraint for, 1336
Urinary catheter placement, analgesia and chemical restraint for, 1348

V

Vanilloid receptor-1 antagonists, for neuropathic pain in cats and dogs, 1403
Vascular innervation, spinal pain due to, in cats and dogs, 1387
Vasculitis, neuropathic pain due to, in cats and dogs, 1389
Vertebral osteomyelitis, in cats and dogs, 1386
Veterinary technician, perspective on pain management, **1415–1428.** See also *Pain management, veterinary technician's perspective on.*
Visceral pain
  analgesia and chemical restraint for, 1346–1348
  defined, 1430
Volvulus
  dilation, analgesia and chemical restraint for, 1346–1347
  gastric, analgesia and chemical restraint for, 1346–1347

W

Washout period, in small animals, 1252–1255
Weight control, for osteoarthritis in dogs, 1457–1458
Weight loss, for osteoarthritis in dogs, 1457–1458
Wind-up, defined, 1430

Z

Zoledronate, 1188, 1196
Zylazine, in cancer pain management, 1439

United States Postal Service

Statement of Ownership, Management, and Circulation
(All Periodicals Publications Except Requestor Publications)

1. Publication Title Veterinary Clinics of North America: Small Animal Practice	2. Publication Number 0 0 3 - 1 5 0	3. Filing Date 9/15/08
4. Issue Frequency Jan, Mar, May, Jul, Sep, Nov	5. Number of Issues Published Annually 6	6. Annual Subscription Price $206.00
7. Complete Mailing Address of Known Office of Publication (*Not printer*) (*Street, city, county, state, and ZIP+4*) Elsevier Inc. 360 Park Avenue South New York, NY 10010-1710		Contact Person Stephen Bushing Telephone (Include area code) 215-239-3688

8. Complete Mailing Address of Headquarters or General Business Office of Publisher (*Not printer*)

Elsevier Inc., 360 Park Avenue South, New York, NY 10010-1710

9. Full Names and Complete Mailing Addresses of Publisher, Editor, and Managing Editor (*Do not leave blank*)

Publisher (*Name and complete mailing address*)

John Schrefer , Elsevier, Inc., 1600 John F. Kennedy Blvd. Suite 1800, Philadelphia, PA 19103-2899

Editor (*Name and complete mailing address*)

John Vassallo, Elsevier, Inc., 1600 John F. Kennedy Blvd. Suite 1800, Philadelphia, PA 19103-2899

Managing Editor (*Name and complete mailing address*)

Catherine Bewick, Elsevier, Inc., 1600 John F. Kennedy Blvd. Suite 1800, Philadelphia, PA 19103-2899

10. Owner (*Do not leave blank. If the publication is owned by a corporation, give the name and address of the corporation immediately followed by the names and addresses of all stockholders owning or holding 1 percent or more of the total amount of stock. If not owned by a corporation, give the names and addresses of the individual owners. If owned by a partnership or other unincorporated firm, give its name and address as well as those of each individual owner. If the publication is published by a nonprofit organization, give its name and address.*)

Full Name	Complete Mailing Address
Wholly owned subsidiary of	4520 East-West Highway
Reed/Elsevier, US holdings	Bethesda, MD 20814

11. Known Bondholders, Mortgagees, and Other Security Holders Owning or Holding 1 Percent or More of Total Amount of Bonds, Mortgages, or Other Securities. If none, check box → ☐ None

Full Name	Complete Mailing Address
N/A	

12. Tax Status (*For completion by nonprofit organizations authorized to mail at nonprofit rates*) (*Check one*)
The purpose, function, and nonprofit status of this organization and the exempt status for federal income tax purposes:
☐ Has Not Changed During Preceding 12 Months
☐ Has Changed During Preceding 12 Months (*Publisher must submit explanation of change with this statement*)

PS Form **3526**, September 2006 (Page 1 of 3 (Instructions Page 3)) PSN 7530-01-000-9931 **PRIVACY NOTICE:** See our Privacy policy in www.usps.com

13. Publication Title: Veterinary Clinics of North America: Small Animal Practice

14. Issue Date for Circulation Data Below: September 2008

15. Extent and Nature of Circulation		Average No. Copies Each Issue During Preceding 12 Months	No. Copies of Single Issue Published Nearest to Filing Date
a. Total Number of Copies (*Net press run*)		3500	3400
b. Paid Circulation (By Mail and Outside the Mail)	(1) Mailed Outside-County Paid Subscriptions Stated on PS Form 3541. (*Include paid distribution above nominal rate, advertiser's proof copies, and exchange copies*)	2137	2035
	(2) Mailed In-County Paid Subscriptions Stated on PS Form 3541 (*Include paid distribution above nominal rate, advertiser's proof copies, and exchange copies*)		
	(3) Paid Distribution Outside the Mails Including Sales Through Dealers and Carriers, Street Vendors, Counter Sales, and Other Paid Distribution Outside USPS®	560	555
	(4) Paid Distribution by Other Classes Mailed Through the USPS (e.g. First-Class Mail®)		
c. Total Paid Distribution (*Sum of 15b (1), (2), (3), and (4)*) ►		2697	2590
d. Free or Nominal Rate Distribution (By Mail and Outside the Mail)	(1) Free or Nominal Rate Outside-County Copies Included on PS Form 3541	98	100
	(2) Free or Nominal Rate In-County Copies Included on PS Form 3541		
	(3) Free or Nominal Rate Copies Mailed at Other Classes Mailed Through the USPS (e.g. First-Class Mail)		
	(4) Free or Nominal Rate Distribution Outside the Mail (Carriers or other means)		
e. Total Free or Nominal Rate Distribution (Sum of 15d (1), (2), (3) and (4)		98	100
f. Total Distribution (Sum of 15c and 15e) ►		2795	2690
g. Copies not Distributed (See instructions to publishers #4 (page #3)) ►		705	710
h. Total (Sum of 15f and g)		3500	3400
i. Percent Paid (15c divided by 15f times 100) ►		96.49%	96.28%

16. Publication of Statement of Ownership

☐ If the publication is a general publication, publication of this statement is required. Will be printed in the **November 2008** issue of this publication. ☐ Publication not required

17. Signature and Title of Editor, Publisher, Business Manager, or Owner

Jean Fanucci – Executive Director of Subscription Services — Date: September 15, 2008

I certify that all information furnished on this form is true and complete. I understand that anyone who furnishes false or misleading information on this form or who omits material or information requested on the form may be subject to criminal sanctions (including fines and imprisonment) and/or civil sanctions (including civil penalties).

PS Form **3526**, September 2006 (Page 2 of 3)